Larynx Cancer

T0263587

Editors

KAREN M. KOST
GINA D. JEFFERSON

OTOLARYNGOLOGIC CLINICS OF NORTH AMERICA

www.oto.theclinics.com

Consulting Editor
SUJANA S. CHANDRASEKHAR

April 2023 • Volume 56 • Number 2

ELSEVIER

1600 John F. Kennedy Boulevard • Suite 1800 • Philadelphia, Pennsylvania, 19103-2899

http://www.oto.theclinics.com

OTOLARYNGOLOGIC CLINICS OF NORTH AMERICA Volume 56, Number 2
April 2023 ISSN 0030-6665, ISBN-13: 978-0-443-18222-8

Editor: Stacy Eastman
Developmental Editor: Diana Grace Ang

Otolaryngologic Clinics of North America (ISSN 0030-6665) is published bimonthly by Elsevier, Inc., 360 Park Avenue South, New York, NY 10010-1710. Months of issue are February, April, June, August, October, and December. Business and Editorial Offices: 1600 John F. Kennedy Blvd., Suite 1800, Philadelphia, PA 19103-2899. Customer Service Office: 6277 Sea Harbor Drive, Orlando, FL 32887-4800. Periodicals postage paid at New York, NY and additional mailing offices. Subscription prices are $468.00 per year (US individuals), $1117.00 per year (US institutions), $100.00 per year (US & Canadian student/resident), $599.00 per year (Canadian individuals), $1416.00 per year (Canadian institutions), $653.00 per year (international individuals), $1416.00 per year (international institutions), $270.00 per year (international student/resident). Foreign air speed delivery is included in all *Clinics'* subscription prices. All prices are subject to change without notice. **POSTMASTER:** Send address changes to *Otolaryngologic Clinics of North America*, Elsevier Health Sciences Division, Subscription Customer Service, 3251 Riverport Lane, Maryland Heights, MO 63043. **Telephone: 1-800-654-2452 (U.S. and Canada); 314-447-8871 (outside U.S. and Canada). Fax: 314-447-8029. E-mail: journalscustomerservice-usa@elsevier.com (for print support); journalsonlinesupport-usa@elsevier.com (for online support).**

Reprints. For copies of 100 or more of articles in this publication, please contact the Commercial Reprints Department, Elsevier Inc., 360 Park Avenue South, New York, NY 10010-1710. Tel.: 212-633-3874; Fax: 212-633-3820; E-mail: reprints@elsevier.com.

Otolaryngologic Clinics of North America is also published in Spanish by McGraw-Hill Interamericana Editores S.A., P.O. Box 5-237, 06500 Mexico D.F., Mexico.

Otolaryngologic Clinics of North America is covered in *MEDLINE/PubMed (Index Medicus), Current Contents/Clinical Medicine, Excerpta Medica, BIOSIS, Science Citation Index,* and *ISI/BIOMED.*

Contributors

CONSULTING EDITOR

SUJANA S. CHANDRASEKHAR, MD, FACS, FAAOHNS
Past President, American Academy of Otolaryngology–Head and Neck Surgery,
Secretary-Treasurer, and President-Elect, American Otological Society, Eastern Section,
Vice President, Triological Society, Partner, ENT & Allergy Associates, LLP, Clinical
Professor, Department of Otolaryngology–Head and Neck Surgery, Donald and Barbara
Zucker School of Medicine at Hofstra/Northwell, Hempstead, New York, USA; Clinical
Associate Professor, Department of Otolaryngology–Head and Neck Surgery, Icahn
School of Medicine at Mount Sinai, New York, New York, USA

EDITORS

KAREN M. KOST, MD, FRCSC
Professor, Department of Otolaryngology–Head and Neck Surgery, McGill University
Health Centre, Montreal, Quebec, Canada

GINA D. JEFFERSON, MD, MPH, FACS
Department of Otolaryngology–Head and Neck Surgery, University of Mississippi Medical
Center, Jackson, Mississippi, USA

AUTHORS

SARAH ADAMS, MS, CCC-SLP
Voice and Swallowing Center, Thomas Jefferson University Hospitals, Philadelphia,
Pennsylvania, USA

SOFIA AFANASIEVA (SONIA), MHSc, S-LP
Department of Speech-Language Pathology, McGill University Health Centre, Glen Site

RONDA ALEXANDER, MD
Assistant Professor of Otolaryngology–Head and Neck Surgery, Albert Einstein College of
Medicine, Director, Division of Laryngology, Montefiore Medical Center, Bronx, New York,
USA

OLUWASEYI O. AWAONUSI
Indiana University, School of Medicine, Indianapolis, Indiana, USA

ANCA M. BARBU, MD
Division of Otolaryngology–Head and Neck Surgery, Cedars-Sinai Medical Center,
Los Angeles, California, USA

MONICA H. BODD, MTS
Duke University, School of Medicine, Durham, North Carolina, USA

NATHANIEL BOUGANIM, MD
Medical Oncology, McGill University, Montreal, Quebec, Canada

MAUDE BRISSON-MCKENNA, MSC(A), S-LP
Department of Speech-Language Pathology, McGill University Health Centre, Glen Site, Montreal, Quebec, Canada

JESSE BURNS, MSc, S-LP(C)
Department of Speech-Language Pathology, McGill University Health Centre, Glen Site, Montreal, Quebec, Canada

ADAM BURR, MD, PhD
Department of Human Oncology, University of Wisconsin Hospital and Clinics, Madison, Wisconsin, USA

TRINITIA Y. CANNON, MD
Department of Head and Neck Surgery and Communication Sciences, Duke University Health System, Durham, North Carolina, USA; Co-Division Chief, Department of Head and Neck Surgery and Communication Sciences, Associate Professor, Director of Head and Neck Surgical Oncology, Duke Raleigh Hospital, Raleigh, North Carolina, USA

AÏDA CHÉRID, MHSC, S-LP
Department of Speech-Language Pathology, McGill University Health Centre, Glen Site, Montreal, Quebec, Canada

MICHELLE M. CHEN, MD
Assistant Professor, Department of Otolaryngology–Head and Neck Surgery, Stanford University, Stanford, California, USA

NICHOLAS COLWELL, MD
Department of Surgery, Division of Otolaryngology–Head and Neck Surgery, University of Wisconsin Hospital and Clinics, Madison, Wisconsin, USA

CARLA DI GIRONIMO, MS, S-LP(C), CCC-SLP
Department of Speech-Language Pathology, McGill University Health Centre, Glen Site, Montreal, Quebec, Canada

TIFFANY A. GLAZER, MD
Department of Surgery, Division of Otolaryngology–Head and Neck Surgery, University of Wisconsin Hospital and Clinics, Madison, Wisconsin, USA

CHIHUN HAN, MD
Department of Otolaryngology–Head and Neck Surgery, Thomas Jefferson University Hospitals, Philadelphia, Pennsylvania, USA

VICTOR B. HSUE, MD
Division of Otolaryngology–Head and Neck Surgery, Cedars-Sinai Medical Center, Los Angeles, California, USA

KYOHEI ITAMURA, MD
Division of Otolaryngology–Head and Neck Surgery, Cedars-Sinai Medical Center, Los Angeles, California, USA

GINA D. JEFFERSON, MD, MPH, FACS
Department of Otolaryngology–Head and Neck Surgery, University of Mississippi Medical Center, Jackson, Mississippi, USA

WEI JIA, MBchB, BSc, MRCS (ENT), PGcert
ENT Department, Poole Hospital, Poole, United Kingdom

RUSSEL KAHMKE, MD, MMCi
Assistant Professor, Department of Head and Neck Surgery and Communication
Sciences, Duke University Medical Center, Durham, North Carolina, USA

ANNE KANE, MD, FACS
Assistant Professor, University of Mississippi Medical Center, Jackson, Mississippi, USA

NAYEL I. KHAN, MD
Department of Otolaryngology–Head and Neck Surgery, Thomas Jefferson University
Hospitals, Philadelphia, Pennsylvania, USA

EMMA KING, FRCS, PhD
ENT Department, Poole Hospital, Poole, United Kingdom

KAREN M. KOST, MD, FRCSC
Professor, Department of Otolaryngology–Head and Neck Surgery, McGill University
Health Centre, Montreal, Quebec, Canada

ANTHONY B. LAW, MD, PhD
Department of Otolaryngology–Head and Neck Surgery, Winship Cancer Institute, Emory
University School of Medicine

ANDRÉANNE LEBLANC, MD
Medical Oncology, Royal Victoria Hospital/Cedars Cancer Centre, Montreal, Quebec,
Canada

STEPHANIE DANIELLE MACNEIL, MD, MSc, FRCSC
Head and Neck Surgical Oncologist, Assistant Professor, Department of
Otolaryngology–Head and Neck Surgery, Western University, Victoria Hospital, London,
Ontario, Canada

LEILA J. MADY, MD, PhD, MPH
Department of Otolaryngology–Head and Neck Surgery, Thomas Jefferson University
Hospitals, Cancer Risk and Control Program of Excellence, Sidney Kimmel Cancer
Center, Philadelphia, Pennsylvania, USA

HAYLEY MANN, MD
Department of Surgery, Division of Otolaryngology–Head and Neck Surgery, University of
Wisconsin Hospital and Clinics, Madison, Wisconsin, USA

SUSAN D. MCCAMMON, MD, PhD, FACS, FAAHPM
Department of Otolaryngology, Heersink School of Medicine, Birmingham, Alabama, USA

LIANE MCCARROLL, MS, CCC-SLP/L
Senior Speech Pathology and Assistant Research Professor, Fox Chase Cancer Center,
Philadelphia, Pennsylvania, USA

MARY CAROLINE MURRAY, MS, CCC-SLP, BCS-S
Instructor/Speech-Language Pathologist, University of Mississippi Medical Center,
Jackson, Mississippi, USA

ELIZABETH NICOLLI
Assistant Professor, Department of Otolaryngology–Head and Neck Surgery, Miller
School of Medicine, University of Miami Hospital, Miami, Florida, USA

SOMTOCHI OKAFOR, MD
Department of Head and Neck Surgery and Communication Sciences, Duke University
Health System, Durham, North Carolina, USA

CAITLIN OLSON, MD
University of Pittsburgh Medical Center, Eye & Ear Institute, Pittsburgh, Pennsylvania,
USA

RUSHA PATEL, MD, FACS
Oklahoma University, Oklahoma City, Oklahoma, USA

SEERAT K. POONIA
Department of Otolaryngology–Head and Neck Surgery, Miller School of Medicine,
University of Miami Hospital, Miami, Florida, USA

CATHERINE F. ROY, MD
Department of Otolaryngology–Head and Neck Surgery, McGill University Health Centre,
Montreal, Quebec, Canada

MIRABELLE SAJISEVI, MD
Assistant Professor, Department of Surgery, Division of Otolaryngology, University of
Vermont Medical Center, Burlington, Vermont, USA

CECELIA E. SCHMALBACH, MD, MSc, FACS
David Myers, MD Professor and Chair, Department of Otolaryngology–Head and
Neck Surgery, Lewis Katz School of Medicine at Temple University, Director, Temple
Head and Neck Institute, Fox Chase Cancer Center, Philadelphia, Pennsylvania,
USA

NICOLE C. SCHMITT, MD
Department of Otolaryngology–Head and Neck Surgery, Emory University School of
Medicine, Associate Professor of Otolaryngology–Head and Neck Surgery, Head and
Neck Cancer Program, Winship Cancer Institute, Emory University School of Medicine,
Atlanta, Georgia, USA

CAITLIN A. SCHONEWOLF, MD, MS
Adjunct Clinical Assistant Professor, Department of Radiation Oncology, University of
Michigan, Ann Arbor, Michigan,
USA

KRISTEN SELIGMAN, MD
Department of Surgery, Division of Otolaryngology–Head and Neck Surgery, University of
Wisconsin Hospital and Clinics, Madison, Wisconsin, USA

JENNIFER L. SHAH, MD
Clinical Assistant Professor, Department of Radiation Oncology, University of Michigan,
Ann Arbor, Michigan, USA

SANA H. SIDDIQUI, MD
Department of Otolaryngology–Head and Neck Surgery, Thomas Jefferson University
Hospitals, Philadelphia, Pennsylvania, USA

JENNIFER A. SILVER, MD
Department of Otolaryngology–Head and Neck Surgery, McGill University Health Centre,
Montreal, Quebec, Canada

SANDRA STINNETT, MD
University of Pittsburgh Medical Center, Eye & Ear Institute, Pittsburgh, Pennsylvania, USA

JESSICA A. TANG, MD
Head and Neck Fellow, Department of Otolaryngology–Head and Neck Surgery, Johns Hopkins Hospital, Baltimore, Maryland, USA

TOMS VENGALOOR THOMAS, MD
Radiation Oncology, University of Mississippi Medical Center, Jackson, Mississippi, USA

SENA TURKDOGAN, MD, FRCSC
Department of Otolaryngology–Head and Neck Surgery, McGill University Health Centre, Montreal, Quebec, Canada

TAMMARA L. WATTS, MD, PhD
Associate Professor, Department of Head and Neck Surgery and Communication Sciences, Duke University Health System, Durham, North Carolina, USA

Contents

Laryngeal cancer is declining in incidence in many parts of the world, as smoking becomes a less common habit. However, challenging cases of laryngeal cancer still exist and require expertise from otolaryngologists. This article reviews the relevant anatomy and lymphatic drainage pathways of the larynx as they pertain to cancer spread. The molecular and immune landscapes of laryngeal cancer, which are tightly linked to smoking, are also discussed.

 Video content accompanies this article at http://www.oto.theclinics. com.

Head and neck cancer (HNC) survivorship is increasing, and with it, a shift in treatment practices has occurred. Radical surgical resections for the treatment of HNC have decreased, and organ preservation treatments have increased. Although effective in treating HNC, chemoradiation therapy toxicities can be detrimental to a patient's overall health, nutrition status, and quality of life (QOL). Considering that dysphagia is typically a driving element of dysfunction, speech–language pathologists are vital to the prehabilitation phase. Prehabilitation programs include a variety of components, with the primary goal being to improve functional and QOL outcomes posttreatment.

Diagnosis of larynx cancer relies on a detailed history and physical and objective assessment with endoscopy and imaging. Endoscopy is needed to assess for vocal fold function that directly affects staging. Computed tomography and MRI can be used to assess for tumor extent in relation to intra- and extra-laryngeal structures, especially paraglottic and pre-epiglottic space involvement as well as cartilage invasion. Accurate staging is critical for subsequent treatment decision-making regarding larynx preservation.

There have been many advancements in the clinical and histologic diagnosis of laryngeal dysplasia (LD), but diagnosis still necessitates invasive histologic evaluation. Furthermore, despite improved histologic identification of dysplastic lesions, the exact details of pathophysiologic progression and the risk of malignant transformation is still uncertain. These unknowns create a barrier to establishing an ideal grading and classification system, which prevents the establishment of a precise and consistent treatment paradigm. Identifying these gaps in knowledge serves to highlight where further studies are warranted, ideally focusing on a better understanding of the biological behavior of LD. This would ultimately allow for the creation of a reliable grading and classification system and for the formalization of management and treatment guidelines for LD.

Multidisciplinary evaluation of early-stage glottic cancer facilitates optimal treatment with either surgery or radiation therapy. Standard of care radiation treatment of early-stage glottic cancer continues to be three-dimensional conformal treatment targeting the whole glottic larynx. Modern radiation treatment techniques are allowing studies to examine the efficacy and toxicity of altered doses and treatment volumes. Advanced techniques, such as stereotactic body radiation therapy or single-vocal cord irradiation, are not yet considered standard of care for early-stage glottic cancer and should be performed at institutions with clinical trials to ensure adequate expertise and quality assurance.

The incidence of all head and neck malignancies is rising worldwide, with carcinoma of the larynx constituting approximately 1% of all cancers. Early glottic cancer responds quite favorably to surgical intervention due to its early presentation, coupled with the low rate of regional and distant metastases. This article focuses on various approaches to the surgical treatment of early glottic cancer. Details include the clinical and radiological evaluation of laryngeal cancer, the goals of treatment, current surgical options for early disease, approach to surgical resection margins and management of nodal disease, and complications associated with each treatment modality.

In advanced glottic cancer, it is widely known that definitive chemoradiation can result in comparable survival outcomes to primary surgery. This deserves consideration given the immense effects total laryngectomy (TL) has on patients. It is important to consider that not all advanced glottic tumors should be treated in the same way, and surgical management remains a critical consideration for optimization of local control and survival outcomes. Advances in organ preservation surgery and the more developed understanding of the survival benefits of TL in extensive T4 disease further support the importance of surgery in the management of advanced glottic cancer.

Laryngeal preservation with combined modality therapy involving radiotherapy and chemotherapy is usually the treatment of choice for patients with good performance status and with locoregionally advanced laryngeal cancer with a functional larynx. Surgical management with total laryngectomy with neck dissection, followed by adjuvant radiation or chemoradiation, is recommended for patients not eligible for laryngeal preservation. This article provides an overview of the current therapeutic approaches used to treat locoregionally advanced laryngeal cancer and outlines other currently investigated therapies.

Although total laryngectomy continues to be important treatment of supraglottic laryngeal cancer, the management of early-stage disease has evolved from primary radiation/chemoradiation to consideration of partial laryngectomy surgery. Surgeon experience and careful patient selection can lead to excellent oncologic and functional outcomes for these techniques. However, advanced stage tumors and salvage situations are challenging and the ability to eradicate disease and preserve function should be carefully considered. Contraindications to supraglottic laryngectomy depend on surgical approach, as do complications. With adequate patient selection, high rates of cure and function can be achieved with both open and transoral supraglottic laryngectomy procedures.

Primary subglottic carcinoma is a rare subgroup of laryngeal malignancy with exact incidence unknown due to the lack of a standard definition of its anatomic boundaries. Early-stage subglottic carcinoma can be treated with either primary radiation or surgery with similar overall survival rates. Most patients present at an advanced stage due to a paucity of symptoms, and these patients are treated in a multidisciplinary fashion. Particular attention should be paid to the prelaryngeal and pretracheal nodal basins, as well as the stoma region, when managing these patients.

Transoral robotic surgery (TORS) is a growing field in the treatment of head and neck cancers. Its benefits have been proven in the treatment of oropharynx HPV-positive squamous cell carcinoma, replacing chemoradiation as primary treatment of early-stage cancers or reducing the required radiation dosage, leading to improved functional outcomes without compromising oncological outcomes. There is also interest in the application of TORS for larynx cancer with the hope of achieving similar outcomes to replace open surgery or radiation treatments. Specifically, in the larynx, TORS can be used to resect supraglottic or glottic tumors.

Video content accompanies this article at http://www.oto.theclinics.
com.

Dysphagia is a common functional outcome following treatment of laryngeal cancer. Despite curative advances in both nonsurgical and surgical
approaches, preserving and optimizing swallowing function is critical.
Understanding the nature and severity of dysphagia depending on initial
tumor staging and treatment modality and intensity is crucial. This chapter
explores current evidence on the acute and chronic impacts of treatments
for laryngeal cancer on swallow function, as well as the medical and
nonmedical management of dysphagia in this population.

Prognosis is defined as the likely outcome or course of a disease and is the
result of a complex interplay between patient and tumor factors. Unfortunately, the prognosis of patients with laryngeal cancer has not changed
significantly over the past several decades. However, as our understanding of these patient and tumor factors becomes more nuanced and the resulting treatment options become more precise, there is the potential to
improve the prognosis for these patients.

Patients with laryngeal cancer undergo life-changing interventions that
impact their individual and social well-being. There remains to be an in-
depth characterization of the multidimensional symptom burden faced
by patients with laryngeal cancer at the end of life. Care at end of life
must attend to symptoms that manifest earlier in the course of illness.
This article characterizes the suffering experienced by patients with laryngeal cancer, including societal shame, poor mental health, and inequitable
outcomes. For patients with advanced laryngeal cancer, surgical palliative
care provides a necessary and helpful paradigm for caregiver support,
goals-of-care conversations, and treatment counseling.

OTOLARYNGOLOGIC CLINICS
OF NORTH AMERICA

SERIES OF RELATED INTEREST

Facial Plastic Surgery Clinics
Available at: https://www.facialplastic.theclinics.com/

THE CLINICS ARE AVAILABLE ONLINE!
Access your subscription at:
www.theclinics.com

Foreword

Collaborating to Save Lives and Voices

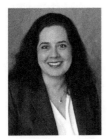

Sujana S. Chandrasekhar, MD, FACS, FAAOHNS
Consulting Editor

Entertainer Sammy Davis Jr. Beatle George Harrison. Author Michael Crichton. Mafia Boss John Gotti. Actor Humphrey Bogart. Three thousand eight hundred people in the United States and 100,000 people in the world per year. They got, and died of, laryngeal carcinoma. An additional 12,000 people per year are diagnosed with laryngeal cancer in the United States. Worldwide, new cases per year number 165,000. The vast majority of cases are in men, due to exposure to the primary risk factor, which is nicotine cigarette smoking, with heavy alcohol consumption aiding and abetting the damage. Due to packaging (**Fig. 1**) and other community outreach measures, the percentage of people who smoke has decreased by 27% in men and 38% in women since 1990; nonetheless, currently up to 1.47 billion people in the world smoke regularly.[1] Currently, over half of the burden of laryngeal cancer is carried by Asia, with 20% carried by Europe, 10% each carried by Latin America and North America, and 5% to 6% carried by Africa.[2]

Even early, or stage 1, laryngeal cancer negatively affects quality of life particularly related to speech, singing, swallowing, and the burdens of either laryngeal microsurgery and/or radiation treatment to the area. Advanced laryngeal cancer may present at a stage whereby the organ cannot be spared, even with multimodality therapy, or even if it is spared, vocal quality and therefore communication with others may suffer significantly. Swallowing and oral nutrition status as well as the social benefits of eating with others are often negatively affected by the tumor and by the treatments. Laryngectomy, of course, results in a permanent stoma in the neck, such as is pictured on the cigarette carton (see **Fig. 1**). This necessitates ongoing humidification and other care, with devices or surgery for communication.

The Guest Editors of this issue of *Otolaryngologic Clinics of North America*, Dr Karen Kost and Dr Gina Jefferson, have compiled an accessible but exhaustive review of Larynx Cancer. Early diagnosis applying knowledge of the complex laryngeal anatomy

Otolaryngol Clin N Am 56 (2023) xv–xvii
https://doi.org/10.1016/j.otc.2023.02.002
0030-6665/23/© 2023 Published by Elsevier Inc.

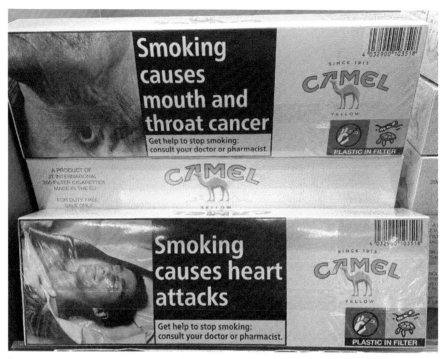

Fig. 1. Cigarette cartons with health warnings at a duty-free shop at the Athens, Greece airport, January 2023.

allows for the best outcomes. Prehabilitation for voice and overall medical status is a recent and robust intervention. Maintaining rigorous staging system protocols allows the otolaryngologist to guide the patient as to the correct treatment plan for them and their cancer. This takes into account tumor stage, nodal involvement, and whether there are distant metastases, as well as the overall condition of the patient. Heavy smokers, particularly those who also drink, must be assessed and managed for all of the myriad potential complications of those lifestyle decisions. Drs Kost and Jerfferson have included articles detailing how to think and highlighting how to do certain operations for certain stages of disease. They point out in their Preface that the large US Veterans Administration study done in 1991, after decades of total laryngectomy for nearly all larynx cancers, led to the current individualized, optimized multidisciplinary, organ-sparing approach.

The issue goes on to cover salvage surgery in case original treatment has failed, and reconstruction options that function but also are esthetically acceptable and try to address voice preservation as well. Most laryngeal cancer is squamous cell cancer, but other cell types can occur, and these are addressed. As otolaryngologists, we are humbled as we take care of patients who have disorders of some of the most accessible, visible, and audible organs. Drs Kost and Jefferson have thoughtfully included articles on rehabilitation of speech and of swallowing in these patients. Finally, knowing how to determine and then deliver the prognosis as well as the care plan to the patient and their family member(s) is highly important, both for survivors and for those who enter end-of-life care, which is also covered beautifully.

Henry Wadworth Longfellow wrote, "The human voice is the organ of the soul." It is our privilege as Otolaryngologists and Head and Neck Surgeons to care for this exquisite musical instrument, in good times and in bad. I commend Drs Kost and Jefferson on providing us readers with this elegantly planned and written issue of *Otolaryngologic Clinics of North America* on Larynx Cancer. I hope that you enjoy reading it and implementing any tweaks that are needed to your care plans in your practice.

Sujana S. Chandrasekhar, MD, FACS, FAAOHNS
Consulting Editor
Otolaryngologic Clinics of North America
Past President
American Academy of Otolaryngology–
Head and Neck Surgery
Secretary-Treasurer and President Elect
American Otological Society
Eastern Section Vice President
Triological Society
Partner, ENT & Allergy Associates LLP
18 East 48th Street, 2nd Floor
New York, NY 10017, USA

Clinical Professor
Department of Otolaryngology
Head and Neck Surgery
Zucker School of Medicine at Hofstra–Northwell
Hempstead, NY, USA

Clinical Associate Professor
Department of Otolaryngology, Head and Neck Surgery
Icahn School of Medicine at Mount Sinai
New York, NY, USA

E-mail address:
ssc@nyotology.com

Website:
http://www.ears.nyc

REFERENCES

1. Dai X, Gakidou E, Lopez AD. Evolution of the global smoking epidemic over the past half century: strengthening the evidence base for policy action. Tobacco Control 2022;31:129–37.
2. Available at: https://gco.iarc.fr/today/data/factsheets/cancers/14-Larynx-fact-sheet.pdf. Accessed February 11, 2023.

Preface

Larynx Cancer

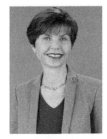
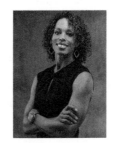

Karen M. Kost, MDCM, FRCSC   Gina D. Jefferson, MD, MPH, FACS
Editors

Laryngeal cancer is the third most prevalent tumor of the respiratory tract in the United States and is the second worldwide.[1] There are an estimated 12,000 incident cases and 3800 annual deaths in the United States.[2] Although there has been a global decline in tobacco use, it remains the most significant risk factor for the predominant laryngeal malignancy, squamous cell carcinoma. The decline in tobacco use has paralleled the decreasing incidence of laryngeal cancer diagnoses by some 2% to 3% yearly.[2] Nonetheless, for those patients afflicted with the disease, the impact on quality of life remains nothing short of profound.

The effect of treatment on voice quality is a primary concern for patients with laryngeal cancer.[3] Minimally invasive surgical procedures for early-stage disease have evolved toward increased transoral approaches, while both open and transoral techniques remain part of the surgical armamentarium in managing more advanced stages of laryngeal cancer. Oncologic outcomes for surgery remain comparable to radiation therapy. Debate continues regarding voice quality outcomes following either surgery or radiation treatment paradigms. Swallowing function is another significant concern, particularly for patients with more advanced lesions requiring multimodality therapy.[3,4] The landmark Veterans Administration organ preservation study in 1991[5] led to laryngeal preservation protocols with the aim of curing locoregionally advanced disease with chemotherapy and radiation while also maintaining airway patency, as well as voice and swallow functions of the organ. Follow-up data, as well as experience, have demonstrated that while preservation of the larynx and its function is possible in appropriately selected cases in the early years post treatment, there is frequent functional impairment over the long term as a sequelae of the progressive post radiation scarring which occurs over time.

There are several factors, elucidated throughout the text, that contribute to candidacy and selection to undergo surgical management over radiation-based therapy. The complexity of the care required in treating laryngeal cancer patients highlights

Otolaryngol Clin N Am 56 (2023) xix–xx
https://doi.org/10.1016/j.otc.2023.02.001
0030-6665/23/© 2023 Published by Elsevier Inc.

the importance of a multidisciplinary team, which includes head and neck surgeons, radiation oncologists, medical oncologists, nutritionists, and speech language pathologists.

This collection of *Otolaryngologic Clinics of North America* articles is dedicated to a discussion of the diagnosis and management of both early-stage and late-stage laryngeal disease, including premalignant entities. A comprehensive review of pre-treatment assessment, available treatment options, including surgical and nonsurgical organ preservation strategies, and innovative approaches, such as treatment prehabilitation and posttreatment rehabilitation, is provided. For the particular subset of patients failing organ preservation options or presenting with primary disease not amenable to conservation techniques, we discuss surgical salvage, reconstruction options, emerging molecular targeted treatment, prognosis, and end-of-life care. To this end, we have selected a group of established and emerging talented experts in the field.

Karen M. Kost, MDCM, FRCSC
Department of Otolaryngology–
Head and Neck Surgery
McGill University Health Centre
1001 Decarie Boulevard, H4A 3J1
Montreal, Quebec H4A 3J1, Canada

Gina D. Jefferson, MD, MPH, FACS
Department of Otolaryngology-Head & Neck Surgery
University of Mississippi
2500 N State Street
Jackson, MS 39216 USA

E-mail addresses:
kmkost@yahoo.com (K.M. Kost)
gjefferson@umc.edu (G.D. Jefferson)

REFERENCES

1. World Health Organization. International Agency for Research on Cancer. Larynx. 12/2020. Available at: https://gco.iarc.fr/today/data/factsheets/cancers/14-Larynx-fact-sheet.pdf. Accessed October 4, 2022.
2. American Cancer Society. Laryngeal and Hypopharyngeal Cancer 2022. Available at: https://www.cancer.org/cancer/laryngeal-and-hypopharyngeal-cancer/about/key-statistics.html. Accessed October 4, 2022.
3. Holländer-Mieritz C, Johnsen J, Johansen C, et al. Comparing the patients' subjective experiences of acute side effects during radiotherapy for head and neck cancer with four different patient-reported outcomes questionnaires. Acta Oncol 2019; 58(5):603–9.
4. Raber-Durlacher JE, Brennan MT, Verdonck-de Leeuw IM, et al, Dysphagia Section, Oral Care Study Group, Multinational Association of Supportive Care in Cancer (MASCC)/International Society of Oral Oncology (ISOO). Swallowing dysfunction in cancer patients. Support Care Cancer 2012;20:433–43.
5. Wolf GT, Fisher SG, Hong WK, et al, Department of Veterans Affairs Laryngeal Cancer Study Group. Induction chemotherapy plus radiation compared with surgery plus radiation in patients with advanced laryngeal cancer. N Engl J Med 1991; 324(24):1685–90.

Laryngeal Anatomy, Molecular Biology, Cause, and Risk Factors for Laryngeal Cancer

Anthony B. Law, MD, PhD[a,b], Nicole C. Schmitt, MD[a,b],*

KEYWORDS

- Laryngeal cancer • Genomics • Smoking • Molecular biology

KEY POINTS

- Specific aspects of laryngeal anatomy and lymphatic drainage routes are relevant to the spread of laryngeal cancers.
- Laryngeal cancer incidence continues to decline along with smoking, which is still the main risk factor.
- Laryngeal cancer has distinct molecular and immune characteristics that distinguish it from other cancers of the head and neck.

INTRODUCTION

Laryngeal cancer is decreasing in incidence in many parts of the world where smoking is becoming less common. However, the National Cancer Institute estimates that there will be 12,470 total cases of laryngeal cancer diagnosed in the United States in 2022.[1] Despite the decreasing incidence in North America and Western Europe, the incidences continue to increase in South-East Asia, Africa, and the Western Pacific.[2] In addition, treatment and management of survivorship issues can be challenging, as discussed in other articles within this issue of *Otolaryngology Clinics*. Although a comprehensive review of laryngeal anatomy and physiology is beyond the scope of this article, it is critical to understand key aspects of laryngeal anatomy and lymphatic spread. This article will also discuss advances in our understanding

ª Department of Otolaryngology – Head and Neck Surgery, Emory University School of Medicine, 550 Peachtree Street Northeast, 11th Floor Otolaryngology, Atlanta, GA 30308, USA;
ᵇ Winship Cancer Institute, Emory University School of Medicine, 550 Peachtree Street Northeast, 11th Floor Otolaryngology, Atlanta, GA 30308, USA
* Corresponding author. Department of Otolaryngology – Head and Neck Surgery, Emory University School of Medicine, 550 Peachtree Street Northeast, 11th Floor Otolaryngology, Atlanta, GA 30308.
E-mail address: nicole.cherie.schmitt@emory.edu

Otolaryngol Clin N Am 56 (2023) 197–203
https://doi.org/10.1016/j.otc.2022.12.001
0030-6665/23/© 2022 Elsevier Inc. All rights reserved.

of the molecular biology and immune landscape of laryngeal cancer, which is directly related in most cases to heavy smoking.

LARYNGEAL ANATOMY AND IMPLICATIONS FOR CANCER
Anatomy of the Larynx

Laryngeal cancers are classified according to their location of origin in the glottis, supraglottis, or subglottis, although the latter is far less common. Glottic cancer (below the apex of the ventricle) is most common, outnumbering supraglottic cancer (above the ventricle) by approximately 3 to 1.[3] Supraglottic tumors have ample space for growth and are often quite exophytic and large at diagnosis. Glottic tumors tend to be diagnosed at lower T stages due to a more confined space and higher likelihood of early symptoms such as hoarseness, or dysphonia. Indeed, most glottic tumors at diagnosis are confined to the anterior surface of one true vocal fold.[3] Tumors involving the anterior commissure are notable because they can be more difficult to manage surgically.

For endoscopic approaches to early glottic tumors of the anterior commissure, adequate exposure can be challenging. Inadequate exposure may compromise removal, potentially resulting in poor oncologic outcomes. There is debate on whether the anterior commissure is a potential region for tumor spread and rapid upstaging of disease. The commissure lacks thyroidal perichondrium, is deficient of underlying vocalis muscle, and has increased vascularization due to ossification of the thyroid cartilage during aging. These factors present a fertile environment for primary tumor spread. In addition, without the underlying vocalis muscle, an early superficial T1 tumor may advance in stage (to T3/T4) with only millimeters of growth before cartilage invasion is present.[4] Conversely, the anterior commissure tendon (Broyles' ligament) provides some protection against spread into the thyroid cartilage but these tumors may still spread to the thyroid cartilage by first extending up to the infrahyoid epiglottis.[3] More advanced glottic tumors can result in vocal fold fixation due to tumor bulk, invasion of intrinsic muscles or ligaments, invasion of the cricoarytenoid joint, or by invasion of the recurrent laryngeal nerve.[3,5] Glottic tumors may become "transglottic" by extending to both the supraglottis and subglottis.

Both supraglottic and glottic tumors can invade into the pre-epiglottic or paraglottic space, which is a continuous space containing fat, lymphatic vessels, and nerves. This space is bounded by the thyroid ala, thyrohyoid membrane, hyoid bone, hypoepiglottic ligament, intrinsic laryngeal muscle medially, and conus elasticus inferiorly (**Fig. 1**). Tumors of the infrahyoid epiglottis and false and true vocal folds tend to invade these fat spaces.[3] Invasion of the pre-epiglottic/paraglottic space or the thyroid cartilage are important prognostic signs that are considered in T staging[6] and treatment planning.

For surgical management of early glottic tumors, careful consideration of the layers of the vocal fold must figure into planning. There may be competing goals between optimization of complete oncologic resection and preservation of voice outcomes when managing these tumors. The glottis is broadly divided into 6 layers, which include the epithelium, superficial lamina propria (SLP), the vocal ligament (composed of the intermediate and deep lamina propria), and finally the muscle of the vocalis. Resection of the epithelium only, in cases of carcinoma in situ, generally results in good voice preservation. Poorer voice outcomes are expected with resection of the SLP, the vocal ligament or the vocalis muscle. A very large decline in voice quality occurs with complete resection of the SLP.[7] This is because the SLP provides equalization of the elastic moduli of the vocal ligament and the epithelium of the vocal fold. Destruction of this modulator results in disorganized regrowth and stiffening of the vocal fold.

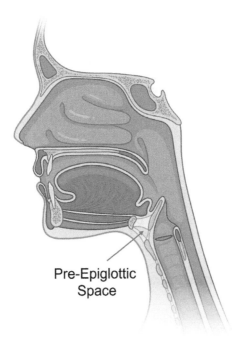

Fig. 1. Laryngeal anatomy showing pre-epiglottic space. (Created with Biorender.com.)

Lymphatic Drainage of the Larynx

The supraglottis has a rich supply of capillary lymphatics. As a result, supraglottic tumors have a high tendency to metastasize to regional lymph nodes, usually levels II and III, and often bilaterally. The vocal folds, in contrast, have a paucity of capillary lymphatics and a much lower tendency to metastasize. The subglottis also has a relatively low supply of capillary lymphatics, which drain to the pretracheal/Delphian lymph nodes, level IV, and paratracheal nodes.[3,5] Based on these characteristics, bilateral elective neck dissection is usually recommended as part of the surgical treatment of supraglottic tumors, even in early stages (T1-T2).

CAUSE AND RISK FACTORS

The vast majority of laryngeal cancers are associated with heavy and prolonged tobacco use.[8] Heavy and prolonged consumption of alcohol is another well-established risk factor, and the risk may be particularly high in patients who heavily use both tobacco and alcohol.[8,9] The risk of laryngeal cancer is influenced by the intensity (packs per day) and duration of tobacco use (including cigarettes, pipes, and cigars), with the highest risk for heavy current smokers and lower risk for ex-smokers.[10] The risk of developing cancer of the larynx and other head and neck subsites seems to be minimal for patients who smoke for less than 10 years.[10] Laryngeal cancer among nonsmokers occurs more commonly in women, with a predominance for the glottis.[11] For alcohol use, the intensity (ie, number of drinks per day) seems to be more important than the duration of alcohol use.[9]

Other patient factors that have been associated with the development of laryngeal cancer include male sex, advanced age, low body mass index, poor diet, type 2 diabetes, and sedentary lifestyle.[12-14] Genetic polymorphisms may be another nonmodifiable risk factor for laryngeal cancer; however, data on genetic risk factors are limited to small studies.[15] Other sources of chronic irritation that have been associated with the risk of laryngeal cancer include gastroesophageal or laryngopharyngeal reflux disease[16,17]; *Helicobacter pylori* infection of the stomach and laryngeal mucosa[18]; occupational exposures to specific chemicals, solvents, sulfuric acid, or asbestos[8,19]; and specific occupations with high exposure to irritants, such as welding or firefighting.[20,21]

The association of most cases of laryngeal cancer with heavy smoking, in contradistinction to other anatomic subsites of the head and neck such as the oropharynx,[13] is reflected in the unique molecular and immune signatures of laryngeal cancer. Although a small proportion of laryngeal tumors do test positive for human papillomavirus (HPV), the significance of this HPV-positivity is unclear, with several prior studies showing no obvious effects on biology or prognosis.[22]

MOLECULAR AND IMMUNE LANDSCAPE OF LARYNGEAL CANCER
Genomic Alterations

Similar to many smoking-related tumors, including those of other anatomic subsites in the head and neck, laryngeal cancers tend to have mutations in p53, cyclin D1, and other tumor suppressors.[23] As might be expected, genetic signatures associated with smoking, including C to A transversions, are prominent in laryngeal cancers.[24] In recent decades, much has been learned about the molecular biology and genomic alterations in head and neck cancer, in part due to analyses of sequencing data from tumor specimens in the Cancer Genome Atlas (TCGA). A recent study comparing genomic alterations among tumors of the larynx versus other HPV-negative sites found a higher number of single nucleotide variations and shallow deletions, with specific alterations that were distinct from those seen in oral cancers.[13] When comparing genomic hypoxia signatures, laryngeal cancer scored lower than oral or hypopharyngeal cancers; in other words, hypoxia seems to be less of a driving factor in laryngeal cancer versus other anatomic sites of the head and neck.[13]

Immune Landscape

Compared with other cancers of the head and neck, laryngeal cancers tend to have a higher tumor mutational burden, which is associated with immune infiltration and better responses to immunotherapy.[25,26] In the genomic alterations study above comparing HPV-negative tumors from different anatomic subsites in TCGA, laryngeal tumors were found to have higher numbers of B lymphocytes and fewer monocytes.[13] Generally, laryngeal cancers with higher density of tumor infiltrating lymphocytes and higher PD-L1 expression have better survival outcomes.[27] Conversely, laryngeal cancers may also be particularly enriched for immunosuppressive cells, such as regulatory T cells or myeloid-derived suppressor cells, which can drive tumor progression and aggressive behavior.[28] A subset of laryngeal cancers with *NOTCH1* gene mutations be "immunologically cold" (with few infiltrating, tumor-targeted immune cells) and poor prognosis.[23] Despite these advances in our knowledge of the genomic and immune aspects of laryngeal cancer, biomarkers of response to different forms or therapy are still needed. Several specific biomarkers, mutations, and prognostic nomograms have been proposed in small studies but large validation studies are still lacking.

CLINICS CARE POINTS

- Although the incidence of laryngeal cancer is decreasing along with tobacco abuse, laryngeal cancers still occur in substantial numbers, with significant morbidity and mortality.
- Due to their locations and patterns of lymphatic spread, glottic cancers may present early with hoarseness, whereas supraglottic tumors tend to present at advanced stage with nodal metastases.
- Heavy smoking and alcohol are, by far, the strongest risk factors for laryngeal cancer. Otolaryngologists should stress smoking cessation and consider screening for other smoking-related cancers, including lung cancer.[29]
- The molecular and immune characteristics of laryngeal cancer, which are in most cases defined by a tobacco signature, are distinct from other cancers of the head and neck. Molecular and immune testing is likely to become an integral part of the workup and treatment planning for laryngeal cancer in the future.

DISCLOSURE

N.C. Schmitt—Consulting: Checkpoint Surgical, Sensorion; Book Royalties: Plural Publishing Research and Clinical Trial Funding: Astex Pharmaceuticals.

REFERENCES

1. National Cancer Institute Surveillance E aERP. Cancer stat facts: Laryngeal cancer. Available at: https://seer.cancer.gov/statfacts/html/laryn.html. Accessed May 22, 2022.
2. Nocini R, Molteni G, Mattiuzzi C, et al. Updates on larynx cancer epidemiology. Chin J Cancer Res 2020;32(1):18–25.
3. Mendenhall WM, Werning JW. Early stage cancer of the larynx. In: Harrison LB, Sessions RB, Hong WK, editors. Head and neck cancer: a multidisciplinary approach. Philadelphia: Lippincott; 2009. p. 339–53.
4. Chone CT, Yonehara E, Martins JE, et al. Importance of anterior commissure in recurrence of early glottic cancer after laser endoscopic resection. Arch Otolaryngol Head Neck Surg 2007;133(9):882–7.
5. Koroulakis A, Agarwal M. Laryngeal cancer. In: StatPearls. Treasure Island (FL): StatPearls Publishing; 2022.
6. Amin MB. AJCC cancer staging manual. 8th edition. New York: Springer; 2017.
7. Xu W, Han D, Hou L, et al. Voice function following CO2 laser microsurgery for precancerous and early-stage glottic carcinoma. Acta Otolaryngol 2007;127(6): 637–41.
8. Lin C, Cheng W, Liu X, et al. The global, regional, national burden of laryngeal cancer and its attributable risk factors (1990-2019) and predictions to 2035. Eur J Cancer Care (Engl) 2022;31(6):e13689.
9. Di Credico G, Polesel J, Dal Maso L, et al. Alcohol drinking and head and neck cancer risk: the joint effect of intensity and duration. Br J Cancer 2020;123(9): 1456–63.
10. Nam IC, Park JO, Kim CS, et al. Association of smoking status, duration and amount with the risk of head and neck cancer subtypes: a national population-based study. Am J Cancer Res 2022;12(10):4815–24.

11. Shoffel-Havakuk H, O'Dell K, Johns MM 3rd, et al. The rising rate of nonsmokers among laryngeal carcinoma patients: Are we facing a new disease? Laryngoscope 2020;130(3):E108–15.
12. Goyal N, Hennessy M, Lehman E, et al. Risk factors for head and neck cancer in more and less developed countries: Analysis from the INHANCE consortium. Oral Dis 2022.
13. Kim HAJ, Zeng PYF, Shaikh MH, et al. All HPV-negative head and neck cancers are not the same: Analysis of the TCGA dataset reveals that anatomical sites have distinct mutation, transcriptome, hypoxia, and tumor microenvironment profiles. Oral Oncol 2021;116:105260.
14. Yan P, Wang Y, Yu X, et al. Type 2 diabetes mellitus and risk of head and neck cancer subtypes: a systematic review and meta-analysis of observational studies. Acta Diabetol 2021;58(5):549–65.
15. Escalante P, Barria T, Cancino M, et al. Genetic polymorphisms as non-modifiable susceptibility factors to laryngeal cancer. Biosci Rep 2020;40(5). BSR20191188.
16. Parsel SM, Iarocci AL, Gastanaduy M, et al. Reflux Disease and Laryngeal Neoplasia in Nonsmokers and Nondrinkers. Otolaryngol Head Neck Surg 2020; 163(3):560–2.
17. Parsel SM, Wu EL, Riley CA, et al. Gastroesophageal and Laryngopharyngeal Reflux Associated With Laryngeal Malignancy: A Systematic Review and Meta-analysis. Clin Gastroenterol Hepatol 2019;17(7):1253–64, e1255.
18. Pajic Matic I, Jelic D, Matic I, et al. Presence of Helicobacter Pylori in the Stomach and Laryngeal Mucosal Linings in Patients with Laryngeal Cancer. Acta Clin Croat 2018;57(1):91–5.
19. Barul C, Fayosse A, Carton M, et al. Occupational exposure to chlorinated solvents and risk of head and neck cancer in men: a population-based case-control study in France. Environ Health 2017;16(1):77.
20. Barul C, Matrat M, Auguste A, et al. Welding and the risk of head and neck cancer: the ICARE study. Occup Environ Med 2020;77(5):293–300.
21. Langevin SM, Eliot M, Butler RA, et al. Firefighter occupation is associated with increased risk for laryngeal and hypopharyngeal squamous cell carcinoma among men from the Greater Boston area. Occup Environ Med 2020;77(6): 381–5.
22. Schmitt NC. HPV in non-oropharyngeal head and neck cancer: does it matter? Ann Transl Med 2020;8(18):1120.
23. Gong XY, Chen HB, Zhang LQ, et al. NOTCH1 mutation associates with impaired immune response and decreased relapse-free survival in patients with resected T1-2N0 laryngeal cancer. Front Immunol 2022;13:920253.
24. South AP, den Breems NY, Richa T, et al. Mutation signature analysis identifies increased mutation caused by tobacco smoke associated DNA adducts in larynx squamous cell carcinoma compared with oral cavity and oropharynx. Sci Rep 2019;9(1):19256.
25. Burcher KM, Lantz JW, Gavrila E, et al. Relationship between Tumor Mutational Burden, PD-L1, Patient Characteristics, and Response to Immune Checkpoint Inhibitors in Head and Neck Squamous Cell Carcinoma. Cancers (Basel) 2021; 13(22):5733.
26. Cui J, Wang D, Nie D, et al. Difference in tumor mutation burden between squamous cell carcinoma in the oral cavity and larynx. Oral Oncol 2021;114:105142.
27. Alessandrini L, Franz L, Ottaviano G, et al. Prognostic role of programmed death ligand 1 (PD-L1) and the immune microenvironment in laryngeal carcinoma. Oral Oncol 2020;108:104836.

28. Trivedi S, Rosen CA, Ferris RL. Current understanding of the tumor microenvironment of laryngeal dysplasia and progression to invasive cancer. Curr Opin Otolaryngol Head Neck Surg 2016;24(2):121–7.

29. Cramer JD, Grauer J, Sukari A, et al. Incidence of Second Primary Lung Cancer After Low-Dose Computed Tomography vs Chest Radiography Screening in Survivors of Head and Neck Cancer: A Secondary Analysis of a Randomized Clinical Trial. JAMA Otolaryngol Head Neck Surg 2021;147(12):1071–8.

Perioperative Assessment/ Prehabilitation in Larynx Cancer

Mary Caroline Murray, MS, CCC-SLP, BCS-S*, Anne Kane, MD, FACS

KEYWORDS

- Head and neck cancer • Prophylactic swallowing exercises • Cancer prehabilitation
- Deglutition • Dysphagia

KEY POINTS

- Dysphagia is a common consequence of chemoradiotherapy (CRT) that negatively impacts the overall health and quality of life of head and neck cancer (HNC) survivors.
- Swallow-focused prehabilitative programs often involve exercise-based regimens that focus on maintaining the strength and mobility of the oropharyngeal musculature before and during CRT.
- Treatments for HNC can result in complex, multifaceted consequences, with improved patient outcomes best achieved through a multidisciplinary team approach.
- Variability in prehabilitative program protocols and their outcomes is noted throughout the literature.

 Video content accompanies this article at http://www.oto.theclinics.com.

INTRODUCTION

Owing to advances in surgical techniques and chemoradiotherapy (CRT) treatment acuity, survivorship of patients with laryngeal cancer has increased to an impressive 61%.[1] However, survival rates do not consider the ways in which cancer treatments may negatively impact a patient's overall quality of life (QOL), despite granting survivorship. Laryngeal cancer commonly impacts the functions of deglutition, voice, and airway status. Surgical resection or CRT to structures vital to these functions can cause head and neck cancer (HNC) survivors to experience varying levels of dysphagia, dysphonia, or airway compromise. Dysphagia is considered one of the most common complications patients experience as a result of their treatments or surgical interventions.[2] With respect to voice and airway;dysphonia, tracheostomy

University of Mississippi Medical Center, 2500 North State Street, Jackson, MS 39216, USA
* Corresponding author.
E-mail address: mmurray@umc.edu

Otolaryngol Clin N Am 56 (2023) 205–214
https://doi.org/10.1016/j.otc.2022.12.003

dependence, and laryngectomy status are consequences that negatively impact patient function and QOL.

An increase in patients opting for organ preservation treatments in lieu of surgical treatment options has been noted in the literature. It has been documented that up to 85% of patients diagnosed with HNC will undergo radiotherapy as part of their primary cancer treatment plan.[3] It is important to note that organ preservation does not necessarily translate to preservation of function. The adverse effects organ preservation poses to the laryngeal system commonly results in acute and chronic toxicities that can negatively impact the aforementioned functions of swallowing, voicing, and breathing.[4]

Although tobacco and alcohol abuse are common risk factors associated with laryngeal cancer, the recent increase in the prevalence of human papillomavirus (HPV)-related oropharyngeal cancers, which has risen from 20.9% in the pre-1990s[5] to an estimated 70%[6] in recent years, has caused the patient demographic to shift. The mean age of patients at the time of laryngeal cancer diagnosis has decreased; HNC survivors are thus younger and healthier, but presenting with chronic CRT toxicities that negatively impact QOL outcomes.[7] It is therefore imperative that HNC providers explore means to dampen the burden of acute and long-term toxicities associated with CRT treatments.

IMPACT OF CHEMORADIOTHERAPY TOXICITIES

Attaining adequate nutritional intake during treatment can become an arduous task secondary to the toxicities associated with CRT.[8] Common acute toxicities that impact swallowing include mucositis, xerostomia, dysgeusia, and odynophagia.[9] Acute toxicities often resolve with time; however, chronic treatment side effects such as radiation-induced fibrosis, permanent xerostomia, permanent dysgeusia, neuropathy, and lymphedema negatively impact function of the oropharyngeal musculature and increase the risk for chronic dysphagia.[9,10] Please refer to **Fig. 1** for an endoscopic image example of a normal larynx. **Fig. 2** presents the endoscopic image examples of four individual patients who were subjected to CRT toxicity insult, ranging from 3 months to 3 years post-CRT.

Patients who present with minimal to no difficulty swallowing before CRT can experience oral diet regression during treatment.[11] Considerable regression, often

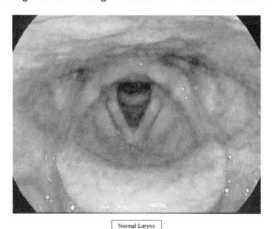

Normal Larynx

Fig. 1. Endoscopic image of a normal larynx.

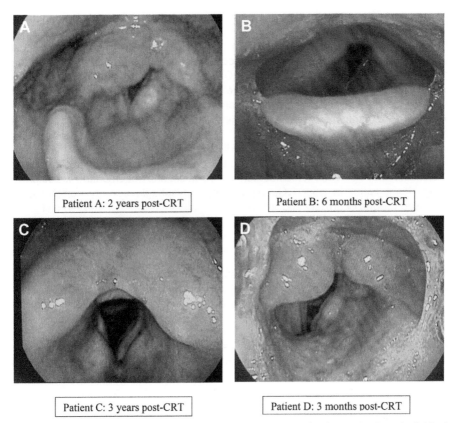

Patient A: 2 years post-CRT

Patient B: 6 months post-CRT

Patient C: 3 years post-CRT

Patient D: 3 months post-CRT

Fig. 2. Endoscopic image examples ofpost CRT changes to the larynx in four individual patients.

warranting gastronomy tube (g-tube) placement, is noted in patients who begin CRT with more severe preexisting elements of dysphagia.[12]

Severe acute or chronic dysphagia secondary to toxicity load has been shown to increase the likelihood of g-tube dependence in HNC survivors.[8] In a study completed by Hutcheson and colleagues,[9] 66% of HNC patients presented with chronic dysphagia and g-tube dependency 5 years posttreatment, as a result of persistent CRT toxicities.[9] Please refer to Video 1 for imaging of a functional oropharyngeal swallow attained through videofluoroscopy. In comparison, please refer to Video 2, which includes videofluoroscopy imaging of a patient who is 10 years post-CRT. The differences in both the safety and efficiency aspects of the respective swallows can be appreciated.

LARYNGEAL CANCER PREHABILITATION

Rehabilitation practices are generally put in place after a decline in function is observed,[13] but in recent years, the practice of prehabilitation has been increasingly used.[14] Prehabilitation includes a multidisciplinary team approach incorporating the skills and knowledge base of a variety of disciplines to start interventions before a patient's cancer treatment. It has been shown to improve patient outcomes in other cancer types,[14] which have led to an increase in the number of studies looking at efficacy of prehabilitation in the HNC patient population.[15,12,16]

The goal of cancer prehabilitation is to increase patient function and decrease severity of potential decline related to upcoming cancer treatments.[14] The increase in HNC survival rates, paired with poor QOL reports,[17] reinforces the importance of prehabilitation and adequate perioperative assessment. The disciplines involved in HNC prehabilitation often include, though are not limited to, speech–language pathologists (SLPs), nutritionists, physiatrists, dieticians, physical therapists, occupational therapists, and rehabilitation nurses.[14]

Deglutition is often the primary focus of HNC-related prehabilitation as it has such a profound impact on daily health and QOL. Dysphagia is a potentially life-threatening dysfunction that can result in malnutrition, dehydration, and pneumonia.[18] It also plays a significant factor in poor QOL reports, with dysphagia severity correlating to increased reports of anxiety and depression.[19]

PRETREATMENT ASSESSMENT

Before surgical or CRT treatments are pursued, it is necessary to complete a comprehensive pretreatment assessment.[20] This assessment enables the surgeon or oncologist to fully appreciate the functional status of the patient before CRT or surgical interventions. Toxicities acquired during CRT can exacerbate preexisting medical issues.[20] The information gained during the pretreatment assessment provides insight to a patient's prognosis following CRT or surgical intervention. This is a necessary component to consider when determining the most viable treatment plan for the patient.

A multidisciplinary team approach is required to fully assess a patient's current medical standing. Areas such as pulmonology, dental, cerebrovascular, and cardiovascular health should be considered for workup and appropriate outgoing referrals completed.[20] Potential comorbidities, such as diabetes, should also be acknowledged and referred appropriately for management.

Prehabilitation Swallow Assessments

Prehabilitation programs necessitate an evaluation to establish baseline function of a patient before any treatment.[16] The evaluation of swallowing function is completed by an SLP. The three assessments SLPs use to establish baseline swallow function are clinical swallow evaluations (CSE), modified barium swallow studies (MBSS), or fiberoptic endoscopic evaluations of swallowing (FEES). The examination chosen often depends on the equipment available to the treating SLP. Flexible endoscopy (FEES) or videofluoroscopy (MBSS) allows clinicians to directly visualize the anatomy and physiology of the oropharyngeal musculature throughout the act of swallowing. It is recommended that patients undergo MBSS or FEES in addition to a CSE, as more objective data can be attained.[21] For example, the presence of silent aspiration that occurs "before" a swallow can be confirmed with MBSS or FEES imaging but is unable to be verified during a CSE. Please refer to **Fig. 3** for a photo example of confirmed aspiration achieved through videofluoroscopy (MBSS) imaging.

Obtaining swallow assessments before the start of CRT allows clinicians to evaluate a patient's baseline swallow status and track potential regression of function. Depending on the severity of the patient's dysphagia before treatment, the placement of a g-tube may be recommended to provide an alternative but safe avenue for nutritional support throughout treatment.[18] Of note, despite the presence of a g-tube, the act of

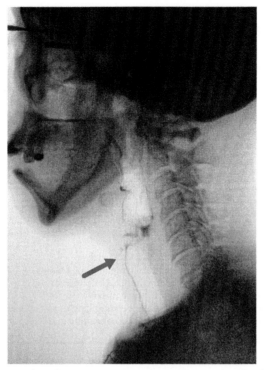

Fig. 3. Photo example of confirmed aspiration achieved through videofluoroscopy (MBSS) imaging. (*Red arrow*) indicates presence of aspirated barium beneath level of the true vocal folds.

deglutition is still often recommended for patients undergoing CRT to help maintain the integrity of the oropharyngeal musculature,[22] if cleared by the treating SLP.

Additional important components commonly included within the pretreatment swallow evaluation include baseline maximum interincisal opening (MIO) measures for trismus tracking, documentation of current body mass index or weight, feeding tube dependency status, and patient-reported QOL questionnaires.[12,23,3] A summary of elements commonly included in swallow-focused prehabilitative programs is presented in **Table 1**.

PROPHYLACTIC SWALLOWING EXERCISES

Following the recommended baseline assessment of a patient's swallow function thorough counseling on anticipated acute and long-term CRT toxicities is completed, and prehabilitative swallowing exercises are taught.[23,3,12,15] These exercises are designed to be completed before and throughout CRT.[23] Swallow-specific prehabilitation exercises, otherwise known as "prophylactic" swallowing exercises, are put in place to increase or preserve strength and mobility of the oropharyngeal musculature, imperative to a safe and efficient swallow.

Prophylactic swallowing exercises commonly practice the "use-it-or-lose-it" philosophy seen in other exercise paradigms.[12] Periods of immobility or disuse of skeletal muscle result in rapid muscle atrophy.[24,25] With the anticipated decline in swallow

Table 1
Common timeline and components of speech–language pathologist prehabilitative programs

Pre-CRT	• Evaluation of the swallow: Establish baseline function
	  ○ Clinical swallow evaluation
	  ○ Modified barium swallow study (MBSS)
	  ○ Fiberoptic endoscopic evaluation of swallowing (FEES)
	• Baseline QOL questionnaires
	• Maximal interincisal opening (MIO) measures/trismus status
	• Weight/body mass index (BMI)
	• Feeding tube status
	• Education/counseling on CRT toxicities
	• Teaching of prophylactic swallowing exercises

During CRT	• Follow-ups with SLP weekly or biweekly
	  ○ Reassess swallow function
	  ○ Monitor/adjust diet as needed
	  ○ Monitor/adjust swallow exercise regimen as needed

Post-CRT	• Evaluation of the patient's swallow function via instrumental examination ○ MBSS or FEES • Updated QOL questionnaires • Updated MIO, weight, BMI, feeding tube status • Reinforce potential for chronic CRT toxicities • Discuss swallow maintenance plan • Refer for swallow therapy pending dysphagia status post-CRT • Additional referrals placed as needed (ie, nutrition, physical therapy, psychology)

Data from Refs.[3,9,12,15,18,23]

function secondary to CRT toxicity burden, the goal is to increase muscle loading of the oropharyngeal musculature and work against the notion of disuse atrophy.[12]

Numerous studies have looked at the efficacy prehabilitative swallowing regimens offer, with high variability noted in the standardization and effectiveness of the reviewed protocols.[26,23,3] A literature review completed by Loewen and colleagues[23] compiled the results of 29 research articles that examined prehabilitation programs for patients with head and neck cancer undergoing CRT, published between the years 2006 and 2020. A high degree of variance was noted in the specific swallow exercises used and the dosing, frequency, and duration of the prescribed exercises.[23,27] In sum, the review concluded that most programs consisted of stretching/range of motion exercises, trismus exercises, and swallow-specific exercises with the most common dosing at 10 repetitions three times per day, for the length of CRT treatment.[23]

In a systematic review completed by Brady and colleagues,[3] the results of eight separate studies that evaluated the impact of dysphagia prehabilitation programs on swallow outcomes post-CRT, found minimal evidence to support prophylactic exercises before CRT. However, the investigators reported that benefits of implementing swallow-specific prehabilitation programs before CRT were demonstrated, though findings in most of the studies included in the review did not show statistical significance.[3]

Some studies have reported an increase in muscle mass preservation, reduced feeding tube dependency and notable improvement in QOL scores following the implementation of prophylactic swallowing exercises,[12,28,29,30,15] with other studies denoting no statistically significant improvements.[23,3,26] Although there is some promise in reducing CRT-induced dysphagia in the acute phases of treatment,[29,12,15] little

Table 2
Common prophylactic swallowing exercises

Swallow Exercise	Target
Effortful swallow	Improve strength of pharyngeal constrictors and base of tongue musculature[1]
Falsetto	Improve strength of pharyngeal constrictors, shortening of pharynx[2]
Gargle	Improve tongue base retraction[3]
Lingual, labial, jaw range of motion (ROM), and resistance exercises	Improve mobility and strength of lips, tongue, and jaw musculature[4]
Masako (Tongue Hold) Maneuver	Improve strength of superior pharyngeal constrictor and base of tongue musculature[5]
Mendelsohn maneuver	Improve hyolaryngeal elevation and excursion, upper esophageal sphincter (UES) opening[6]
Shaker exercise	Improve hyolaryngeal excursion, UES opening, suprahyoid musculature[7]
Super-supraglottic swallow	Improve laryngeal vestibule closure[8]

Data from Refs.[31–38]

evidence exists on the long-term effects prophylactic exercises pose to the swallow mechanism.[9,26] Please refer to **Table 2** for commonly prescribed swallow exercises used in prehabilitative swallow programs,[23,15,18,12,28] based on this author's review of the literature.

SUMMARY

Perioperative assessment and prehabilitation, using a multidisciplinary approach, are integral components that should be included in laryngeal cancer patient care pathways. Dysphagia being a frequent, detrimental side effect commonly acquired or exacerbated by CRT toxicities is often the focus of HNC prehabilitation. Instrumental examinations of MBSS or FEES provide optimal means for establishing baseline swallow function and tracking diet regression or improvement before and post-CRT.

Prehabilitative programs should be multipronged, consisting of instrumental examinations, patient education on anticipated CRT toxicities, prophylactic swallowing exercises, and patient-reported QOL tracking. QOL is an important factor to consider within this patient population. High variability is noted throughout the literature in respect to which prehabilitative swallow-specific protocols yield the most optimal outcomes. In sum, the evidence noted within the literature is promising, yet more research is needed to improve the efficacy and standardization of prophylactic swallowing interventions.

CLINICS CARE POINTS

- Acute and chronic chemoradiotherapy (CRT) toxicities can exacerbate deglutition, voice, or airway dysfunction, all of which commonly produce negative quality of life (QOL) outcomes in patients with laryngeal cancer.

- Prehabilitative swallowing programs should be multifaceted, consisting of instrumental examinations (Modified Barium Swallow Studies or Fiberoptic Endoscopic Evaluations of Swallowing), objective measures (ie, maximum interincisal opening), patient education on anticipated CRT toxicities, prophylactic swallow exercise implementation, and QOL monitoring through patient-reported outcome measures.
- The swallow-specific exercises included in most prehabilitation programs are based around the concept of muscular neuroplasticity.
- No specific set of prophylactic swallowing exercises, dosing, or frequency has been shown to exceed another in respect to effectiveness in the acute stages of CRT or in respect to long-term swallow improvement.
- More research is required to evaluate organ-preserving treatment protocols and their potential to dampen acute and long-term dysphagia severity.

DISCLOSURE

M.C. Murray and A. Kane declare no conflicts of interest and have no financial disclosures.

SUPPLEMENTARY DATA

Supplementary data related to this article can be found online at https://doi.org/10.1016/j.otc.2022.12.003.

REFERENCES

1. American Society of Clinical Oncology (ASCO). Laryngeal and Hypopharyngeal Cancer: Statistics, Cancer.Net Website. Available at: https://www.cancer.net/cancer-types/laryngeal-and-hypopharyngeal-cancer/statistics. Last updated February 2022. Accessed July 1, 2022.
2. Wilson JA, Carding PN, Patterson JM. Dysphagia after nonsurgical head and neck cancer treatment: patients' perspectives. Otolaryngol Head Neck Surg 2011;145(5):767–71.
3. Brady R, McSharry L, Lawson S, et al. The impact of dysphagia prehabilitation on swallowing outcomes post-chemoradiation therapy in head and neck cancer: A systematic review. Eur J Cancer Care (Engl) 2022;31(3):e13549.
4. Patterson JM. Late Effects of Organ Preservation Treatment on Swallowing and Voice; Presentation, Assessment, and Screening. Front Oncol 2019;9:401.
5. Stein AP, Saha S, Yu M, et al. Prevalence of human papillomavirus in oropharyngeal squamous cell carcinoma in the United States across time. Chem Res Toxicol 2014;27(4):462–9.
6. Centers for Disease Control and Prevention (CDC). Division of Cancer Prevention and Control: HPV and Oropharyngeal Cancer. Available at: https://www.cdc.gov/cancer/hpv/basic_info/hpv_oropharyngeal.htm. Last updated December 13, 2021. Accessed July 24, 2022.
7. Schlichting JA, Pagedar NA, Chioreso C, et al. Treatment trends in head and neck cancer: Surveillance, Epidemiology, and End Results (SEER) Patterns of Care analysis. Cancer Causes Control 2019;30(7):721–32.
8. Baijens LWJ, Walshe M, Aaltonen LM, et al. European white paper: oropharyngeal dysphagia in head and neck cancer. Eur Arch Otorhinolaryngol 2021;278(2):577–616.

9. Hutcheson KA, Lewin JS, Barringer DA, et al. Late dysphagia after radiotherapy-based treatment of head and neck cancer. Cancer 2012;118(23):5793–9.
10. Martin M, Lefaix J, Delanian S. TGF-beta1 and radiation fibrosis: a master switch and a specific therapeutic target? Int J Radiat Oncol Biol Phys 2000;47(2): 277–90.
11. Logemann JA, Pauloski BR, Rademaker AW, et al. Swallowing disorders in the first year after radiation and chemoradiation. Head Neck 2008;30(2):148–58.
12. Carnaby-Mann G, Crary M, Schmalfuss I. Pharyngocise": Randomized controlled trial of preventative exercises to maintain muscle structure and swallowing function during head-and-neck-chemoradiothereapy. Int J Radiat Oncol Biol Phys 2012;83(1):210–9.
13. Silver JK, Baima J, Mayer RS. Impairment-driven cancer rehabilitation: an essential component of quality care and survivorship. CA Cancer J Clin 2013;63(5): 295–317.
14. Silver JK, Baima J. Cancer prehabilitation: an opportunity to decrease treatment-related morbidity, increase cancer treatment options, and improve physical and psychological health outcomes. Am J Phys Med Rehabil 2013;92(8):715–27.
15. Kotz T, Federman AD, Kao J, et al. Prophylactic swallowing exercises in patients with head and neck cancer undergoing chemoradiation: a randomized trial. Arch Otolaryngol Head Neck Surg 2012;138(4):376–82.
16. Roe JW, Ashforth KM. Prophylactic swallowing exercises for patients receiving radiotherapy for head and neck cancer. Curr Opin Otolaryngol Head Neck Surg 2011;19(3):144–9.
17. Patterson J. Psychological Interventions for the Head and Neck Cancer Population Who Are Experiencing Dysphagia. SIG 13 Perspect Swallowing Swallowing Disord (Dysphagia) 2019;5:1049–54.
18. Paleri V, Roe JW, Strojan P, et al. Strategies to reduce long-term postchemoradiation dysphagia in patients with head and neck cancer: an evidence-based review. Head Neck 2014;36(3):431–43.
19. Nguyen NP, Frank C, Moltz CC, et al. Impact of dysphagia on quality of life after treatment of head-and-neck cancer. Int J Radiat Oncol Biol Phys 2005;61(3): 772–8.
20. Sahai SK. Perioperative assessment of the cancer patient. Best Pract Res Clin Anaesthesiol 2013;27(4):465–80.
21. Sassi FC, Medeiros GC, Zilberstein B, et al. Screening protocol for dysphagia in adults: comparison with videofluoroscopic findings. Clinics (Sao Paulo). 2017; 72(12):718–22.
22. Mortensen HR Jensen K, Aksglaede K, et al. Prophylactic Swallowing Exercises in Head and Neck Cancer Radiotherapy. Dysphagia 2015;30(3):304–14.
23. Loewen I, Jeffery CC, Rieger J, et al. Prehabilitation in head and neck cancer patients: a literature review. J Otolaryngol - Head Neck Surg 2021;50:2.
24. Berg HE, Tesch PA. Changes in muscle function in response to 10 days of lower limb unloading in humans. Acta Physiol Scand 1996;157:63–70.
25. Piquet F, Stevens L, Butler-Browne G, et al. Differential effects of a six-day immobilization on newborn rat soleus muscles at two developmental stages. J Muscle Res Cell Motil 1998;19:743–55.
26. Messing BP, Ward EC, Lazarus CL, et al. Prophylactic Swallow Therapy for Patients with Head and Neck Cancer Undergoing Chemoradiotherapy: A Randomized Trial. Dysphagia 2017;32(4):487–500.
27. Krekeler BN, Rowe LM, Connor NP. Dose in Exercise-Based Dysphagia Therapies: A Scoping Review. Dysphagia 2021;36(1):1–32.

28. Ohba S, Yokoyama J, Kojima M, et al. Significant preservation of swallowing function in chemoradiotherapy for advanced head and neck cancer by prophylactic swallowing exercise. Head Neck 2016;38(4):517–21.

29. Starmer H. Swallowing exercises in head and neck cancer. SIG 13 Perspect Swallowing Swallowing Disord (Dysphagia) 2017;13:21–6.

30. Kulbersh BD, Rosenthal EL, McGrew BM, et al. Pretreatment, preoperative swallowing exercises may improve dysphagia quality of life. Laryngoscope 2006; 116(6):883–6.

31. Bahia MM, Lowell SY. A Systematic Review of the Physiological Effects of the Effortful Swallow Maneuver in Adults With Normal and Disordered Swallowing. Am J Speech Lang Pathol 2020;29(3):1655–73.

32. Miloro KV, Pearson WG, Langmore SE. Effortful pitch glide: a potential new exercise evaluated by dynamic MRI. J Speech Lang Hear Res 2014;57(4):1243–50.

33. Veis S, Logemann JA, Colangelo L. Effects of three techniques on maximum posterior movement of the tongue base. Dysphagia 2000;15(3):142–5.

34. Logemann JA, Pauloski BR, Rademaker AW, et al. Speech and swallowing rehabilitation for head and neck cancer patients. Oncology (Williston Park) 1997; 11(5):651–64.

35. Hammer MJ, Jones CA, Mielens JD, et al. Evaluating the tongue-hold maneuver using high-resolution manometry and electromyography. Dysphagia 2014;29(5): 564–70.

36. Kahrilas PJ, Logemann JA, Krugler C, et al. Volitional augmentation of upper esophageal sphincter opening during swallowing. Am J Physiol 1991;260(3 Pt 1):G450–6.

37. Shaker R, Kern M, Bardan E, et al. Augmentation of deglutitive upper esophageal sphincter opening in the elderly by exercise. Am J Physiol 1997;272(6 Pt 1): G1518–22.

38. Martin BJ, Logemann JA, Shaker R, et al. Normal laryngeal valving patterns during three breath-hold maneuvers: a pilot investigation. Dysphagia 1993;8(1): 11–20.

Diagnostic Assessment (Imaging) and Staging of Laryngeal Cancer

Kyohei Itamura, MD[a], Victor B. Hsue, MD[a], Anca M. Barbu, MD[a],
Michelle M. Chen, MD MHS[a,b],*

KEYWORDS

- Larynx cancer • Endoscopy • Imaging • Staging • Laryngeal imaging
- Videostroboscopy • Biologic endoscopy • Narrow band imaging

KEY POINTS

- Direct laryngoscopy and biopsy in the operating room are the gold standards for definitive diagnosis of laryngeal cancer, but multiple imaging modalities exist and are in development that aid in the identification of glottic cancers and recurrences.
- Videostroboscopy, high-speed imaging, and videokymography are tools that can better assess vocal fold motion and identify lesions that disrupt the normal mucosal wave.
- Optical coherence tomography, autofluorescence, and biologic endoscopy techniques noninvasively provide information about superficial and deep tissue structures of the glottis.
- Computed tomography and MRI used in conjunction are sensitive and specific tools to accurately assess tumor extent. PET has a known role in assessing for distant metastatic spread.
- Tumor staging of laryngeal carcinoma relies on an accurate assessment of tumor involvement of laryngeal spaces and adjacent cartilage.

ENDOSCOPY AND ADVANCED LARYNGEAL IMAGING TECHNIQUES
Indirect Laryngoscopy

The most accessible examination tool in the general otolaryngologic practice is the indirect laryngoscopy, which allows for visual assessment of the larynx for signs of malignancy. With this method, identifying small epithelial changes and differentiating benign from malignant tumors *in vivo is difficult*; as such, all suspicious lesions require biopsy confirmation.[1,2] There are a few options for indirect laryngoscopy: laryngeal

[a] Division of Otolaryngology–Head and Neck Surgery, Cedars-Sinai Medical Center, 8635 West Third Street #590W, Los Angeles, CA 90048, USA; [b] Department of Otolaryngology–Head and Neck Surgery, Stanford University, 900 Blake Wilbur Drive Rm W3045, Stanford, CA 94305, USA
* Corresponding author.
E-mail address: michelle.chen@stanford.edu

Otolaryngol Clin N Am 56 (2023) 215–231
https://doi.org/10.1016/j.otc.2022.12.006
0030-6665/23/© 2022 Elsevier Inc. All rights reserved.
oto.theclinics.com

mirror examination, flexible fiber-optic laryngoscopy (FFL), and rigid transoral laryngoscopy.

Laryngeal mirror examination provides an adequate overview of the larynx and tongue base. However, it is difficult to visualize the anterior commissure, especially in patients with a strong gag reflex.

FFL and rigid transoral laryngoscopy provide a more detailed look at individual subsites of the larynx using white light and allow for video/photographic documentation of visible pathology. In addition, office indirect laryngoscopy allows for the assessment of laryngeal anatomy, cricoarytenoid joint function, and airway patency, which helps with future planning for intubation and surgery. The ability to record scope examinations and play them back helps facilitate better patient education. The larynx is assessed in a stepwise manner, typically from supraglottis to glottis. Vocal fold motion is also assessed in detail, making careful differentiation between paraglottic space invasion resulting in vocal fold fixation and recurrent laryngeal nerve paralysis. With adequate topical anesthetic administration, FFL can be passed through the vocal folds to visualize the subglottis and proximal trachea to identify subglottic extension. Rigid laryngoscopy uses 70° or 90° endoscopes transorally and can provide a magnified view of the vocal folds when compared with FFL. This method can limit visualization of certain areas of the base of tongue and be limited by patient intolerance or excessive gagging.

Videostroboscopy

Videostroboscopy is a well-established, noninvasive in-office examination of the vocal folds allowing assessment of vocal fold movement and vibration. A stroboscopic light emits flashes of light desynchronized with vocal fold vibrations to create an image of a slower mucosal wave. This effect is particularly helpful in the evaluation of laryngeal structural abnormalities, vibratory asymmetry, and decreased or absent vibration, for the assessment of glottic gaps or other glottic closure abnormalities.[3]

In addition, changes in vocal fold vibration and mucosal wave propagation do not reliably predict the presence of malignancy or depth of invasion in the lamina propria, the vibratory surface of the vocal folds.[4] On the contrary, research has indicated the benefit of stroboscopy in assessing vocal fold vibratory changes to help evaluate early glottic cancer preoperatively; the presence of a flexible mucosal wave has been found to predict the absence of vocal ligament invasion and invasive carcinoma.[4,5] Ultimately, the ability of stroboscopy to detect abnormalities, while not inherently diagnostic of malignancy, can alert the practitioner of potential pathology present and lead to further workup.

High-Speed Imaging

High-speed digital imaging (HSI) is a frequency-independent laryngeal imaging technique that allows for thousands of images (2000 to 4000 fps) of the vibrating vocal folds to be taken per second, usually during rigid transoral laryngoscopy.[6] An example of a series of images captured with HSI in a patient with a vocal fold scar can be seen in **Fig. 1**. This method overcomes the shortcomings of videostroboscopy, such as the latter's dependence on periodic vibration and an optimal minimum phonation time of 2 s.[7] HSI can capture recordings of mucosal waves in cases of severe dysphonia, such as those with very short or aperiodic mucosal vibrations. Indeed, studies have shown HSI to be more accurate and interpretable than stroboscopy in such cases.[8–10] HSI also has the potential to reveal more about vibratory patterns of the vocal folds, such as subtle features indicating vocal fold paresis that were not detected with laryngoscopy or videostroboscopy.[11] Although HSI is not yet widely available in clinical

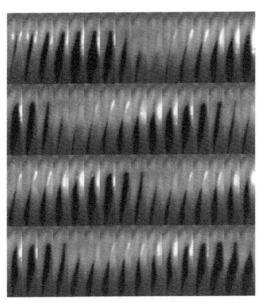

Fig. 1. High-speed imaging montage demonstrating five glottic cycles with vibratory cycle asynchrony from a patient with left vocal fold scar. (*Courtesy of* Peak Woo MD PLLC, New York, NY.)

practice and is very costly, its practical applications continue to be defined. Current challenges with HSI include managing and reviewing the vast amount of data generated with this imaging. A 2-s-long video records up to 8000 frames, and at a typical playback of 20 frames per second, would take ~7 min to review.

Videokymography

Videokymography is an additional method to measure the vibratory capability of the vocal fold and can be considered a one-dimensional version of HSI. In this method, images from a single line transverse to the glottis are recorded; successive line images are shown in real time on a monitor, with the time dimension displayed in the vertical direction. Once these pixel lines are extracted, they are processed consecutively side-by-side based on frame number to create a kymogram. This kymogram visualizes the motion of the mucosal wave, displaying the open and closed phases, periodicity, left-to-right symmetry, phase difference, and amplitude. Current versions of videokymography can juxtapose a kymogram and a laryngoscopic image in a single view. A digital kymograph generated from a patient with a vocal fold polyp is displayed in **Fig. 2**.

Videokymography has the potential to assist with the evaluation of early glottic cancer. Schutte and colleagues[12] described the case of a patient who had previously undergone partial cordectomy and radiation therapy for laryngeal cancer and subsequently presented with persistent dysphonia. Vocal fold mobility was limited and stroboscopic evaluation revealed low-amplitude vibration. Videokymography revealed the absence of mucosal waves, suggesting tumor infiltration, which was later confirmed with a biopsy.

Optical Coherence Tomography

Optical coherence tomography (OCT) is a noninvasive light-based optical tool that can provide high-resolution cross-sectional images of tissue using a near-infrared light

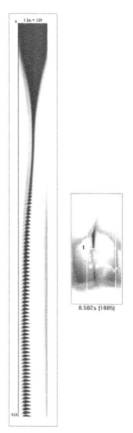

Fig. 2. A digital kymograph generated from a patient with a vocal fold polyp at vocal onset. (*Courtesy of* Peak Woo MD PLLC, New York, NY.)

beam. Originally uses in ophthalmology, the technology has now been adapted for use in otolaryngology with probes placed through endoscopes and laryngoscopes. The main components of the system involve a light source, an interferometer, a detector, and an application system. Using low-coherence interferometry, the basic principle of OCT is the measurement of backscattered light from a tissue probe at approximate resolutions of 10 μm and penetration depths of 2 to 3 mm.[12] Light from the optical source is split into two arms: one arm directed at the tissue sample and one arm at a reference mirror. Light reflected back from the two arms are compared for coherence (if the reflections are identical) and interference (if the optical paths are discordant). As the sample beam is scanned across a tissue surface at a fixed depth, a two-dimensional profile image can be created, providing information regarding the structure of the vocal folds analogous to a vertical histologic section.[13]

Polarization-sensitive OCT (PS-OCT) is an enhanced form of OCT imaging that measures both the intensity and polarization of state changes of reflected light within the tissue to simultaneously characterize tissue structure and birefringence. Collagen fibers, a birefringent material, can change the polarization state of reflected light, allowing PS-OCT to differentiate the collagen-rich vocal ligament from the overlying SLP as well as areas of vocal fold scarring from normal epithelium.[13]

OCT and PS-OCT have been shown to provide information regarding the thickness of the epithelium, integrity of the basement membrane, and structure of the lamina propria as key factors in distinguishing between microinvasive cancer, premalignant lesions, and benign disorders. Kraft and colleagues[14] examined 217 laryngeal lesions in patients undergoing elective microlaryngoscopy and were able to accurately predict the grade of dysplasia in 71% and malignancy in 93% of their cases based on the above factors. This notion was repeatedly confirmed, and the accuracy rate improved upon, in later studies.[15–17] In addition, PS-OCT can help identify the presence of scar tissue, which can guide more accurate biopsies and resections by distinguishing potentially malignant areas from scar tissue or inflammation. Currently, no laryngoscopic imaging systems with integrated OCT components are commercially available on the market; most published studies on the technology use self-constructed in-house systems focused on research purposes.[12,13] As such, OCT and PS-OCT imaging are not currently included in the standard work-up of patients with laryngeal lesions, but show great promise for future use in both the clinic and operating room setting.

Autofluorescence

Autofluorescence (AF) is the natural fluorescence emission of endogenous fluorophores, primarily nicotinamide adenine dinucleotide (NADH) and flavin adenine dinucleotide (FAD), without the addition of any chemical substance, from tissue. Autofluorescence imaging (AFI) is an imaging modality that helps visualize the AF spectrum; when normal tissues are illuminated by ultraviolet and visible light, they emit fluorescent light, whereas neoplastic tissues appear darker due to AF loss caused by metabolic alterations and epithelial thickening.[18]

Zargi and colleagues[19] performed AFI in 108 patients and found sensitivities and specificities of 86.9% and 82.8%, respectively, for identifying malignant lesions in the larynx. When combined with white-light microlaryngoscopy, these two methods yielded a sensitivity of 97.1% for malignant lesions and 61.5% for premalignant lesions, with an overall specificity of 71.8%. AFI can also help identify positive margins intraoperatively, which can lead to improved local control and disease-specific survival. Succo and colleagues[20] performed a prospective cohort study with 73 patients undergoing CO_2 laser resection of early glottic cancers. The use of AFI was also associated with disease-free margins in 97.2% of cases and close margins in 2.8%. Diagnostic accuracy was improved in 16.4% of cases and another 8.2% of cases were upstaged because of AFI use. They reported a sensitivity of 96.5% and a specificity of 98.5%.

Even though the studies mentioned above found high specificities for AFI in controlled settings, the high potential rate of false positives with this technology in the clinical setting should not be overlooked.[21] False positives are typically related to tissues with rich microvascularity causing scattering and AF loss, as is seen in granulation tissue, inflammation, and edema. Bleeding and hyperemia can also diminish underlying tissue AF and lead to false positives. Overgrowth of bacteria (bacteria may produce extra-fluorophores), hyperkeratosis (keratin is strongly fluorescing), and leukoplakia (emits strong AF) lead to potential false negatives. Even though multiple AFI modalities and systems are in production, they are not commonly used as part of the initial screening workup for laryngeal lesions due to this potential for low specificity. Still, the benefits of being a practical, cost-effective, and noninvasive system make AFI a great candidate for future screening systems.

Biologic Endoscopy Techniques: Contact Endoscopy

Contact endoscopy (CE) is a technique allowing surgeons to conduct direct *in vivo* and *in situ* examinations of epithelial cells. The basic technique of CE involves staining superficial cells of the mucosa with 1% nontoxic methylene blue along with magnification of the suspected areas through direct contact of the tip of an endoscope to the mucosal surface to obtain cytologic images.[22] CE enables in vivo visualization of cells and blood vessels with high magnification without requiring tissue biopsy; neoplastic cells and angiogenesis will stain more strongly with methylene blue.

CE images, however, have been shown to be less sensitive than histologic analysis by frozen section in diagnosing invasive carcinoma when directly comparing the two modalities with analysis of paraffin-fixed tissue samples (78% and 100%, respectively).[23] False negatives may occur in cases of incomplete penetration of the stain throughout the epithelial thickness thus hindering the identification of the grade of dysplasia. Another major limitation is the distinction between carcinoma in situ (CIS) and invasive carcinoma, as CE cannot determine whether neoplastic cells breach the basement membrane. These false negatives bring hesitation on the part of the clinician to substitute CE for biopsy in routine clinical practice at present. Overall, the reliability of CE in literature is reported to range from 70% to 88%.[24–26] It remains a promising but underutilized technology in the diagnosis of the laryngeal malignancies.

Biologic Endoscopy Techniques: Narrow Band Imaging

Narrow band imaging (NBI) is an optical enhancement technique that illuminates the intraepithelial papillary capillary loop (IPCL) using narrow bandwidth filters in a red-green-blue sequential illumination system.[27] As the blue light wavelength (415 nm) is absorbed by hemoglobin, the capillary vessels are clearly visualized as brown. The green light wavelength (540 nm) penetrates deeper tissues to enhance subepithelial vessels. In this manner, NBI allows for the visualization of structures of intraepithelial blood vasculature which cannot be seen with conventional white light. The detection of surface mucosal changes that are characteristic of neoplastic lesions (eg, dysplasia, in situ carcinoma, and carcinoma), epithelial abnormalities (thickening and changes in the surface layer), and vascular changes can be best achieved with NBI.

Abnormalities of the IPCL, located beneath the basement membrane of epithelium, have been classified in accordance with their shape changes in NBI by Ni and colleagues; these changes have been found to predict the depth of superficial cancer invasion and are classified into five categories (I to V).[28,29] Type V corresponds to high-grade dysplasia and cancer, type IV suggests a suspicious lesion, whereas types I, II, and III are related to benign lesions.[28] This Ni classification system has been tested by Bertino and colleagues,[30] with 98% of malignant lesions by histopathologic examination corresponding to a type V NBI pattern, and 84.8% of benign lesions corresponding to a type I to IV pattern.

Saraniti and colleagues,[31] in a recent review, found relatively high accuracy rates of NBI in both a preoperative setting (82.9% to 97.8%) and an intraoperative setting (85.7% to 95%) in identifying premalignant and malignant laryngeal lesions. In head-to-head studies against white light endoscopy, NBI has been found to have a higher sensitivity, positive predictive value (PPV), and accuracy in detecting proper resection margins during transoral laser microsurgery.[32] It has also been found to be more accurate in the preoperative assessment and identification of vocal fold lesions.[33–35]

NBI has shown great promise as an adjunct tool to white light endoscopy in preoperatively detecting malignant lesions as an "optical biopsy," and intraoperatively in identifying proper surgical margins. Importantly, as it illuminates prominent vascularity, NBI can highlight the angiogenesis vascularizing cancers hidden on white light sources, especially those in the early stages. **Fig. 3** showcases the angiogenesis highlighted by NBI pointing toward the cancer in both an early- and late-stage laryngeal malignancy. The main limitation with this method is that acute inflammation and chronic post-radiation changes may lead to increased false positives and unjustified biopsies. Zurek and colleagues[36] showed that after 65 to 70 NBI examinations, the plateau of the learning process is reached, suggesting that the incidence of false positives is mainly related to initial experience of the examiners.

IMAGING

Imaging serves an important adjunct role in the workup of laryngeal cancer, characterizing tumor extent, cervical lymphadenopathy, and distant metastasis. The primary imaging modalities employed include computed tomography (CT), MRI, and nuclear studies. More novel imaging technologies include OCT, NBI, and biologic endoscopy techniques described above.

Computed Tomography

CT is an accessible, informative tool in the initial imaging work-up of laryngeal tumors. A CT scan with administration of iodinated contrast agent is performed from the skull

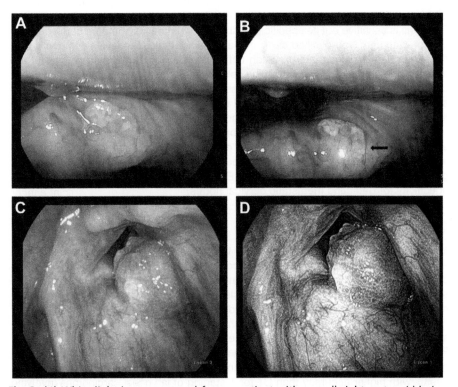

Fig. 3. (A) White light image captured from a patient with a small right arytenoid lesion concerning for malignancy. (B) The same view under narrow band imaging highlighting angiogenesis, with vessels (*black arrow*) feeding into the lesion not seen with white light. (C) White light image captured from a patient with a large exophytic cancer based in the left true vocal fold. (D) The same view under narrow band imaging highlighting the diffuse angiogenesis surrounding the tumor as well as the hypervascularity on the tumor itself. (*Courtesy of* Anca M. Barbu, MD, Los Angeles, CA.)

base to the level of the aortic arch. Particular attention must be paid to acquiring the scan in an axial plane parallel to the plane of the hyoid bone to attain parallel axial cuts through the vocal folds. Thinner submillimeter sections are reconstructed at the level of the larynx for higher resolution in the final reconstructed images for analysis.

Morphologic characterization of tumor includes soft tissue asymmetry, presence of a contrast-enhancing mass, and loss of normal fat and tissue planes.[37] CT imaging is also used to define pre-epiglottic and paraglottic space involvement, which impacts T staging. Sensitivity of CT for paraglottic space invasion has been shown to be 93%. Specificity rates vary from 50% to 76% due to possible presence of peritumoral inflammatory changes without actual invasion.[37] Similarly, prior invasive biopsy procedures at the lesion site may also decrease specificity. Inflammatory reactions at the biopsy site may lead to false positives suggesting further disease spread or invasion on either CT or MRI.

Cartilage invasion is a critical characteristic that must be delineated. The CT characteristics for invasion include sclerosis, lysis, or extra-laryngeal spread.[38] Sclerosis involves bony remodeling of cartilage due to direct invasion or adjacent presence of neoplastic cells. Osteolysis of ossified cartilage may seem as areas of erosion or lysis depending on the size of destruction. A retrospective review by Pietragalla and colleagues[39] studying pretreatment CTs of 40 patients showed diagnostic accuracy of 67.5% to 100% for assessing invasion of the thyroid, cricoid, or arytenoid cartilages. Sclerosis is sensitive but its specificity is limited by natural asymmetric cartilage ossification with age. Non-ossified cartilage has similar attenuation levels compared with the tumor itself, making interpretation difficult. Lysis and extralaryngeal spread are specific signs however not as sensitive as they are seen more in advanced laryngeal cancers.[40] Cancers of the anterior commissure are particularly prone to cartilage invasion as there is no perichondrium around Broyle's ligament and cancers can extend directly from the ligament into the cartilage.

CT imaging can also provide information on nodal spread of disease to help with staging. Generally accepted radiologic criteria for concerning nodal metastases include size greater than 1 cm, round shape, necrosis, and irregular or spiculated margins suggestive of extranodal extension (ENE).[41] CT has a 90% sensitivity and 75% specificity for detecting metastatic cervical nodes.

Magnetic Resonance Imaging

MRI is known for providing superior soft tissue resolution and can be an important adjunct if CT is inconclusive.[42] Anatomic components specific to the larynx with implications on tumor staging, including submucosal space involvement, cartilage invasion, extension into the laryngeal ventricle, and anterior-to-posterior glottic extent, may be better delineated when CT is used in conjunction with MRI.[43]

In assessing the primary tumor, MRI exhibits characteristic intermediate T1 and T2 signal intensity with moderate contrast enhancement and restricted diffusion.[44,45] Furthermore, MRI has an accuracy of 90% in assessing the involvement of the submucosal spaces including the pre-epiglottic and paraglottic spaces.[46,47] MRI is especially useful, with higher accuracy than CT for T staging of laryngeal carcinomas involving the anterior commissure.[48] Although controversy remains regarding the role of MRI in the detection of early glottic cancers, some argue that MRI provides higher diagnostic accuracy (80%) compared with CT (70%) for T1–T2 glottic carcinomas, especially when diffusion-weighted imaging is used.[49,50]

Owing to the aforementioned inherent limitations of CT, MRI can have an important adjunct role in clarifying cartilage invasion from peritumoral inflammation. Because of its high sensitivity (89% to 95%), the negative predictive value of excluding cartilage invasion on MRI has been shown to be 94% to 96%.[51]

Nuclear Imaging

Nuclear imaging relies on functional uptake of radioactive tracers by specific tissue types within the body. The most commonly used modality is PET. PET relies on uptake and detection of fluorine-18-fluorodeoxy-D-glucose (FDG) by highly metabolic cells, which includes neoplasms and also some benign tumors, thyroid nodules, inflammatory tissue, infection, and normal tissue with baseline increased physiologic activity.[52]

The principal indication for FDG-PET is in the evaluation of nodal metastasis. A retrospective review of 47 patients with head and neck squamous cell carcinoma showed that for nodal classification, PET combined with CT had a diagnostic accuracy of 97%, superior to either PET or CT alone.[53] Furthermore, in a prospective study of 91 patients with a clinically negative neck on palpation, FDG-PET showed a sensitivity of 71% compared with 50% for CT/MRI in detecting cervical metastases undetected on physical examination.[54] Although the literature generally supports the superiority of PET/CT for nodal metastasis, the spatial resolution of the scan, typically 4 to 6 mm, does limit its sensitivity for microscopic disease in smaller, subcentimeter lymph nodes.[55]

Another recognized role of FDG-PET in the work-up of laryngeal malignancy is the detection of distant metastasis as well as synchronous or metachronous tumors. At initial diagnosis, the rate of distant metastasis for primary laryngeal carcinoma is within the range of 5% to 15%. Although large-scale studies are not available to assess the diagnostic accuracy of FDG-PET for distant metastases specifically for laryngeal cancer, for head and neck malignancy in general its sensitivity and specificity are thought to be within the range of 80% to 90%.[56] As approximately 8% of patients with laryngeal cancer develop synchronous or metachronous tumors, most typically in the lungs, FDG-PET has been shown to be a useful tool in detecting these additional lesions.[57,58] Although the individual cost of FDG-PET is relatively high, it has been shown to be cost-effective in avoiding futile radical treatment due to its diagnostic utility for metastatic disease.[59]

STAGING
American Joint Committee on Cancer Eighth Edition Staging Manual

The American Joint Committee on Cancer (AJCC) in collaboration with the Union for International Cancer Control (UICC) provides a gold standard staging classification system for all cancers based on anatomic site. Since the publication of its first edition in 1977, the AJCC staging manual has been updated periodically about every 5 to 7 years to its most current form, the eighth edition, published in 2016. The eighth edition classification system was put into effect for new cancers diagnosed from January 1, 2018 onwards.[60]

Clinical Staging

Clinical staging involves a full work-up including history, physical examination, endoscopy, biopsy, and imaging. With regards to laryngeal cancer, the classification system is organized into anatomic subsites including the subglottis, glottis, and supraglottis with attention to vocal fold function in addition to tumor (T), nodal (N), and distant metastatic (M) characteristics (**Table 1**). Of note, a separate AJCC classification system exists for non-epithelial tumors, such as lymphoid, soft tissue, bone, and cartilaginous neoplasms.

T Staging

Accurate determination of vocal fold function is a key criterion specific for laryngeal staging. By definition, glottic function is normal for T1 staging of any subsite. Impaired

Table 1
American Joint Committee on Cancer eighth edition TNM staging

T Stage		Supraglottis	Glottis	Subglottis	Vocal Cord Function
Tis		Carcinoma in situ			
1	a	one supraglottic subsite	One vocal cord involved	One subglottic subsite	Normal
	b		Both vocal cords involved		Normal
2		>1 adjacent subsite or extension to glottis or region outside of supraglottis	Extension to supraglottis or subglottis	Extension to glottis	Impaired mobility
3		Invasion into inner cortex of thyroid cartilage, pre-epiglottic, paraglottic, or postcricoid space			Fixation
4	a	Moderately advanced local disease: Invasion into outer cortex of thyroid cartilage and/or extra-laryngeal structures (thyroid, esophagus, neck soft tissue, trachea)			Any
	b	Very advanced local disease: carotid artery encasement, prevertebral fascia invasion, mediastinal invasion			

N Stage					Extra-nodal Extension
0		No clinically evident nodes			No
1		Single ipsilateral node <3 cm			
2	a	Single ipsilateral node 3-6 cm			
	b	Multiple ipsilateral nodes 3-6 cm			
	c	Any contralateral or bilateral <6 cm			
3	a	Any node >6 cm			
	b	Any node at any size			Yes

M stage					
0	No distant metastasis				
1	Distant metastasis present				

Table 2
Overall prognostic staging based on TNM classification

	N0	N1	N2	N3	
Tis	0	–	–	–	M0
T1	I	III	IVa	IVb	
T2	II	III	IVa	IVb	
T3	III	III	IVa	IVb	
T4a	IVa	IVa	IVa	IVb	
T4b	IVb	IVb	IVb	IVb	
Any T	IVc				M1

mobility upstages to a T2 and any vocal fold fixation is classified as T3. In contrast to other head and neck cancer sites, the exact size of the laryngeal tumor is of less importance but more so its extension into adjacent structures and intra- and extra-laryngeal spaces. Correct determination of invasion of the thyroid, arytenoid, or cricoid cartilages with CT/MRI is critical as any involvement of cartilage is defined as T3. If invasion goes beyond the outer cortex of the thyroid cartilage, the tumor is classified as T4a.

N Staging

N staging depends on the size, number, and laterality of clinically evident cervical lymph nodes. In the AJCC 8th edition, there was a notable update with the introduction of ENE status and the N3b stage. Clinically overt ENE can be determined by physical examination including overlying skin fixation, "matted" nodes, and functional deficits of any or all of the following structures: cranial nerve(s), the sympathetic trunk, brachial plexus, or phrenic nerve. Imaging via CT or MRI can also show ill-defined nodal margins, capsular enhancement as well as adjacent fat or muscle invasion. Accurate assessment of ENE is important because its presence upstages the N status to N3b and overall stage to IVb.

M Staging

Distant metastasis is defined by clinical evidence of disease spread beyond the head and neck region and is seen in 10% to 20% of laryngeal cancers.[61] As the most common distant metastatic site for the larynx is the lungs, imaging of the chest is a very component of the workup of laryngeal cancer. Other metastatic sites include the brain, bone, liver, and skin. Mediastinal lymph nodes are considered distant metastatic spread, though particular attention must be paid to level VII, anterior superior mediastinal nodes, as this is still considered regional disease and would be staged as such.

Overall Prognostic Grouping

The clinical TNM stage is grouped into an overall prognostic stage ranging from stage I to IVc (**Table 2**). Increasing T and N stage upstage the overall stage group. All M1 disease is considered Stage IVc. This staging system is consistent across all head and neck mucosal carcinomas other than p16+ oropharyngeal cancer.

Pathologic Staging

The AJCC sets forth a separate staging system based on pathologic analysis. The main difference between clinical and pathologic TNM staging lies in the nodal analysis. The difference between clinical and pathologic nodal staging is summarized in **Table 3**. For pathologic staging, ENE does not upstage automatically to N3b. If there

Table 3
American Joint Committee on Cancer clinical versus pathologic nodal staging

N Stage		Clinical	Clinical ENE	Pathologic	Pathologic ENE
0		No clinically evident nodes	No	No regional lymph node metastasis	No
1		Single ipsilateral node <3 cm		Single ipsilateral node, <3 cm	No
2	a	Single ipsilateral node 3 to 6 cm		Single ipsilateral node, <3 cm	Yes
				Single, ipsilateral node, >3 cm	No
	b	Multiple ipsilateral nodes 3 to 6 cm		Multiple ipsilateral nodes, <6 cm	No
	c	Any contralateral or bilateral nodes <6 cm		Any contralateral or bilateral nodes <6 cm	No
3	a	Any node >6 cm		Any node >6 cm	No
	b	Any node at any size	Yes		Yes

is only one node that is positive for carcinoma with ENE and is less than 3 cm in size, the final stage is pN2a.

PEARLS AND PITFALLS

Imaging of the larynx, especially with early mucosal lesions, presents a challenge due to the inherent small size of laryngeal structures and spaces, as well as the risk of motion artifact caused by respiration and swallowing. Staging, therefore, may be affected by the quality and interpretation of these studies. Overstaging tumors may lead to unnecessary surgery and understaging may lead to inadequate primary treatment. A retrospective review of 29 patients with supraglottic carcinoma who had undergone surgery showed that 21% had been over-staged and 4% had been under-staged when comparing preoperative staging with pathologic staging.[62] Baugnon and colleagues[63] in their 2013 article reviewed the common pitfalls of laryngeal cancer staging based on site.

With regard to glottic tumors, evaluation of the anterior commissure is critical. Involvement of the anterior commissure in T1 or T2 glottic tumors has been shown to increase the risk of understaging and ultimately of recurrence after primary surgery.[64] Within the supraglottis, careful evaluation of the base of tongue on sagittal images is important in distinguishing T1 from T2 tumors. Submucosal extension into the pre-epiglottic space must be assessed accurately by imaging as involvement upstages the tumor to T3. Extension into the paraglottic space, another tumor characteristic that leads to upstaging to T3, must also be carefully evaluated as tumor extension into this space has been associated with lower local control rate with radiation therapy alone.[65] Inferior extension into the laryngeal ventricle renders the tumor "transglottic," and has implications for T staging as well as surgical options.

Baungon and colleagues[63] argue that perhaps the most challenging yet consequential pitfall of laryngeal cancer staging is determining the extent of cartilage invasion. Status of the cartilage has been the most notable update to laryngeal cancer T staging in the modern era as any involvement upstages to a T3 and extension to the outer cortex to a T4a, or moderately advanced local disease. The role of CT and MRI in assessing cartilage invasion is described earlier in this article.

FUTURE DIRECTIONS

Cancer classification systems such as the AJCC TNM staging aim to provide a universal and common language among multidisciplinary specialists to describe and study cancers. With an increasing interest in precision oncologic medicine, the role of advanced imaging and molecular markers may, in the future, both be integrated into clinical staging as high-quality studies become available.[60]

CLINICS CARE POINTS

- Direct laryngoscopy and biopsy is the gold standard method of diagnosing laryngeal cancer.
- Videostroboscopy is useful for assessing vocal fold vibration. Though not inherently diagnostic of malignancy; it can help decrease suspicion for invasive cancer preoperatively if a normal flexible mucosal wave is visualized.
- Optical coherence tomography is a noninvasive optical tool using near-infrared light beams that can assess the epithelium, basement membrane, and lamina propria to accurately detect dysplasia and malignancy. It can also identify scar tissue to help guide biopsies.

- Autofluorescence is a practical, cost-effective, and noninvasive optical technique that has high sensitivity for identifying malignant lesions in the larynx, but suffers from low specificity due to bleeding, granulation, and inflammation causing false positives.
- Biologic endoscopy techniques are promising adjuncts for diagnosing laryngeal cancer and monitoring for recurrence. Narrow band imaging, specifically, has a five-stage classification and has been found to have high accuracy rates both preoperatively and intra-operatively in identifying premalignant and malignant lesions.
- Primary tumor staging of laryngeal carcinoma requires vocal fold function assessment with endoscopy in addition to determination of extent of laryngeal and extra-laryngeal structures, namely the paraglottic, pre-epiglottic, and post-cricoid spaces.
- Cartilage invasion is critical for tumor staging and can be relatively accurately assessed with a combination of computed tomography and MRI.
- Nuclear imaging with PET is used in assessing nodal involvement and distant metastasis

DISCLOSURE

The authors have no commercial or financial conflicts of interest and any funding sources for all authors.

REFERENCES

1. Manfredi C. Models and analysis of vocal emissions for biomedical applications: 10th International Workshop. Florence: Firenze University Press; 2017. p. 13–5.
2. Iakovidis DK. Sensors, Signal and Image Processing in Biomedicine and Assisted Living. Sensors (Basel) 2020;20(18):5071.
3. Verikas A, Uloza V, Bacauskiene M. Advances in laryngeal imaging. Eur Arch Otorhinolaryngol 2009;266(10):1509–20.
4. Colden D, Zeitels SM, Hillman RE, et al. Stroboscopic assessment of vocal fold keratosis and glottic cancer. Ann Otol Rhinol Laryngol 2001;110(4):293–8.
5. van Balkum M, Buijs B, Donselaar EJ, et al. Goulin Lippi Fernandes E, Wegner I, Grolman W, Janssen LM. Systematic review of the diagnostic value of laryngeal stroboscopy in excluding early glottic carcinoma. Clin Otolaryngol 2017;42(1): 123–30. https://doi.org/10.1111/coa.12678.
6. Woo P. Objective Measures of Laryngeal Imaging: What Have We Learned Since Dr. Paul Moore. J Voice 2014;28(1):69–81. https://doi.org/10.1016/j.jvoice.2013. 02.001.
7. Kitzing P. Stroboscopy–a pertinent laryngological examination. J Otolaryngol 1985;14(3):151–7.
8. Bonilha HS, Deliyski DD, Gerlach TT. Phase asymmetries in normophonic speakers: visual judgments and objective findings. Am J Speech Lang Pathol 2008;17(4):367–76.
9. Bonilha HS, Deliyski DD. Period and glottal width irregularities in vocally normal speakers. J Voice 2008;22(6):699–708.
10. Patel R, Dailey S, Bless D. Comparison of high-speed digital imaging with stroboscopy for laryngeal imaging of glottal disorders. Ann Otol Rhinol Laryngol 2008; 117(6):413–24.
11. Mortensen M, Woo P. High-speed imaging used to detect vocal fold paresis: a case report. Ann Otol Rhinol Laryngol 2008;117(9):684–7.
12. Wittig L, Betz C, Eggert D. Optical coherence tomography for tissue classification of the larynx in an outpatient setting-a translational challenge on the verge of a

resolution? Translational Biophotonics 2021;3(1). https://doi.org/10.1002/tbio. 202000013.

13. Sharma GK, Wong BJF. Optical Coherence Tomography of the Larynx: Normative Anatomy and Benign Processes. Biomed Opt Otorhinolaryngol 2016;573–88. https://doi.org/10.1007/978-1-4939-1758-7-35.

14. Kraft M, Glanz H, von Gerlach S, et al. Clinical value of optical coherence tomography in laryngology. Head Neck 2008;30(12):1628–35.

15. Volgger V, Sharma GK, Jing JC, et al. Long-range Fourier domain optical coherence tomography of the pediatric subglottis. Int J Pediatr Otorhinolaryngol 2015; 79(2):119–26.

16. Englhard AS, Betz T, Volgger V, et al. Intraoperative assessment of laryngeal pathologies with optical coherence tomography integrated into a surgical microscope. Lasers Surg Med 2017;49(5):490–7.

17. Just T, Lankenau E, Hüttmann G, et al. Intra-operative application of optical coherence tomography with an operating microscope. J Laryngol Otol 2009; 123(9):1027–30.

18. Wu C, Gleysteen J, Teraphongphom NT, et al. In-vivo optical imaging in head and neck oncology: basic principles, clinical applications and future directions. Int J Oral Sci 2018;10(2):10.

19. Žargi M, Fajdiga I, Šmid L. Autofluorescence imaging in the diagnosis of laryngeal cancer. Eur Arch Oto-Rhino-Laryngology 2000;257(1):17–23. https://doi. org/10.1007/pl00007506.

20. Succo G, Garofalo P, Fantini M, et al. Direct autofluorescence during CO2 laser surgery of the larynx: can it really help the surgeon? Acta Otorhinolaryngol Ital 2014;34(3):174–83.

21. Sweeny L, Dean NR, Magnuson JS, et al. Assessment of tissue autofluorescence and reflectance for oral cavity cancer screening. Otolaryngol Head Neck Surg 2011;145(6):956–60.

22. Mannelli G, Cecconi L, Gallo O. Laryngeal preneoplastic lesions and cancer: challenging diagnosis. Qualitative literature review and meta-analysis. Crit Rev Oncol Hematol 2016;106:64–90.

23. Cikojević D, Gluncić I, Pesutić-Pisac V. Comparison of contact endoscopy and frozen section histopathology in the intra-operative diagnosis of laryngeal pathology. J Laryngol Otol 2008;122(8):836–9.

24. Wardrop PJ, Sim S, McLaren K. Contact endoscopy of the larynx: a quantitative study. J Laryngol Otol 2000;114(6):437–40.

25. Carriero E, Galli J, Fadda G, et al. Preliminary experiences with contact endoscopy of the larynx. Eur Arch Otorhinolaryngol 2000;257(2):68–71.

26. Warnecke A, Averbeck T, Leinung M, et al. Contact endoscopy for the evaluation of the pharyngeal and laryngeal mucosa. Laryngoscope 2010;120(2):253–8.

27. Cohen J. Comprehensive atlas of high resolution endoscopy and narrowband imaging. West Sussex, UK: John Wiley & Sons; 2008.

28. Ni XG, He S, Xu ZG, et al. Endoscopic diagnosis of laryngeal cancer and precancerous lesions by narrow band imaging. J Laryngol Otol 2011;125(3): 288–96.

29. Kumagai Y, Inoue H, Nagai K, et al. Magnifying endoscopy, stereoscopic microscopy, and the microvascular architecture of superficial esophageal carcinoma. Endoscopy 2002;34(5):369–75.

30. Bertino G, Cacciola S, Fernandes WB, et al. Effectiveness of narrow band imaging in the detection of premalignant and malignant lesions of the larynx: Validation

of a new endoscopic clinical classification. Head & Neck 2015;37(2):215–22. https://doi.org/10.1002/hed.23582.

31. Saraniti C, Chianetta E, Greco G. Mat Lazim N, Verro B. The Impact of Narrow-band Imaging on the Pre- and Intra- operative Assessments of Neoplastic and Preneoplastic Laryngeal Lesions. A Systematic Review. Int Arch Otorhinolaryngol 2021;25(3):e471–8.

32. Klimza H, Jackowska J, Piazza C, et al. The role of intraoperative narrow-band imaging in transoral laser microsurgery for early and moderately advanced glottic cancer. Braz J Otorhinolaryngol 2019;85(2):228–36. https://doi.org/10.1016/j.bjorl.2018.01.004.

33. Popek B, Bojanowska-Poźniak K, Tomasik B, et al. Clinical experience of narrow band imaging (NBI) usage in diagnosis of laryngeal lesions. Otolaryngologia Polska 2019;73(6):18–23. https://doi.org/10.5604/01.3001.0013.3401.

34. Piazza C, Cocco D, De Benedetto L, et al. Narrow band imaging and high definition television in the assessment of laryngeal cancer: a prospective study on 279 patients. Eur Arch Oto-Rhino-Laryngology 2010;267(3):409–14. https://doi.org/10.1007/s00405-009-1121-6.

35. Ni XG, Zhu JQ, Zhang QQ, et al. Diagnosis of vocal cord leukoplakia: The role of a novel narrow band imaging endoscopic classification. Laryngoscope 2019;129(2):429–34.

36. Żurek M, Rzepakowska A, Osuch-Wójcikiewicz E, et al. Learning curve for endoscopic evaluation of vocal folds lesions with narrow band imaging. Braz J Otorhinolaryngol 2019;85(6):753–9.

37. Castelijns JA, Hermans R, van den Brekel MW, et al. Imaging of laryngeal cancer. Semin Ultrasound CT MR 1998;19(6):492–504.

38. Becker M, Zbären P, Laeng H, et al. Neoplastic invasion of the laryngeal cartilage: comparison of MR imaging and CT with histopathologic correlation. Radiology 1995;194(3):661–9. https://doi.org/10.1148/radiology.194.3.7862960.

39. Pietragalla M, Nardi C, Bonasera L, et al. Current role of computed tomography imaging in the evaluation of cartilage invasion by laryngeal carcinoma. Radiol Med 2020;125(12):1301–10.

40. Becker M, Monnier Y, de Vito C. MR Imaging of Laryngeal and Hypopharyngeal Cancer. Magn Reson Imaging Clin N Am 2022;30(1):53–72.

41. Castelijns JA, van den Brekel MW. Imaging of lymphadenopathy in the neck. Eur Radiol 2002;12(4):727–38. https://doi.org/10.1007/s003300101102.

42. Becker M, Burkhardt K, Dulguerov P, Allal A. Imaging of the larynx and hypopharynx. Eur J Radiol 2008;66(3):460–79.

43. Jain A, Anand SS. Imaging in Carcinoma of the Larynx. Carcinoma of the Larynx and Hypopharynx 2019;13–24. https://doi.org/10.1007/978-981-13-3110-7-2.

44. Becker M, Burkhardt K, Dulguerov P, et al. Imaging of the larynx and hypopharynx. Eur J Radiol 2008;66(3):460–79.

45. Mundada P, Varoquaux AD, Lenoir V, et al. Utility of MRI with morphologic and diffusion weighted imaging in the detection of post-treatment nodal disease in head and neck squamous cell carcinoma. Eur J Radiol 2018;101:162–9.

46. Zbären P, Becker M, Läng H. Pretherapeutic staging of laryngeal carcinoma. Clinical findings, computed tomography, and magnetic resonance imaging compared with histopathology. Cancer 1996;77(7):1263–73.

47. Ravanelli M, Paderno A, Del Bon F, et al. Prediction of Posterior Paraglottic Space and Cricoarytenoid Unit Involvement in Endoscopically T3 Glottic Cancer with Arytenoid Fixation by Magnetic Resonance with Surface Coils. Cancers 2019;11(1):67. https://doi.org/10.3390/cancers11010067.

48. Wu JH, Zhao J, Li ZH, et al. Comparison of CT and MRI in Diagnosis of Laryngeal Carcinoma with Anterior Vocal Commissure Involvement. Sci Rep 2016;6:30353.

49. Allegra E, Ferrise P, Trapasso S, et al. Early Glottic Cancer: Role of MRI in the Pre-operative Staging. Biomed Res Int 2014;2014:1–7. https://doi.org/10.1155/2014/890385.

50. Shang DS, Ruan LX, Zhou SH, et al. Differentiating Laryngeal Carcinomas from Precursor Lesions by Diffusion-Weighted Magnetic Resonance Imaging at 3.0 T: A Preliminary Study. PLoS ONE 2013;8(7):e68622. https://doi.org/10.1371/journal.pone.0068622.

51. Becker M, Zbären P, Casselman JW, et al. Neoplastic invasion of laryngeal carti-lage: reassessment of criteria for diagnosis at MR imaging. Radiology 2008; 249(2):551–9.

52. Purohit BS, Ailianou A, Dulguerov N, et al. FDG-PET/CT pitfalls in oncological head and neck imaging. Insights Imaging 2014;5(5):585–602.

53. Jeong HS, Baek CH, Son YI, et al. Use of integrated 18F-FDG PET/CT to improve the accuracy of initial cervical nodal evaluation in patients with head and neck squamous cell carcinoma. Head Neck 2007;29(3):203–10.

54. Roh JL, Park JP, Kim JS, et al. 18F fluorodeoxyglucose PET/CT in head and neck squamous cell carcinoma with negative neck palpation findings: a prospective study. Radiology 2014;271(1):153–61.

55. Castaldi P, Leccisotti L, Bussu F, et al. Role of (18)F-FDG PET-CT in head and neck squamous cell carcinoma. Acta Otorhinolaryngol Ital 2013;33(1):1–8.

56. Gourin CG, Watts T, Williams HT, et al. Identification of distant metastases with PET-CT in patients with suspected recurrent head and neck cancer. Laryngo-scope 2009;119(4):703–6.

57. Strobel K, Haerle SK, Stoeckli SJ, et al. Head and neck squamous cell carcinoma (HNSCC) – detection of synchronous primaries with 18F-FDG-PET/CT. Eur J Nucl Med Mol Imaging 2009;36(6):919–27. https://doi.org/10.1007/s00259-009-1064-6.

58. Nikolaou AC, Markou CD, Petridis DG, et al. Second Primary Neoplasms in Pa-tients With Laryngeal Carcinoma. The Laryngoscope 2000;110(1):58–64. https://doi.org/10.1097/00005537-200001000-00012.

59. Kurien G, Hu J, Harris J, et al. Cost-effectiveness of positron emission tomogra-phy/computed tomography in the management of advanced head and neck can-cer. J Otolaryngol Head Neck Surg 2011;40(6):468–72.

60. Amin MB, Greene FL, Edge SB, et al. AJCC Cancer Staging Manual: Continuing to build a bridge from a population-based to a more "personalized" approach to cancer staging. CA: A Cancer J Clinicians 2017;67(2):93–9. The 8h Edition.

61. Milano MT, Peterson CR 3rd, Zhang H, et al. Second primary lung cancer after head and neck squamous cell cancer: population-based study of risk factors. Head Neck 2012;34(12):1782–8.

62. Kim JW, Yoon SY, Park IS, et al. Correlation between radiological images and pathological results in supraglottic cancer. J Laryngol Otol 2008;122(11):1224–9.

63. Baugnon KL, Beitler JJ. Pitfalls in the staging of cancer of the laryngeal squa-mous cell carcinoma. Neuroimaging Clin N Am 2013;23(1):81–105.

64. Rödel RMW, Steiner W, Müller RM, et al. Endoscopic laser surgery of early glottic cancer: Involvement of the anterior commissure. Head & Neck 2009;31(5): 583–92. https://doi.org/10.1002/hed.20993.

65. Murakami R, Nishimura R, Baba Y, et al. Prognostic factors of glottic carcinomas treated with radiation therapy: value of the adjacent sign on radiological examina-tions in the sixth edition of the UICC TNM staging system. Int J Radiat Oncol Biol Phys 2005;61(2):471–5.

Dysplastic Lesions of the Larynx

Caitlin Olson, MD[a],*, Ronda Alexander, MD[b], Sandra Stinnett, MD[a]

KEYWORDS

- Leukoplakia • Dysplasia • Larynx • Glottis • Vocal folds • Premalignant lesions

KEY POINTS

- Diagnosis of laryngeal dysplasia (LD) relies on endoscopic procedures and histopathologic evaluation.
- New imaging modalities such as narrow band imaging) and the Storz Professional Image Enhancement System hold promise for prehistologic assessment of leukoplakic lesions.
- The factors that encourage the progression of LD to squamous cell carcinoma are not fully elucidated. The risk of malignant transformation increases with increasing grade of dysplasia but this relationship is neither linear nor predictable.
- Preliminary studies suggest a minimum of 6 months follow-up for low-grade dysplasia and 5 years for high-risk or severe dysplasia. Most providers decrease frequency after 2 years, although there is no definitive data to support that this confers any benefit.

DEFINITIONS, FIELD CANCERIZATION, EPIDEMIOLOGY, AND RISK FACTORS

The vocal fold epithelium is nonkeratinized stratified squamous epithelium divided into 2 main layers, the basal layer and the suprabasal layer. Epithelial cells proliferate from the basal layer, mature as they progress more superficially, and eventually desquamate. Normally, the epithelium consists of 5 to 10 layers of cells. A greater than 7-fold increase in the number of layers is considered hyperplastic. Metaplasia can cause abnormal keratin production at the surface of the mucosal epithelium, which results in leukoplakia, also known as laryngeal keratosis.[1,2] Erythroplakia is a manifestation of hyperplasia with an inflammatory reaction at the outermost layer of the epithelium. Erythroleukoplakia, also known as speckled keratosis, is mucosal plaque with intermixed leukoplakia and erythroplakia, with the red portion typically resulting from hypervascularity and vascular dilation. Dysplasia is cytologic and, sometimes, architectural abnormality of the epithelial cells. At the level of the true vocal folds, dysplasia is a precursor to laryngeal squamous cell carcinoma (SCC). Such dysplasia of the

[a] University of Pittsburgh Medical Center, Eye & Ear Institute, 203 Lothrop Street, Suite 500, Pittsburgh, PA 15213, USA; [b] Montefiore Medical Center, Medical Arts Pavilion, 3400 Bainbridge Avenue, Bronx, NY 10467, USA
* Corresponding author.
E-mail address: olsoncp@upmc.edu

Otolaryngol Clin N Am 56 (2023) 233–246
https://doi.org/10.1016/j.otc.2023.01.001
0030-6665/23/© 2023 Elsevier Inc. All rights reserved.

subglottis and supraglottis tends to be asymptomatic and diagnosed incidentally, whereas it will present with dysphonia when present at the glottis. For the purposes of this discussion, we will focus on the glottis when referring to laryngeal dysplasia (LD).[3,4]

It remains unclear how LD progresses to malignancy. Traditionally, carcinogenesis was understood to be a series of stepwise genetic mutations; however, in the setting of SCC of the larynx, the field cancerization model has become more accepted. In this model, carcinogens induce protumorigenic genetic mutations and/or epimutations of cells that predispose these altered cells to eventually progress to a neoplasm. Field cancerization also requires a component of immune escape, where mutations are inherently able to evade the immune response. Of note, the field of abnormal cells may look normal, or it may exhibit various visible morphologic changes. Leukoplakia, erythroplakia, and erythroleukoplakia may all be identified on visual inspection of the larynx.[3,5] However, none of these findings are pathognomonic for LD on histology.[3,6,7] Therefore, the diagnosis of LD relies on endoscopic procedures and histopathologic evaluation (**Fig. 1**).

The incidence of LD is difficult to estimate due to selection bias as most incidence numbers are derived from hospital-based studies and not population studies. However, a population study performed between 1935 and 1984 in Rochester, Minnesota identified an annual incidence of precancerous laryngeal keratosis in the United States of 10.2 lesions per 1,000,000 men and 2.1 lesions per 100,000 women but is based on a total of only 108 cases in those 49 years. This study also showed a strong male predilection, no age-dependence but a peak between 45 and 55 years of age, and rates increasing significantly in parallel to concomitant tobacco use.[4,8]

Histologic changes of the glottis have long been attributed to chronic irritation and inflammation. The most well-known etiologic risk factor for LD is tobacco, in a dose-dependent fashion. Although nonsmokers have a 4.2% chance of developing LD, this increased to 12.4% in light smokers (<10 cigarettes/d) and 47.2% in heavy smokers (<20 cigarettes/d).[9] There is also a synergistic and multiplicative effect when coupled with alcohol consumption, another noted risk factor in 75% of all head and neck SCC.[6,10] The rates of tobacco use have been trending downward since 1984 but it is unclear whether the rates of LD may have followed suit. LD has also been linked to environmental and occupational exposures related to construction, including asbestos, cement dust, and polycyclic aromatic hydrocarbons, which occur naturally in coal, crude oil, and gasoline and are released in combustion. Such industrial exposures increase the odds ratio of developing dysplasia with the progression to laryngeal cancer.[11–13] In 2013, Coca-Pelaz and colleagues reviewed the literature regarding gastroesophageal or laryngopharyngeal reflux as a risk factor for LD and found that

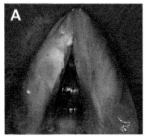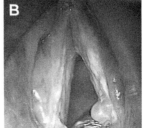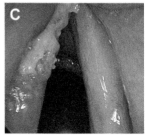

Fig. 1. Intraoperative images of laryngeal leukoplakia depicting mild dysplasia (*A*), moderate-to-severe dysplasia (*B*), and invasive SCC (*C*) confirmed via histopathology.

the evidence was insufficient. The data were confounded by the effect of concurrent tobacco and alcohol consumption as well as the unstandardized and often inaccurate diagnosis of reflux.[14] However, several years later, Parsel and colleagues performed a systematic review and meta-analysis of 18 case-control studies that showed a significantly increased odds ratio for laryngeal malignancy in the setting of gastroesophageal reflux when controlling for tobacco and alcohol.[15] More recently, a small case-control study found elevated levels of pepsin, a marker for laryngopharyngeal reflux, in the saliva of patients with benign and malignant laryngeal neoplasms when compared with a cohort of patients without laryngeal disease.[16]

Past theories that LD was also caused by voice abuse and nutritional deficiency, such as vitamin A or folate, have not been supported by data. Several trials proposed treatment with folate, carotene, and/or retinyl palmitate supplementation but no robust follow-up studies have been performed.[13,17,18] Beta-carotenes and cis-retinoic acid studies have been performed with promising results for oral leukoplakia and oral dysplasia (OD); however, LD is clinically distinct from OD with respect to mutational burden, range of cytologic atypia, and risk of malignant transformation limiting comparisons between the two.[3,19,20]

Finally, we consider the role of human papilloma virus (HPV). Two hundred genotypes of HPV have been identified and stratified according to oncologic risk. High-risk subtypes 16 and 18 are well associated with premalignant lesions in gynecologic and oropharyngeal cancer; however, the association with premalignant lesions of the larynx is weak. Low-risk subtypes 6 and 11 have long been associated with recurrent laryngeal papillomatosis, with dysplasia reported in 5% to 28% and malignant transformation reported in 1% to 7%.[3,21–23] However, the prevalence of HPV low-risk subtypes in low-grade and high-grade dysplasia is estimated to be 50% and 83%, respectively. HPV high-risk subtypes are not consistently identified in the context of LD, ranging from 0% to 56% in reports[24–26]; therefore, its significance remains an area of investigation.

Diagnosis and Diagnostic Procedures

Dysphonia is often the presenting symptom of patients with LD, and the lesion is identified on office laryngoscopic examination. Dysphonia is present in 50.9% to 97.7% of all patients with laryngeal leukoplakia, usually less than 7 months before presentation. At the time of diagnosis, the average lesion is 1.2 cm, unilateral (74%–84% of patients), and commonly involves the medial and superior surfaces of the glottis. Such lesions rarely involve the posterior glottis or false vocal folds. Dysphagia, odynophagia, and dyspnea are uncommon.[3,13,27]

Imaging is not typically useful in LD. Endoscopic evaluation serves to identify the presence of disease and determine the need for further intervention. However, there are modalities that can augment the diagnostic accuracy of office laryngoscopy. Traditional videolaryngoscopic evaluation under white light can identify the presence and absence of lesions but does not produce information about severity/progression. Videolaryngostroboscopy (VLS) has been proposed to parse lesions by assessing mucosal amplitude and vibratory patterns, with the expectation that more invasive lesions would impede the mucosal wave. However, this has inconsistent utility due to inflammatory processes that may alter the mucosal wave, interobserver variation, suboptimal visualization, or other technical difficulties.[28–31] The established advantage of VLS is video recording with frame-by-frame playback and the ability to compare images over time. Combined with bioendoscopic tools such as narrow band imaging (NBI) and the Storz Professional Image Enhancement System (SPIES), VSL can better distinguish between low-risk and high-risk lesions.[32] Other available technologies, including autofluorescence, optical coherence tomography, and contact endoscopy demonstrate limited utility because the presence of leukoplakia obscures the mucosal surface, increasing false negatives.[33]

NBI and SPIES technologies can identify neoangiogenic vascular changes that suggest malignant transformation. NBI (Olympus Corporation, Tokyo, Japan) is an optical image amplification that provides enhanced contrast of the vasculature at the mucosal surface. An optical filter delivers low penetration, narrow band, blue light centered at 415 nm (range 400–430 nm) to penetrate the normal mucosa into the subepithelial tissue, illuminating vasculature just deep to the mucosal surface. A narrow-band green light centered at 540 nm (range 525–555 nm) is also applied to depict the vessels of the submucosa.[34] This modality can augment the workup of LD and is effective for post-intervention surveillance (**Fig. 2**).[35–39] In a meta-analysis by Riffat and colleagues, NBI demonstrated a pooled sensitivity of 85.4% and specificity of 94.9% for differentiating between low-risk and high-risk leukoplakia.[40]

Originally, NBI for LD evaluation was based on a 2011 classification system proposed by Ni and colleagues. This system classified morphologic changes of laryngeal intraepithelial papillary capillary loops (IPCLs) to differentiate among benign, premalignant, and malignant lesions. This was simplified by the European Laryngological Society in 2016, classifying superficial vascular changes into longitudinal and perpendicular in relation to the anteroposterior axis of the vocal cord. Perpendicular vessels are more likely to represent malignancy, premalignancy, or recurrent respiratory papillomatosis.[41] Ni and colleagues then countered with a revised system in 2019 where IPCLs underlying leukoplakia and at the peripheries were classified into 6 different types, I through III were considered benign and IV through VI were considered malignant.[42]

SPIES (Karl Storz, Tuttlingen, Germany) is a digital technique where a high-definition camera system is used to reprocess images for specific enhancements. It enhances the appearance of the vocal fold mucosal surface and can characterize the epithelial vascular architecture using 5 different defined spectral ranges: Spectra A, Spectra B, Clara, Chroma, and Clara+. These modalities use different color filter settings to create contrast by spectral separation. The Clara settings manipulate image brightness, and the Chroma settings increase color contrast; Clara + Chroma combines the manipulation of brightness and color contrast. This technology is newer and not as well studied but reportedly has a sensitivity of 86% and a specificity of 96% for distinguishing between benign low-risk lesions and malignant or high-risk lesions.[32,43,44] Where available, these endoscopic modalities may improve prehistologic diagnosis and more clearly define when a lesion warrants immediate biopsy or resection and

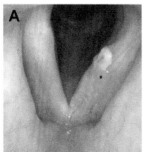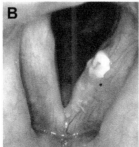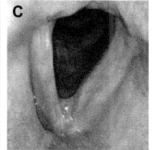

Fig. 2. Laryngeal SCC (*asterisk*) visualized via VLS (*A*), preoperative NBI (*B*), and postoperative NBI (*C*).

which may be monitored, thus decreasing the overall number of biopsies and benign biopsies. The next technological advancement would be optical biopsy capability, where the properties of light would allow a confident diagnosis at endoscopy, mitigating the need for further intervention for histologic analysis.[45] Until that time, when a lesion requires further histopathologic evaluation, the patient must still undergo an operative or office-based biopsy procedure.

For grossly exophytic and suspicious lesions in patients at high risk for general anesthesia, in-office biopsy is a good diagnostic option. Patient selection is paramount, and local anesthesia should be used with caution in those on anticoagulants, lesions that are submucosal or located in areas difficult to access in an awake patient, and in patients at risk for airway compromise. The biopsy is often scheduled and executed in expedited (even same-day) fashion, offering a shorter diagnostic timeline and quick initiation of treatment by avoiding preop workup and OR scheduling constraints. Limitations of in-office biopsy include greater risk for sampling error, especially if it is a small tissue sample from a large lesion with heterogeneous pathologic condition. The specimen may also omit the basement membrane, reducing diagnostic reliability and prompting a more precise biopsy for a suspicious lesion.

Sampling error may occur whether the procedure is done when the patient is awake or under general anesthesia. Depth is an important consideration for thick keratinous lesions where the basal cell layers may be 2 mm or more below the surface. There are also normal variations of the microscopic anatomy of the epithelium that complicate the diagnosis of small samples. There are variations in epithelial thickness, which makes it difficult to grade dysplasia by thickness, complex transition between respiratory and squamous epithelia, and occasionally glands within cords whose ducts can undergo metaplastic changes.[28] Finally, inflammation due to reflux, infection (eg, candida) and irradiation from previous cancer treatment can all also complicate diagnosis. If an office biopsy is nondiagnostic, an operative biopsy should be scheduled.

Historical Basis of Pathologic Laryngeal Dysplasia Classification Systems

Field cancerization is thought to result in a spectrum of cellular changes from epithelial hyperplasia and hyperkeratosis, which progressively transform into dysplasia, SCC in situ, and then, invasive cancer. Despite the unknown molecular steps of the progression of LD to SCC, the risk of malignant transformation increases with the increasing grade of dysplasia. In a large sampling of vocal fold biopsies for leukoplakia, Isenberg and colleagues found dysplasia in only 46.4%; of these, 33.5% showed mild or moderate dysplasia and 15.2% showed severe dysplasia or carcinoma in situ. At long-term follow-up, SCC developed in 3.7% of the patients with no dysplasia, 10.2% of patients with mild-to-moderate dysplasia, and 18.1% of patients with severe dysplasia or carcinoma in situ.[46] This inconsistent biological behavior has been a barrier to creating a widely accepted grading and classification system for LD.

The concept of dysplasia was incorporated in the pathology of the uterine cervix in 1953 but, at that time, laryngeal pathology primarily acknowledged SCC in situ and the various "keratotic" proliferative epithelial laryngeal lesions with the frequency at which they transformed into malignancy. The first laryngeal pathology classification system was presented by Kleinsasser in 1963 and was a 3-tier system based on nuclear atypia within proliferative lesions. Group I encompassed simple hyperplasia, Group II encompassed "restless hyperplasia," and Group III encompassed carcinoma in situ.[47] In 1971, a second 4-tier classification system based on hyperplasia was proposed by Kambič and Lenart. The hyperplasia was graded as simple, abnormal, or atypical, and the last group included carcinoma in situ.[48] Neither of these 2 classification systems were widely adopted because they were published in clinical head and neck journals in their native German and French, respectively. Then, in 1974, 20 years after its adoption in uterine cervical cancer, the term dysplasia was finally incorporated into laryngeal pathology at the Centennial Conference on Laryngeal Cancer workshop held in Toronto. The workshop spurred many clinicopathological studies at that time, resulting in varied nomenclature including squamous intraepithelial neoplasia (SIN) and laryngeal intraepithelial neoplasia (LIN). The 1974 system then became the foundation for the first 2 of 4 World Health Organization (WHO) histologic classifications in 1978 and then 1991. The 1991 WHO classification espoused mild, moderate, and severe dysplasia, with carcinoma in situ as a separate entity.[49] In 1995, the Ljubljana experience, which came to be known as the Ljubljana classification, was published by Kambič and Gale and was a revival of the 1971 Kambič and Lenart classification.[50] Then, in 2005, the third WHO Blue Book on Pathology and Genetics of Head and Neck Tumors was published. It effectively muddied the waters by presenting 3 schemes for classifying laryngeal precursor lesions, although none of them proved superior when assessed for interobserver variability. The first scheme was a 5-grade dysplasia system that included squamous cell hyperplasia, mild, moderate, and severe dysplasia, and carcinoma in situ. The second was a 3-grade SIN featuring mild dysplasia (basal/parabasal hyperplasia), moderate and severe dysplasia, and severe dysplasia and carcinoma in situ. The last was a 4-grade Ljubljana classification including squamous hyperplasia, basal/parabasal hyperplasia, atypical hyperplasia, and carcinoma in situ.[51]

Despite adoption of the dysplasia nomenclature and attempts at a parallel gradation model, LD is histologically different from uterine cervical dysplasia similar to how it has proven to be different from OD. LD has epithelial thickening, surface maturation/keratinization, and dyskeratosis. Uterine carcinoma in situ classically exhibits full epithelial replacement, which is rare in laryngeal lesions. Furthermore, the severe keratinizing dysplasia of the larynx carries a risk of greater frequency of progression to SCC than that of full thickness carcinoma in situ. Consequently, a histologic grading or classification system that fit cervical dysplasia could not be replicated in LD.[49]

The goal of a histologic grading or classification system is to create a reproducible system based on defined morphologic criteria with minimized interobserver variability that can reliably predict biological behavior and prognosis to guide appropriate therapy. With respect to predicting biological behavior, it must reasonably predict the risk of recurrence, the risk of progression, and the development of frank malignancy. It is in predicting the biological behavior that LD has been confounding. In 2012, Ferlito and colleagues proposed a 2-group system based on clinical relevance with regard to treatment. The first group would include metaplastic, hyperplastic, and keratotic lesions that would not require any additional treatment. The second group included dysplastic lesions and carcinoma in situ, which would require either local therapy or repeat surveillance to monitor for progression.[52] This system was appealing but it was difficult to standardize where lesions with moderate histologic dysplasia belonged. The 2017 WHO classification system eradicated the older nomenclature of SIN and LIN in favor of squamous intraepithelial lesions and referred to all dysplastic lesions as precursor lesions. Similar to Ferlito and colleagues' system, it has a 2-grade classification system but with clear histopathological criteria modeled on systems used in other organs such as the esophagus and large intestine. The system separates lesions into low-grade and high-grade dysplasia with the high-grade encompassing moderate and severe dysplasia and carcinoma in situ.[53] This essentially separates lesions at low risk of progression from those with higher risk, providing guidance for intervention. It is important to note that laryngeal aberrations of squamous metaplasia, squamous cell hyperplasia, pseudoepitheliomatous hyperplasia, and simple keratosis without atypia lack potential risk for progression and are often erroneously labeled as premalignant when they do not warrant frequent follow-up. Overall, the 2017 WHO classification is slightly more reproducible and easier for the nonspecialist pathologist to follow; however, it is less precise than earlier systems. Consequently, a surgeon should know the specific pathology grading classification used by their institution and should ideally track their local transformation or progression rates.[49]

The 2017 WHO classification is significant but incomplete progress. Biomarkers or prognosticators to better assess LD risk of progression remain elusive. In 2012, a systematic review by Rodrigo and colleagues reported that no marker had been identified as of that time.[54] However, in 2014, it was suggested that chromosome instability, especially in lower grade lesions, was associated with progression to malignancy.[55] In other studies, immunohistochemistry was used to evaluate genetic expression as a marker for prognosis. Expression of the transcription factor NANOG, a master regulator of embryonic stem cell pluripotency frequently found to be aberrantly expressed in several cancers, has a robust association with elevated laryngeal cancer risk.[56] Expression of the genes CTTN (cortactin) and FAK (focal adhesion kinase) was also associated with an increased risk of progression.[57] A study combining immunohistochemistry and molecular studies proposed SOX2 gene amplification as significantly associated with an increased risk of laryngeal carcinoma.[58] Another study using targeted next-generation sequencing found nonsynchronous mutations in 6 different genes (PIK3CA, FGFR3, TP53, JAK3, MET, and FBXW7). PIK3CA and FGFR3 mutations were seen in progressing dysplastic lesions but not in nonprogressing lesions. Conversely, JAK3, MET, and FBXW7 mutations were seen in nonprogressing dysplastic lesions but not in progressing lesions.[59] MAGE-A, the melanoma-associated antigen A, was also found to be expressed in laryngeal and oral SCCs but absent in healthy mucosal tissues.[60] So far, these biomarkers have shown promise and are being introduced into the diagnostic algorithm.

Prevention and Treatment

As LD is suspected to arise via the field cancerization model, managing exposure to inciting carcinogens is the focus of primary prevention. Smoking and alcohol are strongly associated with LD; therefore, cessation of use is a significant measure for initial prevention. Data show that for early glottic cancer, smoking is also associated with an increased risk of persistence of disease, worse response to treatment, recurrence, and the development of second primaries. Chen and colleagues suggested that the degree of dysplasia and the recurrence rate may depend on reflux as measured by pepsin levels.[61] Therefore, minimization of environmental exposures and strict reflux control should also be recommended preventative measures.[62]

Without a clear, single classification system, treatment paradigms for LD have also been varied and controversial. Current practices have largely been extrapolated from publications focused on early-stage glottic carcinomas, assuming LD is on the same continuum and expecting it to respond similarly to treatments. Options include observation, surgical excision, transoral laser microsurgery, and radiotherapy (RT); there is no meaningful medical treatment of LD. Literature suggests that aspirin and metformin are promising medications to treat dysplasia but no LD-specific studies have been published.[63–67] A limited small case series (3 patients) suggests adjuvant metformin treatment improved outcomes for recurrent LD lesions in patients without diabetes.[68,69]

Ideally, treatment will eradicate the dysplastic disease while preserving the voice function. Patients are often willing to sacrifice vocal quality in the setting of malignancy or high-grade dysplastic lesions but with less severe or benign disease, this is no longer an acceptable trade-off. Allowing the progression of a premalignant process to cancer is unacceptable but aggressive intervention resulting in functional deterioration for a benign process is far from ideal. To further add to the confusion, the transition over time from one treatment paradigm to the next has not been explored relative to outcomes such as oncologic efficacy and voice quality.

The risk of malignant transformation increases with increasing severity of dysplasia.[70–72] Treatment choice may be decided based on 2017 WHO grade (degree and extent of dysplasia), and surgeon preference. Initial histopathologic diagnosis is made with direct laryngoscopy or in-office biopsy. Such biopsy may be a definitive treatment if the lesion is small enough for excisional biopsy. If pathologic condition is consistent with low-grade dysplasia, further options include excision with conventional cold steel microlaryngoscopic surgery or laser excision. For high-grade dysplasia, including carcinoma in situ, transoral laser resection is also an option. Following resection via cold steel or laser, all patients must undergo frequent surveillance, the timing of which is also determined by the severity of dysplasia. RT maintains a role in the treatment of LD for patients with multiple recurrences, persistent or recurrent widespread disease, or high anesthetic risk. Patients may also elect RT if fear of surgery cannot be overcome or if they prefer field treatment in place of repeated biopsies.

Conventional microlaryngoscopic surgery uses cold steel endoscopic instruments to excise lesions. Historically, vocal fold stripping was performed for dysplastic lesions. However, this risks extensive vocal fold damage, so microflap excisions have become the surgical method of choice with the expected improvement in functional outcomes. Compared with transoral laser resection, there may be more bleeding associated with conventional methods. Despite small total blood loss amounts, bleeding in the small surgical field of the larynx can influence visualization of excisional margins and complicate the fine dissection and excision required for this surgery. An article by Schweinfurth and colleagues published in 2001 reported a series of 20 patients with severe dysplasia/*Cacinoma in Situ* (CIS) who underwent microflap excision with a 95% local control rate.[73] A 2006 literature review by Sadri and colleagues reported 77% local control rates with conventional microlaryngoscopic surgery but this included literature for vocal cord stripping in severe dysplasia/CIS.[74] There is a dearth of data examining the role of microlaryngoscopic surgery in LD in comparison to the available information on transoral laser resection.

Transoral laser resection has been primarily performed with either CO_2 or potassium titanyl phosphate (KTP) lasers. CO_2 lasers are widespread and frequently used in tumor surgery, both for malignant and benign tumors. Sadri and colleagues reported a pooled overall local control rate of 81% for CO_2 laser excision of severe dysplasia/CIS, which was greater than the 77% of vocal cord stripping but less than the 95% local control rates achieved by RT.[73] Despite RT having a higher local control rate, CO_2 laser techniques are much less expensive and can be used multiple times in the setting of recurrence. Some also suggest that CO_2 laser surgery results may have improved with time due to improvements in technology and growing familiarity and, therefore, skill in utilization. The angiolytic pulsed KTP laser uses a 532-nm wavelength to target the subepithelial microcirculation, treating the blood supply in addition to the lesion. Studies have showed comparable results regarding long-term disease control with angiolytic laser stripping with KTP laser versus the CO_2 laser excision but superior voice outcomes with the KTP laser.[75] More recently, there has been the introduction of an angiolytic blue light laser with a wavelength of 445 nm, which also targets the subepithelial microcirculation. Some preliminary data shows decreased scarring with the blue laser when compared with KTP in rat vocal cord studies.[76] However, with both angiolytic lasers, larger comparison studies demonstrating any superiority have not been produced.

The risk of recurrence after excision of dysplastic lesions is 20%.[77] The need for follow-up surveillance is widely accepted but the recommended timing varies. Timing, similar to treatment, depends on the degree and extent of dysplasia because it determines risk. Surveillance requires videostrobolaryngoscopy with photo and, ideally, video documentation. In 2010, Weller and colleagues performed a systematic review of case series and attempted a meta-analysis to determine the risk and interval to malignant transformation in LD, and in 2015, Cosway and Paleri created an evidence-based flowchart to help guide the clinical management of LD treatment.[78,79] Both sources recommend a minimum of 6-month follow-up for low-grade dysplasia and 5 years for those with high-risk or severe dysplasia, longer in the setting of progression or recurrence. Despite these recommendations, no data support that they confer any benefit. Currently, most providers follow a surveillance schedule with decreasing frequency after 2 years.

SUMMARY

LD is a precursor of laryngeal SCC. It is proposed that chronic irritation and its consequent inflammation of the nonkeratinized stratified squamous epithelium of the glottis results in dysplastic changes that eventually develop into the genetic and/or epigenetic alterations of field cancerization resulting in malignancy. However, the exact details of this transformation have never been elucidated. Diagnosis begins with the visualization of a laryngeal lesion on examination; however, no morphologic changes, such as leukoplakia, erythroplakia, or erythroleukoplakia, are specifically characteristic for dysplasia. Consequently, biopsy is necessary for histopathologic diagnosis. The NBI and SPIES bioendoscopic imaging modalities have proven to help better differentiate between high-risk and low-risk lesions but they are still incapable of determining the presence or absence of dysplasia. Once biopsy is completed, pathologic assessment also comes with its own controversies. The risk of malignant transformation increases with the increasing grade of dysplasia but not in a linear or predictable manner. This has long confounded the classification and treatment of LD. Consequently, treatment paradigms for dysplastic lesions have been derived data regarding early laryngeal SCC.

The key to solving the puzzle of LD will be in the discovery of understanding its biological behavior, essentially how it transforms from dysplasia to malignancy. This would allow for appropriate predictive prognosis and the appropriate matching of treatment modality. Early study on biomarkers and prognosticators of LD's propensity for malignant transformation is encouraging but requires more research. Until that time, the 2017 WHO classification, which simplistically lumps LD into low-risk and high-risk categories, may be the best facsimile of an LD classification system and guide to treatment options that we have now. It is not ideal and not unanimously accepted but until a better system can be created, the management of LD will likely remain disjointed and managed based on individual institutional and practitioner preference.

CLINICS CARE POINTS

- Histologic changes of the glottis have long been attributed to chronic irritation and inflammation. Well-known risk factors include tobacco, alcohol, gastroesophageal and laryngopharyngeal reflux, as well as environmental and occupational exposures related to construction.

- Dysphonia is present in a substantial proportion of patients with laryngeal leukoplakia. Videolaryngoscopic (VLS) evaluation can identify presence or absence of lesions but does not produce information about severity/progression. VLS, in conjunction with bio endoscopic tools (SPIES/NBI), can better distinguish between low and high-risk lesions.

- Laryngeal dysplasia requires initial histopathologic diagnosis with direct laryngoscopy or in-office biopsy, with the risk of malignant transformation rising with increasing severity of dysplasia. However, there are currently no widely accepted clinical factors or biomarkers to use as prognosticators for progression to malignancy.

- Treatment options tend to be influenced by surgeon preference and institutional pathology classification policies. Treatments include resection via cold steel or laser excision (CO2, KTP, blue light). The goal of therapy is to eradicate dysplastic disease while preserving voice function, with microflap technique largely replacing vocal fold stripping due to improved voice outcomes.

- Recommended post-treatment follow-up surveillance timing includes a minimum of 6-month follow-up for low grade dysplasia, five years for those with high-risk or severe dysplasia, and longer in the setting of progression or recurrence.

REFERENCES

1. Levendoski EE, Leydon C, Thibeault SL. Vocal fold epithelial barrier in health and injury: a research review. J Speech Lang Hear Res 2014;57(5):1679–91.
2. Garrel R, Uro Coste E, Costes-Martineau V, et al. Vocal-fold leukoplakia and dysplasia. Mini-review by the French Society of Phoniatrics and Laryngology (SFPL). Eur Ann Otorhinolaryngol Head Neck Dis 2020;137(5):399–404.
3. Odell E, Eckel HE, Simo R, et al. European Laryngological Society position paper on laryngeal dysplasia Part I: aetiology and pathological classification. Eur Arch Otorhinolaryngol 2021;278(6):1717–22.
4. Bouquot JE, Kurland LT, Weiland LH. Laryngeal keratosis and carcinoma in the Rochester, MN, population 1935-1984. Cancer Detect Prev 1991;15(2):83–91.
5. Park JC, Altman KW, Prasad VMN, et al. Laryngeal Leukoplakia: State of the Art Review. Otolaryngol Head Neck Surg 2021;164(6):1153–9.
6. Argiris A, Karamouzis MV, Raben D, et al. Head and neck cancer. Lancet 2008; 371(9625):1695–709.
7. Curtius K, Wright NA, Graham TA. An evolutionary perspective on field cancerization. Nat Rev Cancer 2018;18(1):19–32.
8. Kostev K, Jacob LEC, Kalder M, et al. Association of laryngeal cancer with vocal cord leukoplakia and associated risk factors in 1,184 patients diagnosed in otorhinolaryngology practices in Germany. Mol Clin Oncol 2018;8(5):689–93.
9. Müller KM, Krohn BR. Smoking habits and their relationship to precancerous lesions of the larynx. J Cancer Res Clin Oncol 1980;96(2):211–7.
10. Wynder EL. Toward the prevention of laryngeal cancer. Laryngoscope 1975; 85(7):1190–6.
11. Santi I, Kroll LE, Dietz A, et al. To what degree is the association between educational inequality and laryngeal cancer explained by smoking, alcohol consumption, and occupational exposure? Scand J Work Environ Health 2014;40(3): 315–22.
12. Dietz A. Epidemiologie des Kehlkopfkarzinoms [Epidemiology of laryngeal cancer]. Laryngorhinootologie 2004;83(11):771–2.
13. Bouquot JE, Gnepp DR. Laryngeal precancer: a review of the literature, commentary, and comparison with oral leukoplakia. Head Neck 1991;13(6):488–97.

14. Coca-Pelaz A, Rodrigo JP, Takes RP, et al. Relationship between reflux and laryngeal cancer. Head Neck 2013;35(12):1814–8.
15. Parsel SM, Wu EL, Riley CA, et al. Gastroesophageal and Laryngopharyngeal Reflux Associated With Laryngeal Malignancy: A Systematic Review and Meta-analysis. Clin Gastroenterol Hepatol 2019;17(7):1253–64, e5.
16. Ž Zubčić, Mendeš T, Včeva A, et al. Presence of pepsin in laryngeal tissue and saliva in benign and malignant neoplasms. Biosci Rep 2020;40(11). BSR20200216.
17. Almadori G, Bussu F, Navarra P, et al. Pilot phase IIA study for evaluation of the efficacy of folic acid in the treatment of laryngeal leucoplakia. Cancer 2006; 107(2):328–36.
18. Issing WJ, Struck R, Naumann A. Long-term follow-up of larynx leukoplakia under treatment with retinyl palmitate. Head Neck 1996;18(6):560–5.
19. Stich HF, Rosin MP, Hornby AP, et al. Remission of oral leukoplakias and micronuclei in tobacco/betel quid chewers treated with beta-carotene and with beta-carotene plus vitamin A. Int J Cancer 1988;42(2):195–9.
20. Stich HF, Mathew B, Sankaranarayanan R, et al. Remission of precancerous lesions in the oral cavity of tobacco chewers and maintenance of the protective effect of beta-carotene or vitamin A. Am J Clin Nutr 1991;53(1 Suppl):298S–304S.
21. Hobbs CG, Birchall MA. Human papillomavirus infection in the etiology of laryngeal carcinoma. Curr Opin Otolaryngol Head Neck Surg 2004;12(2):88–92.
22. Karatayli-Ozgursoy S, Bishop JA, Hillel A, et al. Risk Factors for Dysplasia in Recurrent Respiratory Papillomatosis in an Adult and Pediatric Population. Ann Otol Rhinol Laryngol 2016;125(3):235–41.
23. Preuss SF, Klussmann JP, Jungehulsing M, et al. Long-term results of surgical treatment for recurrent respiratory papillomatosis. Acta Otolaryngol 2007; 127(11):1196–201.
24. Davids T, Muller S, Wise JC, et al. Laryngeal papillomatosis associated dysplasia in the adult population: an update on prevalence and HPV subtyping. Ann Otol Rhinol Laryngol 2014;123(6):402–8.
25. Waters HH, Seth R, Hoschar AP, et al. Does HPV have a presence in diffuse high grade pre-malignant lesions of the larynx? Laryngoscope 2010;120(Suppl 4): S201.
26. Pagliuca G, Martellucci S, Degener AM, et al. Role of Human Papillomavirus in the Pathogenesis of Laryngeal Dysplasia. Otolaryngol Head Neck Surg 2014; 150(6):1018–23.
27. Karatayli-Ozgursoy S, Pacheco-Lopez P, Hillel AT, et al. Laryngeal dysplasia, demographics, and treatment: a single-institution, 20-year review. JAMA Otolaryngol Head Neck Surg 2015;141(4):313–8.
28. Eckel HE, Simo R, Quer M, et al. European Laryngological Society position paper on laryngeal dysplasia Part II: diagnosis, treatment, and follow-up. Eur Arch Otorhinolaryngol 2021;278(6):1723–32.
29. van Balkum M, Buijs B, Donselaar EJ, et al. Systematic review of the diagnostic value of laryngeal stroboscopy in excluding early glottic carcinoma. Clin Otolaryngol 2017;42(1):123–30.
30. Djukic V, Milovanovic J, Jotic AD, et al. Stroboscopy in detection of laryngeal dysplasia effectiveness and limitations. J Voice 2014;28(2):262.e13–21.
31. Peretti G, Piazza C, Berlucchi M, et al. Pre- and intraoperative assessment of midcord erythroleukoplakias: a prospective study on 52 patients. Eur Arch Otorhinolaryngol 2003;260(10):525–8.

32. Staníková L, Walderová R, Jančatová D, et al. Comparison of narrow band imaging and the Storz Professional Image Enhancement System for detection of laryngeal and hypopharyngeal pathologies. Eur Arch Otorhinolaryngol 2018;275(7): 1819–25.

33. Tibbetts KM, Tan M. Role of Advanced Laryngeal Imaging in Glottic Cancer: Early Detection and Evaluation of Glottic Neoplasms. Otolaryngol Clin North Am 2015; 48(4):565–84.

34. Gono K, Obi T, Yamaguchi M, et al. Appearance of enhanced tissue features in narrow-band endoscopic imaging. J Biomed Opt 2004;9(3):568–77.

35. Piazza C, Dessouky O, Peretti G, et al. Narrow-band imaging: a new tool for evaluation of head and neck squamous cell carcinomas. Review of the literature. Acta Otorhinolaryngol Ital 2008;28(2):49–54.

36. Piazza C, Cocco D, De Benedetto L, et al. Narrow band imaging and high definition television in the assessment of laryngeal cancer: a prospective study on 279 patients. Eur Arch Otorhinolaryngol 2010;267(3):409–14.

37. Watanabe A, Taniguchi M, Tsujie H, et al. The value of narrow band imaging for early detection of laryngeal cancer. Eur Arch Otorhinolaryngol 2009;266(7): 1017–23.

38. Staníková L, Kučová H, Walderová R, et al. Využití Narrow Band Imaging v diagnostice časných karcinomů hrtanu [Value of narrow band imaging endoscopy in detection of early laryngeal squamous cell carcinoma]. Klin Onkol 2015; 28(2):116–20.

39. Zabrodsky M, Lukes P, Lukesova E, et al. The role of narrow band imaging in the detection of recurrent laryngeal and hypopharyngeal cancer after curative radiotherapy. Biomed Res Int 2014;2014:175398.

40. Ahmadzada S, Tseros E, Sritharan N, et al. The value of narrowband imaging using the Ni classification in the diagnosis of laryngeal cancer. Laryngoscope Investig Otolaryngol 2020;5(4):665–71. Published 2020 Jun 26.

41. Arens C, Piazza C, Andrea M, et al. Proposal for a descriptive guideline of vascular changes in lesions of the vocal folds by the committee on endoscopic laryngeal imaging of the European Laryngological Society. Eur Arch Otorhinolaryngol 2016;273(5):1207–14.

42. Ni XG, Zhu JQ, Zhang QQ, et al. Diagnosis of vocal cord leukoplakia: The role of a novel narrow band imaging endoscopic classification. Laryngoscope 2019; 129(2):429–34.

43. Emiliani E, Talso M, Baghdadi M, et al. Evaluation of the Spies TM modalities image quality. Int Braz J Urol 2017;43(3):476–80.

44. Puxeddu R, Sionis S, Gerosa C, et al. Enhanced contact endoscopy for the detection of neoangiogenesis in tumors of the larynx and hypopharynx. Laryngoscope 2015;125(7):1600–6.

45. Wang TD, Van Dam J. Optical biopsy: a new frontier in endoscopic detection and diagnosis. Clin Gastroenterol Hepatol 2004;2(9):744–53.

46. Isenberg JS, Crozier DL, Dailey SH. Institutional and comprehensive review of laryngeal leukoplakia. Ann Otol Rhinol Laryngol 2008;117(1):74–9.

47. Kleinsasser O. [The classification and differential diagnosis of epithelial hyperplasia of the laryngeal mucosa on the basis of histomorphological features. II]. Z Laryngol Rhinol Otol 1963;42:339–62. German. PMID: 14033430.

48. Kambic V, Lenart I. Notre classification des hyperplasies de l'épithélium du larynx au point de vue pronostic [Our classification of hyperplasia of the laryngeal epithelium from the prognostic point of view]. J Fr Otorhinolaryngol Audiophonol Chir Maxillofac (1967) 1971;20(10):1145–50.

49. Hellquist H, Ferlito A, Mäkitie AA, et al. Developing Classifications of Laryngeal Dysplasia: The Historical Basis. Adv Ther 2020;37(6):2667–77.
50. Gale N, Kambic V, Michaels L, et al. The Ljubljana classification: a practical strategy for the diagnosis of laryngeal precancerous lesions. Adv Anat Pathol 2000; 7(4):240–51.
51. Barnes L, UniversitatsSpital Zurich International Academy of Pathology World Health Organization International Agency for Research on Cancer. Pathology and genetics of head and neck Tumours. Lyon: IARC Press; 2005.
52. Ferlito A, Devaney KO, Woolgar JA, et al. Squamous epithelial changes of the larynx: diagnosis and therapy. Head Neck 2012;34(12):1810–6.
53. Gale N, Hille J, Jordan RC, et al. Precursor lesions. Dysplasia. In: El-Naggar AK, Chan JKC, Grandis JR, et al, editors. WHO classification of head and neck tumours. Lyon: IARC; 2017. p. 91–3.
54. Rodrigo JP, García-Pedrero JM, Suárez C, et al. Biomarkers predicting malignant progression of laryngeal epithelial precursor lesions: a systematic review. Eur Arch Otorhinolaryngol 2012;269(4):1073–83.
55. Bergshoeff VE, Van der Heijden SJ, Haesevoets A, et al. Chromosome instability predicts progression of premalignant lesions of the larynx. Pathology 2014;46(3): 216–24.
56. Rodrigo JP, Villaronga MÁ, Menéndez ST, et al. A Novel Role For Nanog As An Early Cancer Risk Marker In Patients With Laryngeal Precancerous Lesions. Sci Rep 2017;7(1):11110.
57. Villaronga MÁ, Hermida-Prado F, Granda-Díaz R, et al. Immunohistochemical Expression of Cortactin and Focal Adhesion Kinase Predicts Recurrence Risk and Laryngeal Cancer Risk Beyond Histologic Grading. Cancer Epidemiol Biomarkers Prev 2018;27(7):805–13.
58. Granda-Díaz R, Menéndez ST, Pedregal Mallo D, et al. The Novel Role of SOX2 as an Early Predictor of Cancer Risk in Patients with Laryngeal Precancerous Lesions. Cancers (Basel) 2019;11(3):286.
59. Manterola L, Aguirre P, Larrea E, et al. Mutational profiling can identify laryngeal dysplasia at risk of progression to invasive carcinoma. Sci Rep 2018;8(1):6613.
60. Baran CA, Agaimy A, Wehrhan F, et al. MAGE-A expression in oral and laryngeal leukoplakia predicts malignant transformation. Mod Pathol 2019;32(8):1068–81.
61. Chen YL, Bao YY, Zhou SH, et al. Relationship Between Pepsin Expression and Dysplasia Grade in Patients With Vocal Cord Leukoplakia. Otolaryngol Head Neck Surg 2021;164(1):160–5.
62. Al-Mamgani A, van Rooij PH, Mehilal R, et al. Radiotherapy for T1a glottic cancer: the influence of smoking cessation and fractionation schedule of radiotherapy. Eur Arch Otorhinolaryngol 2014;271(1):125–32.
63. Jacobs EJ, Newton CC, Gapstur SM, et al. Daily aspirin use and cancer mortality in a large US cohort. J Natl Cancer Inst 2012;104(16):1208–17.
64. Algra AM, Rothwell PM. Effects of regular aspirin on long-term cancer incidence and metastasis: a systematic comparison of evidence from observational studies versus randomised trials. Lancet Oncol 2012;13(5):518–27.
65. Rothwell PM, Price JF, Fowkes FG, et al. Short-term effects of daily aspirin on cancer incidence, mortality, and non-vascular death: analysis of the time course of risks and benefits in 51 randomised controlled trials. Lancet 2012;379(9826): 1602–12.
66. Curry J, Johnson J, Tassone P, et al. Metformin effects on head and neck squamous carcinoma microenvironment: Window of opportunity trial. Laryngoscope 2017;127(8):1808–15.

67. Rêgo DF, Elias ST, Amato AA, et al. Anti-tumor effects of metformin on head and neck carcinoma cell lines: A systematic review. Oncol Lett 2017;13(2):554–66.
68. Lerner MZ, Mor N, Paek H, et al. Metformin Prevents the Progression of Dysplastic Mucosa of the Head and Neck to Carcinoma in Nondiabetic Patients. Ann Otol Rhinol Laryngol 2017;126(4):340–3.
69. Mesolella M, Iengo M, Testa D, et al. Chemoprevention using folic acid for dysplastic lesions of the larynx. Mol Clin Oncol 2017;7(5):843–6.
70. Sarioglu S, Cakalagaoglu F, Elagoz S, et al. Inter-observer agreement in laryngeal pre-neoplastic lesions. Head Neck Pathol 2010;4(4):276–80, published correction appears in Head Neck Pathol. 2010;4(4):281. Ersoy, Unsal [corrected to Han, Unsal].
71. Fleskens SA, Bergshoeff VE, Voogd AC, et al. Interobserver variability of laryngeal mucosal premalignant lesions: a histopathological evaluation. Mod Pathol 2011;24(7):892–8.
72. Yang SW, Chao WC, Lee YS, et al. Treatment outcome of vocal cord leukoplakia by transoral laser microsurgery. Lasers Med Sci 2017;32(1):19–27.
73. Schweinfurth JM, Powitzky E, Ossoff RH. Regression of laryngeal dysplasia after serial microflap excision. Ann Otol Rhinol Laryngol 2001;110(9):811–4.
74. Sadri M, McMahon J, Parker A. Management of laryngeal dysplasia: a review. Eur Arch Otorhinolaryngol 2006;263(9):843–52.
75. Lim JY, Park YM, Kang M, et al. Angiolytic laser stripping versus CO2 laser microflap excision for vocal fold leukoplakia: Long-term disease control and voice outcomes. PLoS One 2018;13(12):e0209691.
76. Lin RJ, Iakovlev V, Streutker C, et al. Blue Light Laser Results in Less Vocal Fold Scarring Compared to KTP Laser in Normal Rat Vocal Folds. Laryngoscope 2021;131(4):853–8.
77. Niu YY, Wang J, Huo H, et al. [Clinical analyses of 263 patients with laryngeal leukoplakia]. Zhonghua Er Bi Yan Hou Tou Jing Wai Ke Za Zhi 2018;53(8):575–80.
78. Weller MD, Nankivell PC, McConkey C, et al. The risk and interval to malignancy of patients with laryngeal dysplasia; a systematic review of case series and meta-analysis. Clin Otolaryngol 2010;35(5):364–72.
79. Cosway B, Paleri V. Laryngeal dysplasia: an evidence-based flowchart to guide management and follow up. J Laryngol Otol 2015;129(6):598–9.

Radiation for Early Glottic Cancer

Caitlin A. Schonewolf, MD, MS, Jennifer L. Shah, MD*

KEYWORDS

- Early-stage glottic cancer • Larynx • Radiation treatment • 3D-CRT • IMRT • SBRT
- SVCI

KEY POINTS

- Standard of care radiation treatment of early-stage glottic cancer continues to be three-dimensional opposed lateral fields to include the whole larynx.
- Advanced radiation treatment techniques are allowing studies to examine the efficacy and toxicity of altered doses and treatment volumes.
- Stereotactic body radiation therapy and single-vocal cord irradiation for early-stage glottic cancer are not yet considered standard of care and should be performed at institutions with clinical trials to ensure adequate expertise and quality assurance.

INTRODUCTION

Early glottic cancer is a common head and neck malignancy. Tobacco smoking is the primary risk factor. Other risk factors include alcohol, gastroesophageal reflux disease, and reported occupational exposures, such as asbestos, mustard gas, nickel, soot, and tars.[1] Initial patient workup involves direct laryngoscopy and biopsy. In the presence of clinical T1 or T2 disease, cross-sectional imaging for glottic cancer is not felt to be necessary given the very low, (<5%) risk of nodal involvement.[2] However, for disease-causing impaired mobility, nodal staging with imaging may be prudent and should be strongly considered.[3]

Treatment options for early-stage glottic cancer are broadly categorized as surgical and non-surgical. Non-surgical treatment involves radiation therapy (RT), the details and considerations of which are discussed here. Systemic therapy does not have a role in the management of clinical early-stage (T1-2 N0 Mx) glottic cancer but is used for chemosensitization in Stage III and IV disease and select T2 N0 cases. From the perspective of a radiation oncologist, a biopsy demonstrating invasive disease to justify RT and its sequelae is of paramount concern. However, obtaining a

Department of Radiation Oncology, University of Michigan, 1500 E Medical Center Drive UH B2C490, Ann Arbor MI, USA
* Corresponding author.
E-mail address: jenlobo@med.umich.edu

Otolaryngol Clin N Am 56 (2023) 247–257
https://doi.org/10.1016/j.otc.2022.12.008
0030-6665/23/© 2023 Elsevier Inc. All rights reserved.
oto.theclinics.com

representative tissue sample in early glottic disease may be challenging, and it is important to evaluate a pathology result in the clinical context of the laryngoscopy findings and patient history.

Herein, we will review current standards of care pertaining to radiation treatment of early-stage glottic cancer and explore how advanced technology and treatment techniques are pushing the field toward more focused treatment.

DISCUSSION
Standard Early Glottic Radiation Fields and Treatment

In the era before CT-based RT planning, radiation treatment plans were designed based on two-dimensional imaging—plain films. Knowledge of internal anatomy as it related to landmarks identifiable on plain x-ray was used to guide radiation fields (**Fig. 1**). In the case of early glottic cancer, planning opposed lateral beams to treat the whole larynx was felt to cover the vocal cords easily and adequately, and this simple beam arrangement continues to be used widely today. The field borders are classic: superiorly, the superior border of the thyroid cartilage (T1 disease) or hyoid bone (T2 disease); inferiorly, the caudal border of the cricoid cartilage; posteriorly, the anterior vertebral bodies; and anteriorly, a few centimeters beyond the skin of the neck (flash). Using these traditional field borders, the treatment fields are approximately 5 cm × 5 cm (for T1 disease) or 6 cm × 6 cm (for T2 disease) (**Fig. 2**). Radiation treatment plans are then created using 6 MV photons with the isocenter placed at the anterior edge of the vertebral body and the prescription dose prescribed to the isocenter (**Fig. 3**A).

Typical dose prescriptions for early-stage glottic cancer use a moderate hypofractionated approach of 63 Gy in 2.25 Gy per fraction for T1 disease and 65 Gy in 2.25 Gy per fraction for T2 disease. Several studies have shown the importance of higher doses per fraction in improving local control. One early series from University of California San Francisco (UCSF) evaluated the influence of fraction size, total dose, and other prognostic factors on local control in T1-2 glottic cancer.[4] The analysis included 398 patients treated from 1956 to 1995 with various fraction sizes ranging from <1.8 Gy per fraction to >2.25 Gy per fraction. For T2 lesions, fraction size was prognostic for local control on multivariate analysis. Local control was 100% for fraction size $\geq$ 2.25 Gy compared with only 44% for fraction size < 1.8 Gy. These data and

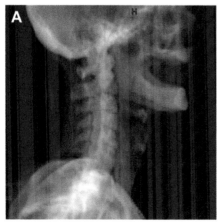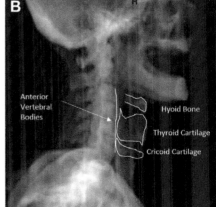

Fig. 1. Lateral x-ray of the head and neck (*A*) demonstrating anatomic landmarks for development of early glottic radiation treatment field borders (*B*).

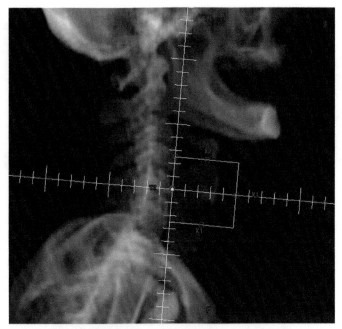

Fig. 2. Field shape (5 cm × 5 cm box) of one lateral beam overlying the lateral x-ray for patient with T1N0M0 early stage glottic cancer.

other institutional series[5–10] led to the development of a randomized trial at the Osaka Medical Center in Japan in the late 1990s.[11] This study included 180 patients with T1 N0 M0 early glottic carcinoma and randomized them to either standard fractionation dosing (2 Gy per fraction) or moderate hypofractionation (2.25 Gy per fraction). Total radiation dose was determined based on extent of disease so that higher total doses were used for those patients with more than two-thirds of the vocal cord involved compared with those with more minimal tumors involving two-thirds or less of the vocal cord. Five-year local control rates were significantly higher in those patients who received 2.25 Gy per fraction without any increase in acute or long-term side effects compared with standard fractionation (92% vs 77%, respectively), thereby establishing 63 Gy in 28 fractions at 2.25 Gy per fraction as a new standard of care dose prescription for radiation treatment of T1 disease. The DAHANCA 6 randomized trial similarly demonstrated that accelerated radiation dose delivered as 6 fractions per week instead of the standard 5 fractions per week resulted in a significant local control benefit for T1-2 N0 patients who comprised most of the patients in this study.[12] As mentioned, every effort should be made to demonstrate invasive disease by biopsy; however, several retrospective studies have demonstrated excellent clinical outcomes with moderate hypofractionation for glottic carcinoma in situ as well.[13–16]

Disease extending to the supraglottis or subglottis and/or with impaired cord mobility is categorized as T2 and has nuanced implications. Although accelerated radiation alone is recognized as a standard of care as described above, the local control is notably inferior compared with T1 disease, and T2 disease has been reported as a poor prognostic factor in series of early glottic cancer patients treated with radiation alone.[4,17–19] Koyfman and colleagues at the Cleveland Clinic sub-categorized their T2 patients treated from 1986 to 2013 into T2a (no impaired mobility) and T2b (with impaired mobility) per AJCC staging in this era. They reported a 3-year local control

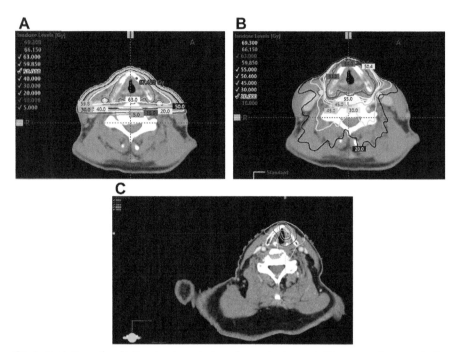

Fig. 3. Evolution of radiation treatment plans for early stage glottic cancer. Representative axial CT slices with isodose lines of radiation treatment plan using (*A*) 3D-CRT opposed lateral fields, (*B*) carotid sparing IMRT, and (*C*) SBRT. Courtesy of David Sher, MD, Dallas, TX.

of 95.1% for T2a N0 patients and 73.2% for T2b N0 patients treated with radiation alone. T2b-3 N0 patients treated with chemoradiation fared better with local control of 91.5% compared with the T2b N0 subset treated with radiation alone, thus arguing for consideration of treatment intensification in this group.[20] The potential benefit of chemoradiation for T2 N0 patients has been reported by other groups as well.[21,22] Increasing immobility implicates paraglottic space involvement and risk of nodal spread and regional recurrence. It is relevant to recognize that the prescription isodose line in the standard opposed lateral fields for early glottic cancer does encompass the anterior regions of cervical nodal levels II and III bilaterally (see **Fig. 3**). In practice, it is commonplace to add a fraction to the 2.25 Gy per fraction regimen and treat patients with T2 N0 disease to 65.25 Gy in 29 fractions based on the experiences at UCSF and University of Florida.[4,17]

A meta-analysis of early glottic cancer patients treated from 1995 - 2014 reported risk factors for local recurrence after RT to include tobacco use during/after treatment, bulky tumors, anterior commissure involvement, and poorly differentiated disease.[19] Despite suspicion that subglottic extension may be a high-risk feature, this variable did not reach statistical significance. Sarcomatoid histology has also raised clinical concern for increased rate of local failure, but the literature would suggest otherwise.[23,24] Despite local failure at 5 years in approximately 10% of patients with T1 disease and 20% to 30% in patients with T2 disease treated with radiation alone, surgical salvage with a total laryngectomy results in 5-year cause-specific survival exceeding 95% for T1 disease and 90% for T2 disease.[17,25] In practice, counseling patients for smoking cessation and offering resources to achieve this goal is strongly advised to minimize the risk of local recurrence.

Impact of Evolving Technology on Early Glottic Cancer Management

In the early 2000s, the ability to plan radiation treatment using computed tomography (CT) scans was developed and constituted the first of two major revolutions in technologic advancement impacting RT. CT-based planning allowed for three-dimensional visualization of radiation isodose lines for each patient, termed 3D conformal radiation therapy (3D-CRT). Although local control rates with standard opposed lateral fields are excellent, some early reports with this technique in the two-dimensional era raised concern over worse local control with anterior commissure involvement and/or posterior vocal cord extension.[19,26,27] 3D-CRT, however, allows adjustment of the beam arrangements, possible use of bolus for anterior commissure disease, and calculation point manipulation to ensure prescription dose coverage of the areas of clinical involvement seen on laryngoscopy, including the anterior and posterior commissures. Imaging capabilities integrated into the linear accelerators, termed image-guided radiation therapy (IGRT), have additionally allowed taking MV or kV films while the patient is positioned for treatment just before dose delivery each day yielding increased accuracy in treatment delivery.

It is prudent to recognize that the studies which have defined the standard of care largely enrolled patients before the early 2000s, before cross-sectional imaging became widely used in health care. These patients were staged and selected based on clinical findings on laryngoscopy and external head/neck exams. In the era of cross-sectional imaging, however, radiographic up-staging due to perceived paraglottic space invasion is not uncommon unless vocal cord mobility is truly unaffected by disease. Volume of disease is a known prognostic factor in locally advanced head and neck cancer,[28,29] and while concurrent chemotherapy is often used for these patients, nuances in the radiation treatment plan to target the cervical nodal regions most at risk and spare the parotid glands, submandibular glands, and oral cavity using modern radiation treatment techniques can and should be used to mitigate toxicity. There is admitted variation in the clinical assessment of early glottic cancer. The role of imaging and the degree of vocal cord mobility is best rendered through multidisciplinary evaluation to achieve consistency between clinical definition and treatment recommendations among the team.

Toxicity of Early Glottic Three-Dimensional Radiation Treatment

Overall, radiation treatment of early-stage glottic carcinoma is very well tolerated and severe complications from treatment are rare. In early series, acute side effects including skin and mucosal reactions occurred in fewer than 10% of patients undergoing traditional opposed lateral fields.[11,18,30] Severe complications requiring surgical intervention were rare overall (1.8%) in another series, and were associated with larger field sizes and older treatment periods (before 1971, during which patients were treated without techniques to improve dose homogeneity).[4] In the cooperative group setting, 5-year cumulative incidence of Grade 3 to 4 late effects was very low at 8.5%.[18] Furthermore, overall voice quality and preservation have been shown to be good following 3DCRT for early-stage glottic cancer in most of the patients.[4,11,18,31,32]

Late laryngeal dysphagia is a concern in patients treated with head and neck RT. Post-RT dysphagia is associated with mean dose to the constrictor muscles and larynx as well as the volume of these structures receiving 50 to 60 Gy.[33] Development of 3D planning in early-stage glottic radiation treatment planning has led to the ability to assess dose to the constrictors and provides an opportunity to used the recommended dose constraints in planning for patients.

Radiation treatment in locally advanced H&N[34–36] and other non-H&N disease sites[37] has been associated with an increased risk of late cardiovascular events secondary to accelerated atherosclerosis. One study sought to examine the role of radiation in the risk of fatal cerebrovascular events in early-stage glottic cancer by comparing surgically treated patients with those who underwent RT.[38] The study used a competing risks survival analysis to show that radiation treatment was associated with an increased risk of fatal cerebrovascular event compared with surgery (odds ratio [OR] 1.75). The difference in the cumulative incidence of fatal cerebrovascular events between surgery and RT was small but statistically significant, 1.5% vs. 2.8%, respectively. Owing to the excellent oncologic outcomes and high likelihood for long-term survival in early glottic cancer, significant interest exists to use modern techniques to create more conformal radiation treatment plans and thereby reduce late long-term complications of treatment.

Use of Modern Treatment Techniques for Early Glottic Radiation Therapy

The second major revolution impacting RT was the development of intensity-modulated radiation therapy (IMRT). This technique involves modulation, the movement of individual tungsten plates that comprise the multileaf collimator during treatment delivery, to shape the treatment beam resulting in a dose distribution that closely matches the shape of the target in three dimensions. In the early version of IMRT, the beam angles relative to the patient were fixed at 9 to 12 positions; however, the modern version, termed volumetric modulated arc therapy (VMAT), allows for dose modulation continuously as the beam rotates around the patient up to 360°. This enables delivering dose from significantly more degrees, resulting in optimally shaped treatment plans that yield not only full prescription dose coverage of targets but also spare normal tissues in the head/neck region from unnecessary radiation dose fall-off. IMRT is now considered the standard of care for locally advanced head and neck cancer management. IGRT is used in addition to VMAT to ensure that these highly conformal radiation treatment plans are delivered accurately.

The role of these techniques in early glottic cancer is evolving. Early dosimetric studies examining the use of IMRT for early-stage glottic cancer demonstrated significant dose reduction to the carotid arteries compared with traditional opposed fields and 3D conformal radiation techniques.[39] In this study comparing radiation treatment plans using opposed laterals, 3D-CRT, and IMRT, the median carotid dose was 38 Gy, 25 Gy and 10 Gy, respectively. The question remains whether this reduction in dose to the carotid arteries from IMRT (see **Fig. 3**B) would translate into a measurable difference in toxicity in the clinic.

In a retrospective case-control study from multiple institutions, oncologic outcomes were examined for 3D-CRT with opposed lateral fields and IMRT for T1 glottic cancers.[40] Patients included in this analysis ($n = 153$) were treated from 2000 to 2013, with most of them (71%) treated with 3D-CRT with opposed lateral beams. There were no significant differences in any oncologic outcomes between 3D-CRT and IMRT; 3-year locoregional control, 3-year overall survival, and ultimate locoregional control following salvage surgery were the same between groups. Other similar modern series have shown equivalence in oncologic outcomes between 3D-CRT and IMRT for early-stage glottic.[41]

Regarding toxicity, long-term side effects were not statistically significantly different between 3D-CRT with IMRT. Need for feeding tube at 6 months post-treatment occurred in 4 patients in the conventional group and none in the IMRT group, but these numerical differences were not statistically significant ($P = 0.5$).[40] In addition, aspiration events post-treatment were not statistically different between 3D-CRT and IMRT

(7% vs 5%, respectively, $P = .4$). Post-RT cerebrovascular events were overall rare and only occurred in 4 patients in the 3D-CRT group (3%) and none in the IMRT cohort (0%). Despite the numerical difference for cerebrovascular events between groups, this was not statistically significant ($P = .7$).

Given the theoretical benefits of reduced risk of stroke by reducing the dose to the carotid arteries and equivalent local control with IMRT compared with 3D-CRT, some institutions are now standardly using IMRT for early glottic cancer.[40,42] One potential pitfall of more conformal techniques is the possibility of nodal recurrence due to lack of incidental dose from the opposed lateral fields covering the anterior lymph node levels II and III (see Fig. 3A and B). This scenario is exemplified in a case report of an 81-year-old man with a T1N0 glottic cancer who had a level III lymph node recurrence following carotid-sparing IMRT.[43] The lymph node likely received 30 Gy with IMRT compared with the full prescription dose in a 3D-CRT plan. Although a case report should not limit the implementation of advanced techniques, understanding the evolution of radiation treatment fields is an important lesson as we select patients for increasingly more conformal treatments.

ALTERATION OF DOSE OR TARGET VOLUMES FOR EARLY GLOTTIC RADIATION THERAPY

A restriction in radiotherapy facilities during World War II led the Christie Hospital in the U.K. to use a 3-week radiation course for early glottic cancer. The British Institute of Radiology later conducted a trial from 1966 to 1975 randomizing 734 patients to short-course versus long-course radiation for early glottic cancer, resulting in no significant difference in local control and less severe late effects in the short-course arm.[44] The Christie and Royal Marsden Hospitals adopted a 3-week regimen as their standard treatment and reported their experience treating 200 patients from 1989 to 1997. They prescribed 50 to 52.5 Gy in 16 fractions over 21 days with fraction size ranging from 3.12 to 3.28 Gy and reported a 5-year local control rate of 93% and 5-year overall survival of 80%.[45] Subsequent reports in the U.K. showed similar results. Queen Elizabeth Hospital in Birmingham reported 2-year and 5-year local control rates of 92% and 88%, respectively, in 100 patients with T1 N0 M0 disease treated from 1993 to 2001 with 50 Gy in 16 fractions.[46] Ermis and colleagues reported a more modern experience of 132 patients with T1 or T2 disease treated to 55 Gy in 20 fractions from 2004 - 2013. 5-year local control was 85%, and ultimate local control after salvage surgery was 97%.[47] Amid the COVID-19 pandemic, published consensus guidelines recognized hypofractionated regimens prescribed over 3 to 4 weeks, and these regimens are also reflected in the NCCN guidelines.[3,48]

The aforementioned studies have all prescribed radiation doses to the entirety of the anatomic larynx as the target volume. However, in an effort to further mitigate toxicity, several studies have investigated altered dose fractionation as well as target volumes for early-stage disease. Levendag and colleagues in the Netherlands initially reported a 5-year local rate of 93% when treating 164 patients with T1a glottic disease with single vocal cord irradiation (SVCI) using a 4D conformal radiation technique accounting for respiratory motion.[49] This group subsequently published their analysis of 30 patients with T1a disease from their prospective registry treated with SVCI to 58.08 Gy in 16 fractions (3.63 Gy per fraction). At a median follow-up of 30 months, 2-year local control was 100% with no grade 3 toxicity, only 17% grade 2 dermatitis or dysphagia, and improvement in voice quality as assessed by the voice-handicap index (VHI) questionnaire.[50] Further validation was reported in an expanded cohort of 111 consecutive patients with a median follow-up of 41 months demonstrating similarly impressive 3-year and 5-year local control rates of 99.1% and 97.1%, respectively, with this technique.[51] This approach may gain traction as other centers report consistent results with SVCI.[52] A multi-institutional prospective clinical trial is currently randomizing T1 N0 glottic cancer patients in a 1:3 ratio to standard complete-larynx RT versus vocal cord RT. The planned target volume in the experimental arm is the involved vocal cord(s) plus a margin to account for respiratory motion and positioning uncertainties[53] (clinicaltrials.gov; NCT03759431).

Reduction in the target volume requiring treatment is the gateway to reducing the number of fractions over which radiation doses can safely be delivered, thus ushering in a role for stereotactic body radiation therapy (SBRT) prescribed over just 5 fractions. Sher and colleagues at the University of Texas Southwestern enrolled 29 patients to a prospective phase I study evaluating tolerability of increasing dose-per-fraction with three regimens: (1) 50 Gy in 15 fractions, (2) 45 Gy in 10 fractions, and (3) 42.5 Gy in 5 fractions (see **Fig. 3**C). Dose-limiting toxicities were reached in two patients, both actively smoking, treated with regimens 1 and 2 due to grade 3 to 4 laryngeal edema, necrosis, and dysphagia.[54] The subsequent phase 2 study of glottic SBRT has recently completed enrollment (clinical trials.gov, NCT03548285).

Although these modern techniques and approaches show promising results, it is critical to emphasize that the delivery of these treatment plans requires extensive patient evaluation to appropriately select patients followed by meticulous radiation treatment planning and quality assurance. Radiation treatment planning requires a skilled team consisting of dosimetrists, physicists, and clinicians to carefully delineate target volumes, optimize treatment plans, and ensure appropriate image guidance and assessment. Notably, the investigators pursuing glottic SBRT have reported on their surface imaging technique to address swallowing motion during the delivery of high dose-per-fraction treatment to the larynx.[55] This highlights the sophisticated thought, skill, and experience in treatment planning that is required for the delivery of these techniques.

SUMMARY

For the past several decades, radiation oncologists have been treating early glottic cancer with simple opposed lateral radiation treatment fields based on anatomic landmarks to encompass the whole larynx with minimal toxicity and excellent disease control rates. Although these simple radiation treatments remain the standard of care, several groups are exploring how advanced technology with refined treatment volumes may help to mitigate the toxicity of treatment while maintaining excellent disease control.

CLINICS CARE POINTS

- Multidisciplinary assessment of patients with early-stage glottic cancer is critical to select treatment and develop optimal radiation treatment plans.
- Standard of care radiation treatment of early-stage glottic cancer continues to be three-dimensional opposed lateral fields to include the whole larynx.
- Advanced radiation treatment techniques are allowing studies to examine the efficacy and toxicity of altered doses and treatment volumes.
- Stereotactic body radiation therapy and single-vocal cord irradiation for early-stage glottic cancer are not yet considered standard of care and should be performed at institutions with clinical trials to ensure adequate expertise and quality assurance.

- Published reports demonstrate that local control in early-stage glottic cancer is excellent with any one of these radiation treatment techniques.

DISCLOSURES

The authors have nothing to disclose.

REFERENCES

1. Gunderson LL, Tepper JE. Clinical radiation oncology. In: Garden AS MW, Ang KK, editors. Larynx and hypopharynx cancer. 3rd edition. Philadelphia: Elsevier; 2012. p. 639–40.
2. Million RR, Cassisi NJ. Management of head and neck cancer: a multidisciplinary approach. Philadelphia: JB Lippincott; 1994.
3. Caudell JJ, et al. NCCN Guidelines(R) Insights: Head and Neck Cancers, Version 1.2022. J Natl Compr Canc Netw 2022;20(3):224–34.
4. Le QT, et al. Influence of fraction size, total dose, and overall time on local control of T1-T2 glottic carcinoma. Int J Radiat Oncol Biol Phys 1997;39(1): 115–26.
5. Fein DA, et al. Do overall treatment time, field size, and treatment energy influence local control of T1-T2 squamous cell carcinomas of the glottic larynx? Int J Radiat Oncol Biol Phys 1996;34(4):823–31.
6. Rudoltz MS, Benammar A, Mohiuddin M. Prognostic factors for local control and survival in T1 squamous cell carcinoma of the glottis. Int J Radiat Oncol Biol Phys 1993;26(5):767–72.
7. van der Voet JC, et al. The impact of treatment time and smoking on local control and complications in T1 glottic cancer. Int J Radiat Oncol Biol Phys 1998;42(2): 247–55.
8. Burke LS, et al. Definitive radiotherapy for early glottic carcinoma: prognostic factors and implications for treatment. Int J Radiat Oncol Biol Phys 1997;38(5): 1001–6.
9. Chatani M, et al. Radiation therapy for early glottic carcinoma (T1N0M0). The adverse effect of treatment interruption. Strahlenther Onkol 1997;173(10):502–6.
10. Yu E, et al. Impact of radiation therapy fraction size on local control of early glottic carcinoma. Int J Radiat Oncol Biol Phys 1997;37(3):587–91.
11. Yamazaki H, et al. Radiotherapy for early glottic carcinoma (T1N0M0): results of prospective randomized study of radiation fraction size and overall treatment time. Int J Radiat Oncol Biol Phys 2006;64(1):77–82.
12. Lyhne NM, et al. The DAHANCA 6 randomized trial: Effect of 6 vs 5 weekly fractions of radiotherapy in patients with glottic squamous cell carcinoma. Radiother Oncol 2015;117(1):91–8.
13. Mendenhall WM, et al. Curative-intent radiotherapy for glottic carcinoma in situ. Head Neck 2020;42(12):3515–7.
14. Spayne JA, et al. Carcinoma-in-situ of the glottic larynx: results of treatment with radiation therapy. Int J Radiat Oncol Biol Phys 2001;49(5):1235–8.
15. Smitt MC, Goffinet DR. Radiotherapy for carcinoma-in-situ of the glottic larynx. Int J Radiat Oncol Biol Phys 1994;28(1):251–5.
16. Le QT, et al. Treatment results of carcinoma in situ of the glottis: an analysis of 82 cases. Arch Otolaryngol Head Neck Surg 2000;126(11):1305–12.

17. Chera BS, et al. T1N0 to T2N0 squamous cell carcinoma of the glottic larynx treated with definitive radiotherapy. Int J Radiat Oncol Biol Phys 2010;78(2): 461–6.
18. Trotti A 3rd, et al. Randomized trial of hyperfractionation versus conventional fractionation in T2 squamous cell carcinoma of the vocal cord (RTOG 9512). Int J Radiat Oncol Biol Phys 2014;89(5):958–63.
19. Eskiizmir G, et al. Risk factors for radiation failure in early-stage glottic carcinoma: A systematic review and meta-analysis. Oral Oncol 2016;62:90–100.
20. Bhateja P, et al. Impaired vocal cord mobility in T2N0 glottic carcinoma: suboptimal local control with Radiation alone. Head Neck 2016;38(12):1832–6.
21. Akimoto T, et al. Radiation therapy for T2N0 laryngeal cancer: a retrospective analysis for the impact of concurrent chemotherapy on local control. Int J Radiat Oncol Biol Phys 2006;64(4):995–1001.
22. Furusaka T, et al. Concurrent chemoradiation therapy with docetaxel (DOC) for laryngeal preservation in T2N0M0 glottic squamous cell carcinomas. Acta Otolaryngol 2013;133(1):99–112.
23. Ballo MT, et al. Radiation therapy for early stage (T1-T2) sarcomatoid carcinoma of true vocal cords: outcomes and patterns of failure. Laryngoscope 1998;108(5): 760–3.
24. Ding L, et al. Sarcomatoid Carcinoma in the Head and Neck: A Population-Based Analysis of Outcome and Survival. Laryngoscope 2021;131(2):E489–99.
25. Mendenhall WM, et al. Management of T1-T2 glottic carcinomas. Cancer 2004; 100(9):1786–92.
26. Zouhair A, et al. Decreased local control following radiation therapy alone in early-stage glottic carcinoma with anterior commissure extension. Strahlenther Onkol 2004;180(2):84–90.
27. Lee JH, et al. Radiotherapy with 6-megavolt photons for early glottic carcinoma: potential impact of extension to the posterior vocal cord. Am J Otolaryngol 2001; 22(1):43–54.
28. Timmermans AJ, et al. Tumor volume as a prognostic factor for local control and overall survival in advanced larynx cancer. Laryngoscope 2016;126(2):E60–7.
29. Strongin A, et al. Primary tumor volume is an important predictor of clinical outcomes among patients with locally advanced squamous cell cancer of the head and neck treated with definitive chemoradiotherapy. Int J Radiat Oncol Biol Phys 2012;82(5):1823–30.
30. Mendenhall WM, et al. T1-T2N0 squamous cell carcinoma of the glottic larynx treated with radiation therapy. J Clin Oncol 2001;19(20):4029–36.
31. Osborn HA, et al. Comparison of endoscopic laser resection versus radiation therapy for the treatment of early glottic carcinoma. J Otolaryngol Head Neck Surg 2011;40(3):200–4.
32. Naunheim MR, et al. Voice Outcomes After Radiation for Early-Stage Laryngeal Cancer. J Voice 2020;34(3):460–4.
33. Wang X, Eisbruch A. IMRT for head and neck cancer: reducing xerostomia and dysphagia. J Radiat Res 2016;57(Suppl 1):i69–75.
34. Sun L, et al. Association Between Up-front Surgery and Risk of Stroke in US Veterans With Oropharyngeal Carcinoma. JAMA Otolaryngol Head Neck Surg 2022; 148(8):740–7.
35. Arthurs E, et al. Stroke after radiation therapy for head and neck cancer: what is the risk? Int J Radiat Oncol Biol Phys 2016;96(3):589–96.
36. Carpenter DJ, et al. The risk of carotid stenosis in head and neck cancer patients after radiation therapy. Oral Oncol 2018;80:9–15.

37. Darby SC, et al. Risk of ischemic heart disease in women after radiotherapy for breast cancer. N Engl J Med 2013;368(11):987–98.
38. Swisher-McClure S, et al. Risk of fatal cerebrovascular accidents after external beam radiation therapy for early-stage glottic laryngeal cancer. Head Neck 2014;36(5):611–6.
39. Chera BS, et al. Carotid-sparing intensity-modulated radiotherapy for early-stage squamous cell carcinoma of the true vocal cord. Int J Radiat Oncol Biol Phys 2010;77(5):1380–5.
40. Mohamed ASR, et al. Outcomes of carotid-sparing IMRT for T1 glottic cancer: comparison with conventional radiation. Laryngoscope 2020;130(1):146–53.
41. Zumsteg ZS, et al. Carotid sparing intensity-modulated radiation therapy achieves comparable locoregional control to conventional radiotherapy in T1-2N0 laryngeal carcinoma. Oral Oncol 2015;51(7):716–23.
42. Amini A, et al. Outcomes between intensity-modulated radiation therapy versus 3D-conformal in early stage glottic cancer. Head Neck 2021;43(11):3393–403.
43. DePaoli B, et al. Regional Recurrence after Carotid Sparing IMRT for Early Stage Glottic Cancer. Pract Radiat Oncol 2022. S1879-8500(22)00264-00268.
44. Wiernik G, et al. Final report of the general clinical results of the British Institute of Radiology fractionation study of 3F/wk versus 5F/wk in radiotherapy of carcinoma of the laryngo-pharynx. Br J Radiol 1990;63(747):169–80.
45. Gowda RV, et al. Three weeks radiotherapy for T1 glottic cancer: the Christie and Royal Marsden Hospital Experience. Radiother Oncol 2003;68(2):105–11.
46. Cheah NL, et al. Outcome of T1N0M0 squamous cell carcinoma of the larynx treated with short-course radiotherapy to a total dose of 50 Gy in 16 fractions: the Birmingham experience. Clin Oncol (R Coll Radiol 2009;21(6):494–501.
47. Ermis E, et al. Definitive hypofractionated radiotherapy for early glottic carcinoma: experience of 55Gy in 20 fractions. Radiat Oncol 2015;10:203.
48. Thomson DJ, et al. Practice recommendations for risk-adapted head and neck cancer radiotherapy during the COVID-19 pandemic: An ASTRO-ESTRO consensus statement. Radiother Oncol 2020;151:314–21.
49. Levendag PC, et al. Single vocal cord irradiation: a competitive treatment strategy in early glottic cancer. Radiother Oncol 2011;101(3):415–9.
50. Al-Mamgani A, et al. Single Vocal Cord Irradiation: Image Guided Intensity Modulated Hypofractionated Radiation Therapy for T1a Glottic Cancer: Early Clinical Results. Int J Radiat Oncol Biol Phys 2015;93(2):337–43.
51. Tans L, et al. Single vocal cord irradiation for early-stage glottic cancer: Excellent local control and favorable toxicity profile. Oral Oncol 2022;127:105782.
52. Chung SY, Lee CG. Feasibility of single vocal cord irradiation as a treatment strategy for T1a glottic cancer. Head Neck 2020;42(5):854–9.
53. Bahig H, et al. Vocal-cord Only vs. Complete Laryngeal radiation (VOCAL): a randomized multicentric Bayesian phase II trial. BMC Cancer 2021;21(1):446.
54. Sher DJ, et al. Phase 1 Fractional Dose-Escalation Study of Equipotent Stereotactic Radiation Therapy Regimens for Early-Stage Glottic Larynx Cancer. Int J Radiat Oncol Biol Phys 2019;105(1):110–8.
55. Zhao B, et al. Surface guided motion management in glottic larynx stereotactic body radiation therapy. Radiother Oncol 2020;153:236–42.

Surgical Treatment of Early Glottic Cancer

Jennifer A. Silver, MD, Sena Turkdogan, MD, FRCSC, Catherine F. Roy, MD, Karen M. Kost, MD, FRCSC*

KEYWORDS

- Vocal fold • Early glottic cancer • Laryngeal cancer • Endoscopic surgery
- Transoral laser microsurgery

KEY POINTS

- Early glottic cancer is highly curable, with 5-year local control rates ranging from 85% to 95% for T1 and 60% to 80% for T2 disease.
- Goals include eradication of disease while maintaining voice, swallowing, and airway patency.
- Surgical approaches include endoscopic minimally invasive surgery versus open techniques.
- Minimally invasive techniques include carbon dioxide laser, potassium titanyl phosphate laser, or transoral robotic surgery.
- Most commonly, transoral laser microsurgery follows the European Laryngological Society classification for endoscopic cordectomies.

INTRODUCTION

Definition, Risk Factors, and Epidemiology

Early glottic cancer is typically defined as Tis, T1a, T1b, and T2 disease with no nodal involvement (ie, stage 0, I, and II disease) and generally carries a favorable prognosis.[1] Classifying this group as *early* has been an area of debate as it is tumoral extent, rather than rate of growth, that ultimately determines staging. Some authors suggest that grouping stage 0 to 2 disease as *localized* may be more accurate, though this may be solely a nomenclature quandary.[2] By convention, this article uses the term *early* to denote lower stage laryngeal cancer (stage 0–2).

Early glottic cancers represent the majority of glottic cancers, largely because even small lesions often result in significant dysphonia, prompting rapid otolaryngology consultation and diagnosis. The most common histopathologic diagnosis is squamous cell carcinoma (SCC). A recent analysis of the National Cancer Database

Department of Otolaryngology–Head and Neck Surgery, McGill University Health Centre, 1001 Decarie Boulevard, Montreal, Quebec H4A 3J1, Canada
* Corresponding author.
E-mail address: kmkost@yahoo.com

Otolaryngol Clin N Am 56 (2023) 259–273
https://doi.org/10.1016/j.otc.2022.12.009
0030-6665/23/© 2023 Elsevier Inc. All rights reserved.

reported that only 1% of all malignant laryngeal cancers were non-SCC (mostly neuro-endocrine tumors and bone/cartilage sarcomas).[3] Early glottic cancer is highly curable, with a reported 5-year local control rate ranging from 85% to 95% for T1 and 60% to 80% for T2 disease.[4]

Well-recognized risk factors are tobacco use and alcohol consumption, as is the case for most cancers of the aerodigestive tract. There are data to support untreated gastroesophageal reflux as a cofactor in the genesis of laryngeal cancer.[5] Low socio-economic status, marijuana and opioid use, red meat, and occupational exposures have been proposed as additional risk factors in the literature, but the causal link is not as clearly defined.[6,7] Although human papilloma virus (HPV) is well established in the etiology of oropharyngeal SCCs,[8] its role in laryngeal cancer is still unclear. Meta-analyses have reported an HPV prevalence in laryngeal SCC of approximately 25%. Acknowledging the mere presence of viral components, however, is not neces-sarily indicative of active viral replication and does not imply a role in tumor develop-ment or progression.[8]

Epidemiologically, primary laryngeal and glottic cancer are uncommon, with an esti-mated lifetime risk of one in 190 for men and one in 830 for women. The most recent estimates for laryngeal cancer for 2022 from the American Cancer Society report about 12,470 new cases yearly, 60% of which arise from the glottis. Both the overall prevalence and mortality from laryngeal cancer have been steadily decreasing at a rate of 2% to 3% per year.[9]

Anatomic Correlates and Locoregional Pattern of Spread

An understanding of laryngeal embryology is critical in appreciating patterns of locore-gional spread. Contrary to the supraglottis, which is derived from a single midline structure (the buccopharyngeal primordium), the glottis and subglottis arise from two laterally based furrows of the tracheobronchial primordium that fuse in the midline with a median-based furrow. The paired embryologic origin accounts for the unilateral lymphatic networks of the glottis and subglottis. The lymphatics to this area follow the inferior laryngeal artery emanating from the inferior thyroid artery to drain into the prel-aryngeal and pretracheal nodes.[2] Lymphatic drainage to the glottis is usually sparse, thus accounting for the low rates of nodal metastases.[10]

The pattern of spread within the larynx and to the extralaryngeal tissues is guided by ligaments, dense connective tissues, and cartilage. The submucosal elastic layer, conus elasticus, quadrangular membrane, ventricular connective tissue, and hyoepi-glottic ligament act as strong natural barriers to tumor spread (**Fig. 1**A). Laryngeal car-tilages are also relatively resistant to tumor invasion, in part due to their poor vascularity and the overlying perichondrium.

The anterior commissure has been postulated to be an area of weakness as the perichondrium is naturally deficient at areas of muscular attachments, yet this remains the subject of controversy. Tumors involving the anterior commissure were hypothe-sized to spread inferiorly to the vocal tendon ligament (also known as Broyles liga-ment)[10] (**Fig. 1**B). Observational studies have shown anterior commissure involvement is associated with a greater risk of local treatment failure and tumor persistence regardless of the chosen treatment modality (surgery or radiotherapy).[11] To the contrary, Kirchner and Carter performed histopathological analyses of laryngeal carcinomas and rather postulated the vocal tendon ligament to be a robust barrier to the adjacent thyroid cartilage.[12] The observed higher failure rates with cancers involving the anterior commissure may thus be a reflection of tumor understaging and undertreatment, as deep invasion may be challenging to identify radiologically in this area.[13]

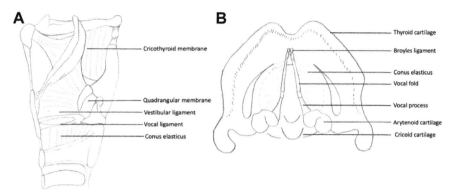

Fig. 1. Laryngeal anatomy, specifically demonstrating (*A*) quadrangular membrane and conus elasticus and (*B*) Broyles ligament.

CLINICAL AND RADIOLOGICAL EVALUATION

Almost all patients with laryngeal cancer present to an otolaryngologist with some degree of hoarseness.[2,14] Given this audible voice change from baseline, many patients are assessed and diagnosed in the early stages of disease.[6,15]

Flexible transnasal laryngoscopy has replaced the indirect mirror examination as the primary modality for in-office glottic assessment.[16,17] During evaluation, the clinician examines the size, location, color, appearance of the lesion, involvement of adjacent structures and specifically notes the mobility of the vocal cords due to its prognostic implications.[18] A reduction in vocal fold mobility stages the tumor as T2 and fixation of the cord stages the tumor as T3.[1,19,20] The change in movement can be due to invasion of the thyroarytenoid muscle, paraglottic space or cricoarytenoid joint, or mass effect from a bulky tumor.

Before obtaining radiological confirmation, certain clinical signs can assist in staging the tumor at the time of presentation. Ulceration of the infrahyoid epiglottis, fullness in the region of the vallecula, or fullness on palpation of the thyrohyoid membrane may indicate pre-epiglottic space invasion. Medial to lateral manual manipulation of the larynx typically elicits a laryngeal click, which may become absent in the presence of postcricoid spread. Last, localized pain or tenderness to palpation over the lamina may suggest the gross invasion of the cartilage.

Clinical examination with flexible laryngoscopy can also be supplemented with videoendoscopy and videostroboscopy.[21] Videoendoscopy is becoming standard practice as recording the examinations allows for better monitoring and aids in treatment-related decisions over time. Videostroboscopy provides even greater detail of fine vocal fold mobility, amplitude of vibration, and mucosal wave, all of which collectively help characterize epithelial lesions.[22] There are conflicting beliefs about the usefulness of stroboscopy in differentiating premalignant versus malignant lesions as multiple studies have demonstrated high sensitivity in the diagnosis of glottic cancer but low specificity in excluding glottic cancer in a patient with a vocal fold lesion.[23–27] However, videostroboscopy provides benefits in terms of follow-up and surveillance, as clinicians are able to identify minute changes in the mucosal wave more accurately.[28]

In-office endoscopic diagnostic procedures, such as laryngeal biopsy, are becoming more widespread as there are multiple benefits with minimal risk compared with biopsies performed in the operating room.[29] For the vast majority of patients in whom the procedure is possible, there are several advantages, which include (i) obviate the need for a general anesthetic, (ii) circumventing operating room delays, and (iii) faster turnaround time for pathologic analysis.[16] In a systematic review of in-office biopsies, a diagnostic accuracy of 81.6% was reported.[29] Occasionally, however, patients are unable to tolerate the procedure, in-office sampling may be insufficient, or the surgeon prefers direct laryngoscopy and biopsy (with or without excision) in the operating room.[30]

Diagnostic imaging studies are most useful in identifying spread to or involvement of deeper structures to stage glottic cancers.[31] A fine-cut computed tomography (CT) scan of the larynx is rapid, minimizes motion artifact, and accurately evaluates possible bony anatomy/cartilage invasion.[31,32] CT scans are also useful in assessing cervical lymphadenopathy, although nodal disease is rare in early glottic cancers. MRI offers better evaluation of the soft tissues and is able to determine involvement of the laryngeal ventricle, anterior commissure, and cartilage involvement.[31] A prospective study comparing CT and MRI reports with the final pathology results in 26 patients with early glottic cancer concluded that MRI may be superior for treatment planning due to better determination of anterior commissure involvement.[33] PET-CT is not often an up-front imaging modality for early glottic neoplasms but remains in the arsenal for assessment in follow-up to identify recurrent or residual disease.[34,35]

GOALS OF TREATMENT

The primary objective in the treatment of early glottic cancer remains cure of disease while maintaining an adequate airway. Secondary goals include preservation of voice and swallowing and reserving treatment options in the event of future recurrences.[36] Specifically, the American Society of Clinical Oncology Clinical Practice Guidelines counsel that patients with early glottic cancer should undergo initial treatment with the intent for laryngeal preservation.[37]

For early glottic cancers, patients require single modality therapy which may consist of radiation therapy (RT) or surgery, be it open or transoral surgery. The modality chosen depends on the tumor location and extent, general health status of the patient, the common practice and resources available at the institution, and patient preference. Although early tumors treated with radiation or surgery have similar oncologic outcomes in multiple systematic reviews of non-randomized studies, the results of voice quality assessments are conflicting.[38–40]

Given this clinical equipoise between surgical treatment and RT in early-stage laryngeal tumors, the published literature recommends that treatment decisions be guided by patient preference after comprehensive discussion of treatment options and long-term secondary effects.[41]

TREATMENT MODALITY APPROACHES

The main treatment approaches for early glottic cancer include RT and surgical excision. NCCN guidelines demonstrate a preference for endoscopic resection of glottic carcinoma in situ and are equivocal concerning RT versus surgical resection in T1–T2, N0 tumors. Adverse features after resection such as a positive margin, close margin, or other high-risk features (perineural invasion or lymphovascular invasion) may require postoperative radiation or re-resection if feasible.[1]

Radiation for early glottic cancer was extensively discussed in the previous article, and consequently the focus here will be on surgical treatments and their complications. Indeed, both approaches have their unique advantages and disadvantages, although application of new surgical approaches and modalities have been shown to result in shorter hospitalization, decreased morbidity, and lower costs.[42] A recent meta-analysis by Vaculik and colleagues[43] comparing T1 glottic cancer outcomes in CO_2 transoral laser microsurgery (TLM) versus RT, suggested that TLM is the superior modality in terms of overall survival, disease-specific survival, and laryngeal preservation. Furthermore, surgery as a primary treatment strategy allows for more treatment options if patients present with recurrent disease.[44,45] Patients who have been primarily treated with RT cannot be re-irradiated, and performing radical laser resection is significantly more difficult in a previously irradiated larynx. Therefore, these patients have a much higher likelihood of requiring a total laryngectomy. Indeed, several studies have demonstrated a lower probability of laryngeal preservation in patients initially treated with RT.[38,46,47] Last, although earlier dogmas suggested that a possible disadvantage of surgery included poorer voice outcomes when compared with RT, recent studies show conflicting evidence, suggesting that voice outcomes may be equivalent if not better in certain cases.[48,49] A randomized-controlled trial comparing voice quality after RT or TLM up to 2 years posttreatment found that there were similar voice outcomes.[50] However, a multimodality voice analysis study assessed RT and TLM patients using objective (Analysis of Dysphonia in Speech and Voice Software CSID Score and assessment by blinded speech language pathologists) and subjective outcomes (Voice Handicap Index).[48] Their findings suggested that there were better long-term voice outcomes in TLM patients on objective measures but no difference on self-perception scores. The investigators hypothesize that this is a result of the progressive fibrosis from RT.

Surgical modalities in early glottic cancer can be categorized as endoscopic minimally invasive surgery, including outpatient laser treatments, transoral microsurgery or transoral robotic surgery (TORS), and open surgical approaches. The risks, benefits, and potential complications associated with each approach will be elaborated below.

Endoscopic Minimally Invasive Surgery

Endoscopic management of premalignant lesions and early-stage glottic carcinomas can be performed during direct laryngoscopy using an operative microscope. Lesions are excised with either microlaryngoscopic instruments or a carbon dioxide laser, often referred to as CO_2 TLM. Because its frequency of light is absorbed by water, CO_2 laser minimizes tissue damage. Transoral laser procedures usually carry less morbidity and allow an earlier return to function. The use of this technique must consider the skill of the operating surgeon and the ability to adequately visualize the larynx during suspension. Several reports have confirmed the efficacy of TLM for the treatment of early glottic cancer. The reported local control rates of TLM in patients with T1a and T1b glottic cancer range from 86% to 93%, with a laryngeal preservation rate of approximately 95%.[51–53]

The potassium titanyl phosphate (KTP) laser has also been used as an alternative to CO_2 for carcinoma in situ or small, selected T1 cancers, as it is thought to better preserve the lamina propria.[54] The KTP laser has better hemostatic properties given that the 532-nm wavelength is preferentially absorbed by hemoglobin and therefore has angiolytic properties.[55] Studies have shown that KTP laser may provide effective treatment of primary early glottic cancers and even patients who failed radiotherapy for T1 and T2 glottic cancers.[56,57] However, because KTP lasers vaporize the specimen, margin analysis is difficult and relies on careful clinical follow-up. The use of the KTP laser has been successful in the outpatient department in patients with CIS or early glottic cancers.[58] The frequent follow-ups for reevaluations allow this to be a safe alternative and obviate the need for GA in these selected cases. Parker and colleagues[59] retrospectively analyzed KTP laser use on 88 cases of T1 and T2 cancers in

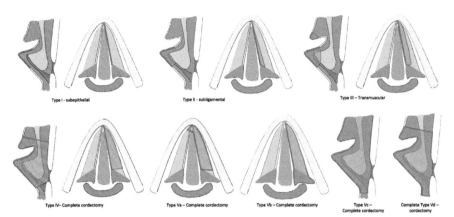

Fig. 2. Classification of endoscopic cordectomies by the European Laryngological Society. (Remacle, M., Eckel, H., Antonelli, A. et al. Endoscopic cordectomy. a proposal for a classification by the Working Committee, European Laryngological Society. European Archives of Oto-Rhino-Laryngology 257, 227–231 (2000). https://doi.org/10.1007/s004050050228.)

the operating room setting. Despite 24 patients requiring repeat treatment, the disease-specific and overall survival rates were 100% and 92.3%, respectively, demonstrating that KTP treatment and close surveillance have positive outcomes. A trial randomizing T1a and T1b patients with laryngeal cancer to CO_2 laser cordectomy or KTP laser ablation found that there were similar oncologic outcomes but those in the KTP cohort were more likely to preserve the vocal fold architecture.[60]

The European Laryngological Society proposed a classification of endoscopic laryngeal cordectomies based on extent of resection in order to ensure consistent definitions and more reliable reporting of postoperative results.[61] This classification has become adopted worldwide and consists of eight types of cordectomies (Fig. 2): a subepithelial cordectomy (type I), which is resection of the epithelium; a subligamental cordectomy (type II), which is a resection of the epithelium, Reinke's space and vocal ligament; transmuscular cordectomy (type III), which proceeds through the vocalis muscle; total cordectomy (type IV); extended cordectomy, which encompasses the contralateral vocal fold and the anterior commissure (type Va); extended cordectomy, which includes the arytenoid (type Vb); extended cordectomy, which encompasses the subglottis (type Vc); and extended cordectomy, which includes the ventricle (type Vd). Indications for performing these cordectomies may vary according to surgeon preference but are usually guided by clinical and radiological evidence of tumor extent.

Open Surgery

Conservation open laryngeal surgery encompasses a broad array of open surgical techniques ranging from a laryngofissure approach with cordectomy to supracricoid laryngectomy.[62] Rarely, the laryngofissure approach with cordectomy might be required for patients with poor transoral exposure. However, both emerging evidence demonstrating the oncological and functional benefits of TLM and specialized instrumentation have resulted in even fewer indications for open partial laryngectomy.[63,64]

Vertical partial laryngectomy, also known classically as a hemilaryngectomy, is indicated in the treatment of tumors that arise on the true vocal cord with limited involvement of the anterior commissure. In this type of resection, the entire ipsilateral glottic larynx is removed including the paraglottic space and corresponding thyroid ala while preserving the ipsilateral arytenoid. Closing the strap muscles over the defect can help to create a pseudocord. All patients undergoing this procedure require a tracheotomy, which is a major disadvantage of this approach compared with endoscopic procedures.

In the case of anterior commissure involvement, a frontolateral partial laryngectomy may be considered. This procedure extends the resection to the contralateral cord, including the anterior commissure. The involvement of the anterior commissure decreases local control with several studies demonstrating decreased control rates from 93% to 75%[65,66] due to the possible hypotheses described above. Contraindications for both types of vertical partial laryngectomy include tumor involvement of the interarytenoid area, subglottic extension greater than 10 mm, and poor medical condition, especially significant pulmonary disease.

Open partial laryngectomy approaches should be considered for selected tumors when the outcomes of radiation are less optional and TLM is not feasible. The latter may be due to local extension to an adjacent site, tumor bulk, or difficulties with access.[67] In addition, specific expertise is needed to ensure reproducible results from open partial laryngectomy, as this technique is associated with several special challenges in terms of patient selection, surgical technique, and postoperative care.

Transoral Robotic Surgery

Although endoscopic and open approaches to the glottis have traditionally been the preferred surgical approach for laryngeal access, TORS has been gaining popularity as its increasing presence and advanced surgeon training has allowed for a novel surgical approach to many head and neck sites. Recently, its feasibility in microlaryngeal surgery has been demonstrated in mannequin, cadaver, and canine models.[68–70]

Limitations in translaryngeal microsurgery exist, including restricted and nonintuitive movement of microlaryngeal instrumentation, limited visualization by the size and position of the laryngoscope, and the distance between the glottic structures and the operating surgeons' hands. Although hand-held endoscopes have been recently applied to provide close and direct visualization through the laryngoscope, this method occupies one hand of the operating surgeon and thus limits many operative laryngeal procedures. Rigid endoscopes also have a limited two-dimensional visualization of the operative field. Certain studies have also quoted a shorter learning curve for robotic use when compared with standard laparoscopic techniques.[71,72]

Recent application of the robot in laryngeal surgery may include several advantages, including a wide exposure, multiplanar transection of tissues, and a three-dimensional view provided by the integrated high-resolution endoscope. Furthermore, the surgeon may repeatedly and instantaneously reposition the robotically controlled camera and instruments to change viewpoint during the procedure.[73] In January 2010, the US Food and Drug Administration approved TORS for use in benign and malignant diseases of the tonsils, pharynx, and larynx.[74]

Despite these advancements, the use of the surgical robot for endolaryngeal and glottic surgery is still controversial with limited availability of controlled human trials.[75,76] Technical disadvantages have been noted with robotic laryngeal surgery and include poor visualization due to a combination of hypertrophied lingual tonsils and the relatively large size of the robotic arms and instruments in vision.[77,78] A recent review of nine published studies suggested that the current robotic systems do not seem adequate for transoral robotic cordectomy and that robotic approaches to these lesions were associated with higher rates of complications and tracheotomy than conventional TLM[77] (**Table 1**).

SURGICAL RESECTION MARGINS

The most important goal during surgical resection is to obtain clear margins. Although most head and neck malignancies require a 5-mm margin as the standard of histologically cancer-free tissue, conservative laryngeal surgery tolerates closer surgical margins.[79,80]

Given the high cure rates for glottic cancer, there has been an emphasis on the preservation of voice as an important measure of surgical success.[81] This is achieved by resecting minimally, but still achieving histologically clear margins around the cancer, all without compromising survival. Zeitels and colleagues[82] published a prospective clinical trial on 32 patients with T1 or T2 unilateral glottic cancer who underwent suspension microlaryngoscopy, subepithelial infusion to assess lesion depth, and narrow margin resection with CO_2 laser or cold steel (if within the superficial lamina propria). Only one patient had recurrence which was re-resected and remained free of disease in over 3 years of follow-up. No patient in this cohort required salvage open surgery or RT. The strategy of using the surgical microscope creates a similar environment to Mohs resection, where the magnification allows the operator to take the minimum tissue around the cancer, a 1-mm peripheral margin and 1 to 2 mm deep margin, to maximally preserve the microstructure of the vocal folds.[81]

Specimens from total laryngectomy resections were analyzed to identify the margin of resection, and these patients were followed for 4 years postoperatively. There were no cases of local recurrence in patients with a resection margin of 2 mm or larger ($n = 40$), but one of nine patients with a 1-mm margin had local recurrence, and 48% of 21 patients who had involved margins recurred.[83]

Some centers use frozen section analysis to confirm intraoperative negative margins before completion of the surgical procedure.[36,84] Five-year locoregional control rates were higher in patients with clear surgical margins from the first surgical procedure, compared with those who underwent a reoperation for positive margins despite the second resection specimen having histopathologically clear margins.[85]

Overall, a 2-mm clear margin is suggested in resection of early glottic cancers.

MANAGEMENT OF THE NECK

Anatomically, nodal metastases of glottic cancers are rare as lymphatic supply to this area is less robust compared with other head and neck regions.[10,67,86] There is some discussion regarding the management of N0 neck in glottic cancer given the divergence from standard algorithms of other head and neck cancer subsites. This is based on the practice that elective treatment of the neck is recommended if the risk of occult nodal disease is greater than 15% to 20%.[87–90] When metastases to the lymph nodes do occur, they are commonly found in levels II, III, and IV. Retrospective studies of patients with glottic cancer who had undergone elective neck dissection with a clinical negative neck have demonstrated occult nodal disease in 0% to 16% of these early cases (T1–T2).[90–93] Another retrospective study of 585 patients only had 4% nodal metastases at follow-up in patients with early glottic cancer who did not receive neck radiation.[94] As well, patients receiving radiation to the neck did not demonstrate better regional control rates than those without neck irradiation (nodal failure rates of 3.7% and 2.6% in irradiated and non-irradiated patients, respectively, $P = .88$).[95]

If the surgical resection specimen demonstrates other poor prognostic factors on pathological examination, elective neck dissection may play a role. In a retrospective cohort study of data from the National Cancer Database from 2004 to 2016, 372/991 patients with cT1N0 or cT2N0 glottic cancer underwent elective neck dissection.[93]

Table 1
Complications associated with different modalities (in increasing order of frequency)

Modality	Complications	
	Early	Late
Radiation	Fatigue	Chronic skin changes
	Skin changes/dermatitis	Thick secretions
	Mucositis	Chronic pain
	Dry mouth	Dysphonia
	Thick secretions	Laryngitis
	Sore throat	Laryngeal edema
	Dysphonia	Hypothyroidism
	Loss of appetite, loss of	Dysphagia
	taste	Esophageal or pharyngeal
	Poor oral intake	stenosis
	Weight loss	Requirement of enteral
	Laryngeal edema	feeding
		Chondronecrosis
		Accelerated carotid stenosis
		Chronic aspiration
		Tracheostomy
		Frozen larynx
		Radiation-induced
		malignancy
Open surgery	Dysphonia	Pain
	Dysphagia	Anterior glottic web
	Wound infection	Laryngeal synechia
	Subcutaneous emphysema	Dysphonia
	Tracheostomy (temporary)	Dysphagia
	Salivary fistula	Prolonged aspiration risk
	Aspiration risk	Tracheostomy (long term)
Transoral minimally invasive surgery including laser, cold steel, or robotic approaches	Dysphonia	Dysphonia
	Dental injury	Anterior glottic web
	Airway edema	Laryngeal synechia
	Hemorrhage	Dysphagia
	Transient/mild inspiratory	Prolonged aspiration risk
	stridor aspiration	
	pneumonia	
	Perichondritis	
	Thermal injury	
	Laser injuries to	
	surrounding structures	
	Airway fire	
	Pneumothorax	
	Post-extubation airway	
	obstruction	
	Tracheostomy (2% risk)	
	Carotid artery exposure or	
	blowout (very rare)	

Among those, 61 patients had positive occult nodal disease and this was associated with higher tumor grade ($P = .004$) and decreased survival ($P<.001$).

Generally, patients with early glottic cancer with a clinically and radiologically negative neck does not require elective neck dissection or RT targeting the neck, and elective contralateral neck dissection is not routinely recommended for ipsilateral N+ glottic cancer.

SUMMARY

Patients diagnosed with early glottic cancer have a good prognosis and should undergo initial treatment with the intent for laryngeal preservation to maintain one's voice and swallowing capabilities. Single modality treatment is generally sufficient for early glottic cancers. Both primary surgery and RT can be offered; however, the surgical approaches have expanded and now include endoscopic minimally invasive surgery and open techniques. The most common surgical treatment is now some type of cordectomy via TLM, as guided by the European Laryngology Society classification system. Surgical resection has comparable results to nonsurgical treatments and reserves RT for possible recurrences or second primary cancers.

CLINICS CARE POINTS

- Early glottic cancer, including Tis, T1a, T1b, and T2 disease with no nodal involvement, is highly curable with a reported 5-year local control rate ranging from 85% to 95% for T1 and 60% to 80% for T2 disease.
- The primary goal of treatment remains eradication of disease. Secondary goals include preservation of voice and swallowing and patency of the airway.
- Primary surgery or radiation therapy may be used for early glottic cancers. The surgical approaches include endoscopic minimally invasive surgery, including transoral microsurgery or transoral robotic surgery, and various open surgical techniques.
- Transoral laser microsurgery is becoming the most common treatment modality, and the European Laryngological Society has published a widely recognized classification system of laryngeal endoscopic cordectomies.
- Clear surgical margins are essential regardless of the operative technique. A 2-mm clear margin is suggested in resection of early glottic cancer as opposed to the majority of head and neck malignancies where a 5-mm margin is standard.
- Nodal metastasis in early glottic cancer is rare. Consequently, elective neck dissection or radiation therapy is unnecessary in patients with no clinical or radiological evidence of nodal disease.

DISCLOSURE

Dr K.M. Kost has an affiliation with Pentax; however, there is no relation or involvement with the current work.

REFERENCES

1. Amin MB, Greene FL, Edge SB, et al. The eighth edition AJCC cancer staging manual: continuing to build a bridge from a population-based to a more "personalized" approach to cancer staging. CA Cancer J Clin 2017;67(2):93–9.
2. Cummings CWFPW. Cummings otolaryngology–head & neck surgery. Philadelphia: Elsevier/Saunders; 2021.
3. Torabi SJ, Cheraghlou S, Kasle DA, et al. Nonsquamous cell laryngeal cancers: incidence, demographics, care patterns, and effect of surgery. Laryngoscope 2019;129(11):2496–505.
4. Wang G, Li G, Wu J, et al. Analysis of prognostic factors for Tis-2N0M0 early glottic cancer with different treatment methods. Braz J Otorhinolaryngol 2022;88(3): 375–80.

5. Zhang D, Zhou J, Chen B, et al. Gastroesophageal reflux and carcinoma of larynx or pharynx: a meta-analysis. Acta Otolaryngol 2014;134(10):982–9.

6. Koroulakis A, Agarwal M. Laryngeal cancer. StatPearls. Treasure Island (FL): Stat-Pearls Publishing; 2022. Copyright © 2022, StatPearls Publishing LLC.

7. Williamson AJ, Bondje S. Glottic cancer. StatPearls [internet]. StatPearls Publishing; 2022.

8. Gama RR, Carvalho AL, Longatto Filho A, et al. Detection of human papillomavirus in laryngeal squamous cell carcinoma: systematic review and meta-analysis. Laryngoscope 2016;126(4):885–93.

9. Laryngeal and hypopharyngeal cancer. American Cancer Society. 2021. Available at: https://www.cancer.org/cancer/laryngeal-and-hypopharyngeal-cancer.html. Accessed.

10. Mor N, Blitzer A. Functional anatomy and oncologic barriers of the larynx. Otolaryngol Clin North Am 2015;48(4):533–45.

11. Mannelli G, Comini LV, Santoro R, et al. T1 glottic cancer: does anterior commissure involvement worsen prognosis? Cancers (Basel) 2020;12(6).

12. Gioacchini FM, Tulli M, Kaleci S, et al. Therapeutic modalities and oncologic outcomes in the treatment of T1b glottic squamous cell carcinoma: a systematic review. Eur Arch Otorhinolaryngol 2017;274(12):4091–102.

13. Kirchner JA, Carter D. Intralaryngeal barriers to the spread of cancer. Acta Otolaryngol 1987;103(5–6):503–13.

14. Merletti F, Faggiano F, Boffetta P, et al. Topographic classification, clinical characteristics, and diagnostic delay of cancer of the larynx/hypopharynx in Torino, Italy. Cancer 1990;66(8):1711–6.

15. Karatzanis AD, Psychogios G, Zenk J, et al. Comparison among different available surgical approaches in T1 glottic cancer. Laryngoscope 2009;119(9):1704–8.

16. Cohen JT, Safadi A, Fliss DM, et al. Reliability of a transnasal flexible fiberoptic in-office laryngeal biopsy. JAMA Otolaryngol Head Neck Surg 2013;139(4):341–5.

17. Cohen JT, Benyamini L. Transnasal flexible fiberoptic in-office laryngeal biopsies-our experience with 117 patients with suspicious lesions. Rambam Maimonides Med J 2014;5(2):e0011.

18. Peretti G, Piazza C, Mensi MC, et al. Endoscopic treatment of cT2 glottic carcinoma: prognostic impact of different pT subcategories. Ann Otol Rhinol Laryngol 2005;114(8):579–86.

19. Hirano M, Kurita S, Matsuoka H, et al. Vocal fold fixation in laryngeal carcinomas. Acta Otolaryngol 1991;111(2):449–54.

20. McCoul ED, Har-El G. Meta-analysis of impaired vocal cord mobility as a prognostic factor in T2 glottic carcinoma. Arch Otolaryngol Head Neck Surg 2009;135(5):479–86.

21. Paul BC, Chen S, Sridharan S, et al. Diagnostic accuracy of history, laryngoscopy, and stroboscopy. Laryngoscope 2013;123(1):215–9.

22. Bless DM, Hirano M, Feder RJ. Videostroboscopic evaluation of the larynx. Ear Nose Throat J 1987;66(7):289–96.

23. Djukic V, Milovanovic J, Jotic AD, et al. Stroboscopy in detection of laryngeal dysplasia effectiveness and limitations. J Voice 2014;28(2):262.e13–21.

24. Gugatschka M, Kiesler K, Beham A, et al. Hyperplastic epithelial lesions of the vocal folds: combined use of exfoliative cytology and laryngostroboscopy in differential diagnosis. Eur Arch Otorhinolaryngol 2008;265(7):797–801.

25. Mehlum CS, Rosenberg T, Groentved AM, et al. Can videostroboscopy predict early glottic cancer? A systematic review and meta-analysis. Laryngoscope 2016;126(9):2079–84.

26. Rzepakowska A, Sielska-Badurek E, Osuch-Wójcikiewicz E, et al. The predictive value of videostroboscopy in the assessment of premalignant lesions and early glottis cancers. Otolaryngol Pol 2017;71(4):14–8.

27. Zhao RX, Hirano M, Tanaka S, et al. Vocal fold epithelial hyperplasia. vibratory behavior vs extent of lesion. Arch Otolaryngol Head Neck Surg 1991;117(9): 1015–8.

28. Casiano RR, Zaveri V, Lundy DS. Efficacy of videostroboscopy in the diagnosis of voice disorders. Otolaryngol Head Neck Surg 1992;107(1):95–100.

29. Owusu-Ayim M, Ranjan SR, Lim AE, et al. Diagnostic accuracy outcomes of office-based (outpatient) biopsies in patients with laryngopharyngeal lesions: a systematic review. Clin Otolaryngol 2022;47(2):264–78.

30. Anis MM. Correlating laryngoscopic appearance of laryngeal lesions with histopathology. Laryngoscope 2019;129(6):1308–12.

31. Tibbetts KM, Tan M. Role of advanced laryngeal imaging in glottic cancer: early detection and evaluation of glottic neoplasms. Otolaryngol Clin North Am 2015; 48(4):565–84.

32. Becker M, Burkhardt K, Dulguerov P, et al. Imaging of the larynx and hypopharynx. Eur J Radiol 2008;66(3):460–79.

33. Allegra E, Ferrise P, Trapasso S, et al. Early glottic cancer: role of MRI in the preoperative staging. Biomed Res Int 2014;2014:890385.

34. Austin JR, Wong FC, Kim EE. Positron emission tomography in the detection of residual laryngeal carcinoma. Otolaryngol Head Neck Surg 1995;113(4):404–7.

35. Brouwer J, Hooft L, Hoekstra OS, et al. Systematic review: accuracy of imaging tests in the diagnosis of recurrent laryngeal carcinoma after radiotherapy. Head Neck 2008;30(7):889–97.

36. Bailey BJ, Johnson JT, Newlands SD. Head & neck surgery–otolaryngology. 4th edition. Philadelphia: Lippincott Williams & Wilkins; 2006. p. 1940–60.

37. Forastiere AA, Ismaila N, Lewin JS, et al. Use of larynx-preservation strategies in the treatment of laryngeal cancer: American Society of Clinical Oncology clinical practice guideline update. J Clin Oncol 2018;36(11):1143–69.

38. Abdurehim Y, Hua Z, Yasin Y, et al. Transoral laser surgery versus radiotherapy: systematic review and meta-analysis for treatment options of T1a glottic cancer. Head Neck 2012;34(1):23–33.

39. Higgins KM, Shah MD, Ogaick MJ, et al. Treatment of early-stage glottic cancer: meta-analysis comparison of laser excision versus radiotherapy. J Otolaryngol Head Neck Surg 2009;38(6):603–12.

40. Feng Y, Wang B, Wen S. Laser surgery versus radiotherapy for T1-T2N0 glottic cancer: a meta-analysis. ORL J Otorhinolaryngol Relat Spec 2011;73(6):336–42.

41. Stoeckli SJ, Schnieper I, Huguenin P, et al. Early glottic carcinoma: treatment according patient's preference? Head Neck 2003;25(12):1051–6.

42. Silver CE, Beitler JJ, Shaha AR, et al. Current trends in initial management of laryngeal cancer: the declining use of open surgery. Eur Arch Otorhinolaryngol 2009;266(9):1333–52.

43. Vaculik MF, MacKay CA, Taylor SM, et al. Systematic review and meta-analysis of T1 glottic cancer outcomes comparing CO_2 transoral laser microsurgery and radiotherapy. J Otolaryngol Head Neck Surg 2019;48(1):44.

44. Warner L, Lee K, Homer JJ. Transoral laser microsurgery versus radiotherapy for T2 glottic squamous cell carcinoma: a systematic review of local control outcomes. Clin Otolaryngol 2017;42(3):629–36.
45. Day AT, Sinha P, Nussenbaum B, et al. Management of primary T1-T4 glottic squamous cell carcinoma by transoral laser microsurgery. Laryngoscope 2017; 127(3):597–604.
46. Mo HL, Li J, Yang X, et al. Transoral laser microsurgery versus radiotherapy for T1 glottic carcinoma: a systematic review and meta-analysis. Lasers Med Sci 2017; 32(2):461–7.
47. Remmelts AJ, Hoebers FJ, Klop WM, et al. Evaluation of lasersurgery and radiotherapy as treatment modalities in early stage laryngeal carcinoma: tumour outcome and quality of voice. Eur Arch Otorhinolaryngol 2013;270(7):2079–87.
48. Ma Y, Green R, Pan S, et al. Long-term voice outcome following radiation versus laser microsurgery in early glottic cancer. J Voice 2019;33(2):176–82.
49. Taylor SM, Kerr P, Fung K, et al. Treatment of T1b glottic SCC: laser vs. radiation–a Canadian multicenter study. J Otolaryngol Head Neck Surg 2013;42(1):22.
50. Aaltonen LM, Rautiainen N, Sellman J, et al. Voice quality after treatment of early vocal cord cancer: a randomized trial comparing laser surgery with radiation therapy. Int J Radiat Oncol Biol Phys 2014;90(2):255–60.
51. Hartl DM, de Monès E, Hans S, et al. Treatment of early-stage glottic cancer by transoral laser resection. Ann Otol Rhinol Laryngol 2007;116(11):832–6.
52. Grant DG, Salassa JR, Hinni ML, et al. Transoral laser microsurgery for untreated glottic carcinoma. Otolaryngol Head Neck Surg 2007;137(3):482–6.
53. Sjögren EV, Langeveld TP, Baatenburg de Jong RJ. Clinical outcome of T1 glottic carcinoma since the introduction of endoscopic CO2 laser surgery as treatment option. Head Neck 2008;30(9):1167–74.
54. Zeitels SM, Burns JA. Oncologic efficacy of angiolytic KTP laser treatment of early glottic cancer. Ann Otol Rhinol Laryngol 2014;123(12):840–6.
55. Hrelec C. Management of laryngeal dysplasia and early invasive cancer. Curr Treat Options Oncol 2021;22(10):90.
56. Barbu AM, Burns JA, Lopez-Guerra G, et al. Salvage endoscopic angiolytic KTP laser treatment of early glottic cancer after failed radiotherapy. Ann Otol Rhinol Laryngol 2013;122(4):235–9.
57. Zeitels SM, Burns JA, Lopez-Guerra G, et al. Photoangiolytic laser treatment of early glottic cancer: a new management strategy. Ann Otol Rhinol Laryngol Suppl 2008;199:3–24.
58. Xie X, Young J, Kost K, et al. KTP 532 nm laser for laryngeal lesions. a systematic review. J Voice 2013;27(2):245–9.
59. Parker NP, Weidenbecher MS, Friedman AD, et al. KTP laser treatment of early glottic cancer: a multi-institutional retrospective study. Ann Otol Rhinol Laryngol 2020;130(1):47–55.
60. Lahav Y, Cohen O, Shapira-Galitz Y, et al. CO(2) laser cordectomy versus KTP laser tumor ablation for early glottic cancer: a randomized controlled trial. Lasers Surg Med 2020;52(7):612–20.
61. Remacle M, Eckel HE, Antonelli A, et al. Endoscopic cordectomy. a proposal for a classification by the Working Committee, European Laryngological Society. Eur Arch Otorhinolaryngol 2000;257(4):227–31.
62. Ogura JH. Selection of patients for conservation surgery of the larynx and pharynx. Trans Am Acad Ophthalmol Otolaryngol 1972;76(3):741–51.

63. Sigston E, de Mones E, Babin E, et al. Early-stage glottic cancer: oncological results and margins in laser cordectomy. Arch Otolaryngol Head Neck Surg 2006; 132(2):147–52.

64. Gallo A, de Vincentiis M, Manciocco V, et al. CO2 laser cordectomy for early-stage glottic carcinoma: a long-term follow-up of 156 cases. Laryngoscope 2002;112(2):370–4.

65. Liu C, Ward PH, Pleet L. Imbrication reconstruction following partial laryngectomy. Ann Otol Rhinol Laryngol 1986;95(6 Pt 1):567–71.

66. Johnson JT, Myers EN, Hao SP, et al. Outcome of open surgical therapy for glottic carcinoma. Ann Otol Rhinol Laryngol 1993;102(10):752–5.

67. Pfister DG, Laurie SA, Weinstein GS, et al. American Society of Clinical Oncology clinical practice guideline for the use of larynx-preservation strategies in the treatment of laryngeal cancer. J Clin Oncol 2006;24(22):3693–704.

68. Hockstein NG, Nolan JP, O'Malley BW Jr, et al. Robot-assisted pharyngeal and laryngeal microsurgery: results of robotic cadaver dissections. Laryngoscope 2005;115(6):1003–8.

69. Hockstein NG, Nolan JP, O'Malley BW Jr, et al. Robotic microlaryngeal surgery: a technical feasibility study using the daVinci surgical robot and an airway mannequin. Laryngoscope 2005;115(5):780–5.

70. Weinstein GS, O'Malley BW Jr, Hockstein NG. Transoral robotic surgery: supraglottic laryngectomy in a canine model. Laryngoscope 2005;115(7):1315–9.

71. Yohannes P, Rotariu P, Pinto P, et al. Comparison of robotic versus laparoscopic skills: is there a difference in the learning curve? Urology 2002;60(1):39–45 [discussion: 45].

72. Chang L, Satava RM, Pellegrini CA, et al. Robotic surgery: identifying the learning curve through objective measurement of skill. Surg Endosc 2003;17(11):1744–8.

73. O'Malley BW Jr, Weinstein GS, Hockstein NG. Transoral robotic surgery (TORS): glottic microsurgery in a canine model. J Voice 2006;20(2):263–8.

74. Wang CC, Lin WJ, Wang JJ, et al. Transoral robotic surgery for early-t stage glottic cancer involving the anterior commissure-news and update. Front Oncol 2022; 12:755400.

75. Hans S, Chebib E, Lisan Q, et al. Oncological, surgical and functional outcomes of transoral robotic cordectomy for early glottic carcinoma. J Voice 2021.

76. Kayhan FT, Koc AK, Erdim I. Oncological outcomes of early glottic carcinoma treated with transoral robotic surgery. Auris Nasus Larynx 2019;46(2):285–93.

77. Lechien JR, Baudouin R, Circiu MP, et al. Transoral robotic cordectomy for glottic carcinoma: a rapid review. Eur Arch Otorhinolaryngol 2022.

78. Remacle M, Prasad VMN. Preliminary experience in transoral laryngeal surgery with a flexible robotic system for benign lesions of the vocal folds. Eur Arch Otorhinolaryngol 2018;275(3):761–5.

79. Beitler JJ, Smith RV, Silver CE, et al. Close or positive margins after surgical resection for the head and neck cancer patient: the addition of brachytherapy improves local control. Int J Radiat Oncol Biol Phys 1998;40(2):313–7.

80. Looser KG, Shah JP, Strong EW. The significance of "positive" margins in surgically resected epidermoid carcinomas. Head Neck Surg 1978;1(2):107–11.

81. Friedman AD, Hillman RE, Landau-Zemer T, et al. Voice outcomes for photoangiolytic KTP laser treatment of early glottic cancer. Ann Otol Rhinol Laryngol 2013; 122(3):151–8.

82. Zeitels SM, Hillman RE, Franco RA, et al. Voice and treatment outcome from phonosurgical management of early glottic cancer. Ann Otol Rhinol Laryngol Suppl 2002;190:3–20.

83. Lam KH, Lau WF, Wei WI. Tumor clearance at resection margins in total laryngectomy. a clinicopathologic study. Cancer 1988;61(11):2260–72.
84. Ossoff RH, Sisson GA, Shapshay SM. Endoscopic management of selected early vocal cord carcinoma. Ann Otol Rhinol Laryngol 1985;94(6 Pt 1):560–4.
85. Jäckel MC, Ambrosch P, Martin A, et al. Impact of re-resection for inadequate margins on the prognosis of upper aerodigestive tract cancer treated by laser microsurgery. Laryngoscope 2007;117(2):350–6.
86. Coskun HH, Medina JE, Robbins KT, et al. Current philosophy in the surgical management of neck metastases for head and neck squamous cell carcinoma. Head Neck 2015;37(6):915–26.
87. Sarno A, Bocciolini C, Deganello A, et al. Does unnecessary elective neck treatment affect the prognosis of N0 laryngeal cancer patients? Acta Otolaryngol 2004;124(8):980–5.
88. Gallo O, Deganello A, Scala J, et al. Evolution of elective neck dissection in N0 laryngeal cancer. Acta Otorhinolaryngol Ital 2006;26(6):335–44.
89. Weiss MH, Harrison LB, Isaacs RS. Use of decision analysis in planning a management strategy for the stage N0 neck. Arch Otolaryngol Head Neck Surg 1994; 120(7):699–702.
90. Yang CY, Andersen PE, Everts EC, et al. Nodal disease in purely glottic carcinoma: is elective neck treatment worthwhile? Laryngoscope 1998;108(7):1006–8.
91. Erdag TK, Guneri EA, Avincsal O, et al. Is elective neck dissection necessary for the surgical management of T2N0 glottic carcinoma? Auris Nasus Larynx 2013; 40(1):85–8.
92. Psychogios G, Mantsopoulos K, Bohr C, et al. Incidence of occult cervical metastasis in head and neck carcinomas: development over time. J Surg Oncol 2013; 107(4):384–7.
93. Patel TR, Eggerstedt M, Toor J, et al. Occult lymph node metastasis in early-stage glottic cancer in the national cancer database. Laryngoscope 2021;131(4): E1139–46.
94. Chera BS, Amdur RJ, Morris CG, et al. T1N0 to T2N0 squamous cell carcinoma of the glottic larynx treated with definitive radiotherapy. Int J Radiat Oncol Biol Phys 2010;78(2):461–6.
95. Fein DA, Hanlon AL, Lee WR, et al. Neck failure in T2N0 squamous cell carcinoma of the true vocal cords: the Fox Chase experience and review of the literature. Am J Clin Oncol 1997;20(2):154–7.

Surgical Management of Advanced Glottic Cancer

Seerat K. Poonia[1], Elizabeth Nicolli*

KEYWORDS

- Advanced glottic cancer • Laryngectomy • Organ preservation
- Primary chemoradiation

KEY POINTS

- Supracricoid partial laryngectomy (SCPL) confers comparable survival and local control outcomes to primary chemoradiation (CRT) for appropriate T3 cancers.
- Given the level of expertise and equipment requirements, the outcomes with transoral laser microsurgery while comparable to SCPL and primary CRT for T3 cancer, may not be replicable.
- There is an overall survival benefit with total laryngectomy over primary chemoradiation in patients with T4a disease.
- In patients with clinically negative necks, elective neck dissection may be considered in T3 glottic disease and is recommended in T4 disease.

INTRODUCTION

This article will present contemporary approaches to the surgical management of advanced glottic cancer. These will be described specifically in the context of primary treatment, whereas salvage cases will be discussed elsewhere.

Definition of Advanced Stage

Glottic cancer refers to malignancy originating from the true vocal folds. Its severity is typically defined by T-stage, which incorporates the tumor size, degree of local invasion, and resectability. The primary tumor in advanced glottic cancer generally correlates with T3 or T4 criteria (Table 1 and Figs. 1 and 2), with or without nodal spread, according to the Eighth Edition AJCC Staging Guidelines.[1] Global staging includes the presence and extent of nodal disease and presence of distant metastases, which also have significant influence on prognosis and treatment planning.

Department of Otolaryngology – Head and Neck Surgery, Miller School of Medicine, University of Miami Hospital, 1121 NW 14th Street, Sylvester Medical Office Building, 3rd Floor, Suite 325 Miami, FL 33136, USA
[1] Present address: 1504 Bay Road, #1609, Miami Beach, FL, 33139, USA
* Corresponding author.
E-mail address: exn164@med.miami.edu

Otolaryngol Clin N Am 56 (2023) 275–283
https://doi.org/10.1016/j.otc.2022.12.007
0030-6665/23/© 2022 Elsevier Inc. All rights reserved.

oto.theclinics.com

Table 1
The primary tumor in advanced glottic cancer generally correlates with T3 or T4 criteria with or without nodal spread, according to the Eighth Edition AJCC Staging Guidelines

T Category	T Criteria
T3	Tumor limited to the larynx with vocal cord fixation and/or invasion of the paraglottic space and/or inner cortex of the thyroid cartilage
T4	Moderately advanced or very advanced
T4a	Tumor invades through outer cortex of the thyroid cartilage and/or invades tissues beyond the larynx (e.g., trachea, cricoid cartilage, soft tissues of neck including deep extrinsic muscle of the tongue, strap muscles, thyroid, or esophagus)
T4b	Tumor invades prevertebral space, encases carotid artery, or invades mediastinal structures

Background

Historically, total laryngectomy (TL) followed by radiation therapy was the gold standard for the treatment of advanced glottic cancer. However, favor shifted toward nonsurgical treatment after the seminal Department of Veteran's Affair study was published showing that in responders with stage 3 and 4 glottic cancer, there was no significant difference in overall survival in patients undergoing primary chemoradiation versus those undergoing TL.[2] This paradigm shift is reasonable given the dramatic impact TL has on the patient and the logical desire for organ preservation if possible. It is critical to note, however, that in this study there was a significantly higher local recurrence in primary chemoradiated patients and that salvage laryngectomy was required for persistent disease or recurrence in 29% of stage 3 patients and 44% of stage 4 patients. Additionally, out of the 64% of patients who underwent primary chemoradiation and were disease free at 2 years, only 39% of them had a functional larynx. Nonetheless, the trial heavily influenced practice patterns and resulted in universally increased the use of definitive chemoradiation to treat advanced laryngeal cancer and a corresponding decrease in the use of TL.[3] Importantly, during the same time period, an increase in mortality among this patient population was also demonstrated in the National Cancer Database, which notably was not associated with an increased incidence of late stage disease.[4]

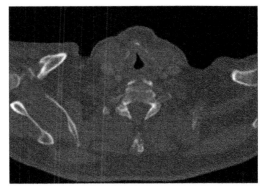

Fig. 1. Preoperative CT scan demonstrating a T3 glottic cancer with fullness of the glottic and paraglottic space and no evidence of cartilage involvement.

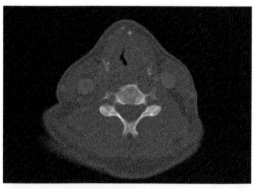

Fig. 2. Preoperative CT scan demonstrating a large T4 glottic mass and irregularity of the thyroid cartilage suggestive of tumor infiltration.

Furthermore, it is important to consider that in many prospective randomized trials that have previously shown acceptable results with primary chemoradiation regimens, patients with particularly advanced tumors exhibiting extensive local invasion tend to be excluded. For example, in the landmark RTOG 91-11 trial, patients with advanced glottic cancer were studied; however, those with thyroid cartilage invasion or more than 1 cm of base of tongue invasion were excluded.[5] Therefore, these results are only applicable to a certain subgroup of patients presenting with advanced disease, and although nonsurgical organ preservation remains a treatment goal, it is imperative to consider not only surgical organ preservation but also TL when indicated. Since these historic trials, studies have followed that focused on advanced laryngeal cancer without exclusion of extensive disease, and their results advocate in many scenarios for surgical management.[6,7] Additionally, surgical organ preservation has evolved immensely as an important consideration in select advanced glottic cancer. Thus, while the Veteran's Affairs trial served as a landmark demonstration that nonsurgical organ preservation is a reasonable goal in the treatment of advanced laryngeal cancer, subsequent data has also highlighted the importance of an approach individualized to the patient and their cancer, specifically with continued consideration of surgical management in patients with advanced glottic disease.

Goals

The primary goal when treating advanced glottic cancer, as with any type of resectable cancer, is long-term disease-free survival.[8] Organ preservation is considered subsequently, and only when it may be prioritized without compromising the oncologic outcome. In this article, we will focus on surgical management only and review current evidence for organ preservation surgery and TL techniques. We will also discuss important surgical considerations pertaining to the management of the neck. Reconstructive considerations are discussed elsewhere.

ORGAN PRESERVATION SURGERY OF THE LARYNX
Background

Organ preservation surgery of the larynx is considered with the goal of retaining enough of the laryngeal complex to allow for speech and swallowing, without a permanent tracheostomy or gastrostomy tube. In the context of advanced glottic cancer, the surgical techniques that may be considered include the supracricoid partial

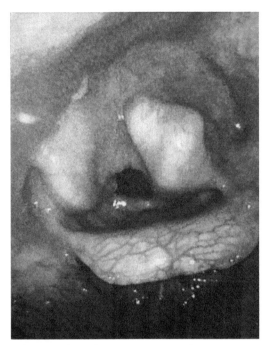

Fig. 3. Postoperative flexible direct laryngoscopy examination status after SCPL demonstrating intact cricoarytenoid units.

laryngectomy with cricohyoidoepiglottopexy (SCPL-CHEP) and transoral laser resection. There have been no studies directly comparing organ preservation surgery to primary chemoradiation for advanced stage glottic cancer; however, there is literature to support the efficacy of these techniques separately.

Supracricoid Partial Laryngectomy

In order to achieve success with this technique certain key structures must be preserved including at least one mobile cricoarytenoid unit (arytenoid cartilage, intact cricoarytenoid joint, posterior and lateral cricoarytenoid muscles, and recurrent and superior laryngeal nerves) and a completely intact cricoid cartilage (**Fig. 3**). Only then will the larynx maintain its essential functions of speech and swallowing.[9] That said, in select cases of T3 glottic cancer, there are specific instances in which the SCPL-CHEP demonstrates utility including those that are anteriorly based and invade the inner cortex of the thyroid cartilage. The technique allows for complete resection of the paraglottic spaces and thyroid cartilage together and thus depending on the tumor, the surgery may be suitable even for advanced cancer. Oncologic contraindications for the surgery include invasion of the preepiglottic space, fixation of the arytenoid cartilage, subglottic extension or cricoid involvement, invasion of the posterior commissure, invasion of the outer cortex of the thyroid cartilage, or extralaryngeal spread.[9,10] Notably, indications for this surgery are also limited by age, performance status, and pulmonary function of the patient.

Transoral laser resection

Transoral laser microsurgery (TLM) utilizing an endoscopic approach to the larynx and a carbon dioxide, potassium titanyl phosphate (KTP) (or similar wavelength) laser is

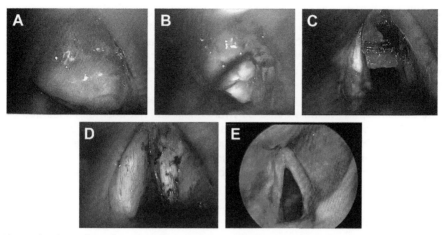

Fig. 4. (*A-B*): In direct laryngoscopy preoperatively demonstrating T3 glottic carcinoma of the right vocal fold with involvement of the anterior commissure but no cartilage invasion. (*C-D*): In direct laryngoscopy intraoperatively as the patient underwent TLM, demonstrating serial division until clearance of the cancer was achieved. (*E*): Postoperative flexible indirect laryngoscopy examination demonstrating no evidence of recurrence and well-healed glottis.

widely used to resect early stage laryngeal cancer (**Fig. 4**A-E). Its applications are limited in advanced stage glottic cancer. With this technique, the tumor is removed piecemeal. The tumor is divided repeatedly, and the margins are assessed in multiple planes. Thus, the surgeon is able to accurately map the cancer, assuring clearance but also minimizing loss of healthy tissue.[11,12] In the setting of advanced cancer, the technique may have merit provided the exposure is adequate but it is important to note that for more extensive lesions TLM can be significantly equipment and experience intensive.[13] As with the SCPL-CHEP, TLM seeks to avoid tracheostomy and allow for early speech and swallow rehabilitation, with the added advantage of eliminating the morbidity associated with open surgery.

Current Evidence

Retrospective studies have demonstrated effective local control and organ preservation for selected T3 patients treated with SCPL-CHEP. The 5-year local control was estimated at 90% in a series of 20 patients with fixation of the true vocal fold thus classified as T3.[14] In another study, which included T2 tumors with impaired vocal fold motion (n = 90) and T3 tumors with fixation (n = 22), the group reported 94.6% 5-year local control and an estimated 86.7% absolute survival.[15] Finally, in a cohort of 118 patients with T3 disease, local control was estimated at 98.3% with organ preservation in 89.8% but it is important to note that in this study 100 patients also received a platin-based induction chemotherapy regimen.[16]

Although TLM shows utility in early stage tumors, data for its efficacy in locally advanced tumors with cartilage or base of tongue invasion, for example, is less robust. In one series of 117 patients in which 28% had T4 glottic tumors, the 5-year local control rate was 74%; however, it is unclear what percentage of the patients who recurred were T3 versus T4.[13] Vilaseca and colleagues reported a series of 147 patients, 35% with T3 glottic disease (none with T4), which demonstrated 5-year larynx preservation of 59%. In this study, the local recurrence rate was 38%, and although it is unclear what the rate was in patients with advanced glottic cancer specifically, vocal fold fixation and laryngeal cartilage invasion were cited as significant prognostic factors association with decreased local control.[17] These factors are critical to consider when assessing whether a patient with locally advanced cancer is suitable for this approach, noting that while its use has been reported in the literature, the outcomes may not be replicable by less-experienced surgeons.

Although nonsurgical and surgical means of organ preservation confer similar survival outcomes, it is notable that a survival benefit has not been demonstrated by SCPL-CHEP versus TLM or when either is compared with the overall survival rates for CRT in RTOG 91-11.[5,18] Thus, an individualized focus on patient selection, technical considerations and on optimizing functional outcomes remains an important key to treatment planning in the setting of advanced glottic disease that may be amenable to organ preservation.

TOTAL LARYNGECTOMY
Background

At one time, TL followed by adjuvant radiation therapy was considered a standard treatment of advanced laryngeal cancer. The treatment paradigm has continued to evolve through nonsurgical approaches and organ preservation surgery owing to the unfortunate fact that patients who undergo TL experience complete loss of voice and impaired swallow function, which heavily influenced quality of life and social functioning.[19] Nonetheless, it is apparent that for select patients with advanced glottic cancer, there is a survival benefit with TL, and thus, the surgery will continue to be considered in this setting.

Indications

TL involves surgical removal of the larynx. In the oncologic setting, advanced glottic cancer is a common indication for TL. As previously discussed, the decision to proceed with TL is not a trivial one, and the extent of the cancer and its resultant impact on the functionality of the larynx is an important consideration. Extensive tumor involvement of the larynx seen in T4a tumors, specifically penetration of tumor through the thyroid cartilage and involvement of extralaryngeal tissue is an indication for TL. TL may also be considered in cT3 glottic tumors when laryngeal function is already compromised. When this is the case, nonsurgical organ preservation no longer has the desired impact on the functional outcome and may in fact result in worse swallowing.

Current Evidence

As previously discussed, the survival outcomes of patients undergoing TL are comparable to primary chemoradiation,[2,4,18] and neither has been shown to be superior. Importantly though, an overall survival advantage with TL when compared with definitive chemoradiation has been demonstrated in patients with extensive stage 4 tumors. In one database study of 7019 patients with advanced laryngeal cancer, those with stage 4 disease treated with TL had significantly better overall survival than those who underwent primary chemoradiation (hazard ratio for death = 1.43, $P > .001$).[6] In another retrospective study of 451 patients, 195 with stage 4 laryngeal cancer, survival was better in patients with stage 4 who were treated surgically (49%) compared with those treated with chemoradiation (21%) ($P < .0001$).[7] By primary tumor stage in this same study, T4 patients again had significantly better survival with surgery (55%) than those treated with chemoradiation (25%).

In patients with stage 3 laryngeal cancer who are not amenable to organ preservation surgery, survival outcomes between definitive chemoradiation and TL are comparable. It is reasonable to tailor the treatment plan to the patient, most often considering organ preservation in the case of a functional larynx. However, in stage 4 and specifically T4 disease, the data demonstrate significantly improved survival with primary surgical treatment.

MANAGING THE NECK

In laryngeal squamous cell carcinoma, cervical lymph node metastases largely influence survival outcomes, and treatment of the neck in advanced glottic cancer is critical.[20–22] This may be accomplished with surgery or irradiation; however, radiation therapy is often reserved for cases in which the modality will be used for the primary tumor as well.[23] The surgical recommendation when considering whether to treat the neck (therapeutically or electively) includes a selective lateral neck dissection (levels 2–4) and a central neck dissection (level 6).[24–27] If the disease is lateralized, a unilateral neck dissection is reasonable; however, in an advanced disease that is often nearing or crossing the midline, a bilateral dissection must be considered.[21,28]

Despite relatively reduced lymphatic drainage of the vocal folds when compared with supraglottic and subglottic sites, elective treatment of the clinically node negative neck is recommended for advanced glottic tumors staged T3 or higher.[23] In one study of 212 patients with glottic cancer treated with elective neck dissection, occult lymph node metastasis was noted at a rate of 13.4% for T3 lesions and 23.4% for T4 lesions.[24] Similar findings for T3 and T4 glottic cancer have been demonstrated elsewhere.[29,30]

The National Comprehensive Cancer Network (NCCN) recommendations for cT3cN0 glottic cancer being treated with primary TL include pretracheal and ipsilateral paratracheal dissection. For cT3cN1-3 disease, the recommendation is ipsilateral or bilateral neck dissection with pretracheal and ipsilateral paratracheal dissection. For cT4a cN0-3 disease, the NCCN recommends ipsilateral or bilateral neck dissection with pretracheal and ipsilateral paratracheal node dissection.[31]

SUMMARY

In advanced glottic cancer, it is widely known that definitive chemoradiation can result in comparable survival outcomes to primary surgery. This deserves consideration given the immense effects TL has on the patient. That said it is important to consider that not all advanced glottic tumors should be treated the same and thus surgical management must remain a critical consideration for optimization of local control and survival outcomes. Advances in organ preservation surgery and the more developed understanding of the survival benefits of TL in extensive T4 disease further support the importance of surgery in management of advanced glottic cancer.

CLINICS CARE POINTS

- Advanced glottic cancer refers most generally to T3 and T4 lesions arising from the true vocal folds
- SCPL may be considered in select T3 lesions when at least one mobile cricoarytenoid unit and a completely intact cricoid cartilage can be preserved
- SCPL confers comparable survival and local control outcomes to primary CRT for appropriate T3 cancers

- Applications of TLM in advanced glottic cancer are limited to select T3 cancers, with worse local control outcomes in the setting of laryngeal cartilage invasion and vocal fold fixation
- Given the level of expertise and equipment requirements, the outcomes with TLM while comparable to SCPL and primary CRT for T3 cancer, may not be replicable
- There is an overall survival benefit with TL over primary chemoradiation in patients with extensive T4a disease
- Treatment of the neck is mandatory in patients with clinically positive neck disease and includes ipsilateral or bilateral neck dissection with pretracheal and ipsilateral paratracheal node dissection
- In patients with clinically negative necks, elective neck dissection may be considered in T3 glottic disease and is recommended in T4 disease

DISCLOSURE

We have no financial disclosures to report.

REFERENCES

1. Amin MB, Green FL, Edge SB, et al. The Eighth Edition AJCC Cancer Staging Manual: continuing to build a bridge from a population-based to a more "personalized" approach to cancer staging. CA Cancer J Clin 2017;67(2):93–9.
2. Department of Veterans Affairs Laryngeal Cancer Study, Wolf GT, Fisher SG, Hong WK, et al. Induction chemotherapy plus radiation compared with surgery plus radiation in patients with advanced laryngeal cancer. N Engl J Med 1991; 324(24):1685–90.
3. Chen AY, Schrag N, Hao Y, et al. Changes in treatment of advanced laryngeal cancer 1985-2001. Otolaryngol Head Neck Surg 2006;135(6):831–7.
4. Hoffman HT, Porter K, Karnell LH, et al. Laryngeal cancer in the United States: changes in demographics, patterns of care, and survival, Laryngoscope. Laryngoscope 2006;116(9 Pt 2 Suppl 111):1–13.
5. Forastiere AA, et al. Long-term results of RTOG 91-11: a comparison of three nonsurgical treatment strategies to preserve the larynx in patients with locally advanced larynx cancer. J Clin Oncol 2013;31(7):845–52.
6. Chen AY, Halpern M. Factors predictive of survival in advanced laryngeal cancer. Arch Otolaryngol Head Neck Surg 2007;133(12):1270–6.
7. Gourin CG, Conger BT, Sheils WT, et al. The effect of treatment on survival in patients with advanced laryngeal carcinoma. Laryngoscope 2009;119(7):1312–7.
8. Hartl DM. Evidence-based practice: management of glottic cancer. Otolaryngol Clin North Am 2012;45(5):1143–61.
9. Weinstein GS LO, Brasnu D, Laccourreye H. Organ preservation surgery for laryngeal cancer. San Diego, CA: Singular Publishing Group; 2000.
10. Holsinger FC, Weinstein GS, Laccourreye O. Supracricoid partial laryngectomy: an organ-preservation surgery for laryngeal malignancy. Curr Probl Cancer 2005; 29(4):190–200.
11. Pearson BW, Salassa JR. Transoral laser microresection for cancer of the larynx involving the anterior commissure. Laryngoscope 2003;113(7):1104–12.
12. Steiner W. Results of curative laser microsurgery of laryngeal carcinomas. Am J Otolaryngol 1993;14(2):116–21.
13. Hinni ML, Salassa JR, Grant DG, et al. Transoral laser microsurgery for advanced laryngeal cancer. Arch Otolaryngol Head Neck Surg 2007;133(12):1198–204.

14. Laccourreye O, Salzer SJ, Brasnu D, et al. Glottic carcinoma with a fixed true vocal cord: outcomes after neoadjuvant chemotherapy and supracricoid partial laryngectomy with cricohyoidoepiglottopexy. Otolaryngol Head Neck Surg 1996;114(3):400–6.
15. Chevalier D, Laccourreye O, Brasnu D, et al. Cricohyoidoepiglottopexy for glottic carcinoma with fixation or impaired motion of the true vocal cord: 5-year oncologic results with 112 patients. Ann Ann Otol Rhinol Laryngol 1997;106(5):364–9.
16. Dufour X, Hans S, Mones ED, et al. Local control after supracricoid partial laryngectomy for "advanced" endolaryngeal squamous cell carcinoma classified as T3. Arch Otolaryngol Head Neck Surg 2004;130(9):1092–9.
17. Vilaseca I, Bernal-Sprekelsen M, Blanch JL. Transoral laser microsurgery for T3 laryngeal tumors: Prognostic factors. Head Neck 2010;32(7):929–38.
18. Rades D, Schroeder U, Bajrovic A, et al. Radiochemotherapy versus surgery plus radio(chemo)therapy for stage T3/T4 larynx and hypopharynx cancer - results of a matched-pair analysis. Eur J Cancer 2011;47(18):2729–34.
19. Gillison ML, Forastiere AA. Larynx preservation in head and neck cancers. A discussion of the National Comprehensive Cancer Network Practice Guidelines. Hematol Oncol Clin North Am 1999;13(4):699–718, vi.
20. Gallo O, Deganello A, Scala J, et al. Evolution of elective neck dissection in N0 laryngeal cancer. Acta Otorhinolaryngol Ital 2006;26(6):335–44.
21. Fiorella R, Nicola VD, Fiorella ML, et al. Conditional" neck dissection in management of laryngeal carcinoma. Acta Otorhinolaryngol Ital 2006;26(6):356–9.
22. Shah JP. Cervical lymph node metastases–diagnostic, therapeutic, and prognostic implications. Oncology (Williston Park) 1990;4(10):61–9 [discussion: 72, 76].
23. Ferlito A, Silver CE, Rinaldo A, et al. Surgical treatment of the neck in cancer of the larynx. ORL J Otorhinolaryngol Relat Spec 2000;62(4):217–25.
24. Ma H, Lian M, Feng L, et al. Management of cervical lymph nodes for cN0 advanced glottic laryngeal carcinoma and its long-term results. Acta Otolaryngol 2014;134(9):952–8.
25. Zhang B, Xu ZG, Tang PZ. Elective lateral neck dissection for laryngeal cancer in the clinically negative neck. J Surg Oncol 2006;93(6):464–7.
26. Katilmis H, Ozturkcan S, Ozdemir I, et al. Is dissection of levels 4 and 5 justified for cN0 laryngeal and hypopharyngeal cancer? Acta Otolaryngol 2007;127(11): 1202–6.
27. Shah JP. Patterns of cervical lymph node metastasis from squamous carcinomas of the upper aerodigestive tract. Am J Surg 1990;160(4):405–9.
28. Bottcher A, Olze H, Thieme N, et al. A novel classification scheme for advanced laryngeal cancer midline involvement: implications for the contralateral neck. J Cancer Res Clin Oncol 2017;143(8):1605–12.
29. Campora ED, Radici M, Camaioni A, et al. Clinical experiences with surgical therapy of cervical metastases from head and neck cancer. Eur Arch Otorhinolaryngol 1994;251(6):335–41.
30. The N0 neck in head and neck cancer patients. Eur Arch Otorhinolaryngol 1993; 250(8):423.
31. Caudell JJ, Gillison ML, Maghami E, et al. NCCN Guidelines(R) Insights: Head and Neck Cancers, Version 1.2022. J Natl Compr Canc Netw 2022;20(3):224–34.

Chemoradiation for Locoregionally Advanced Laryngeal Cancer

Andréanne Leblanc, MD[a],*, Toms Vengaloor Thomas, MD[b],
Nathaniel Bouganim, MD[a]

KEYWORDS

- Functional organ preservation • Locoregionally advanced • Laryngeal cancer
- Combined modality • Chemotherapy • Radiotherapy

KEY POINTS

- Functional organ preservation with concurrent chemotherapy and radiotherapy is the treatment of choice for fit patients with locoregionally advanced laryngeal cancer with functional larynx.
- Concurrent chemoradiation with weekly cisplatin is a new standard option.
- For older patients and those with poor functional status, definitive radiotherapy alone is more appropriate to avoid treatment-related morbidity and mortality.
- For patients undergoing primary surgical management, adjuvant radiotherapy is indicated for all T3 and T4 tumors. The addition of concurrent chemotherapy is indicated for patients with high-risk features, such as positive resection margins or lymph nodes with extracapsular extension.
- Studies are ongoing to evaluate the use of immunotherapy with concurrent chemoradiation but have failed to show a benefit in progression-free survival and overall survival so far.

INTRODUCTION

Patients with early-stage laryngeal cancer (stage I or II) are treated with surgical resection or definitive radiation therapy (RT) to the primary site. For locoregionally advanced disease (T2N+, T3, and selected patients with T4 disease), functional organ preservation with combined modality therapy involving radiotherapy and chemotherapy is the treatment of choice. Combined modality approaches include chemotherapy given at the same time as radiotherapy (concurrent chemoradiotherapy [CCRT]), induction chemotherapy (IC) followed by definitive radiotherapy, or IC followed by CCRT (sequential chemoradiation). Radiation alone is reserved for elderly patients and those

[a] Medical Oncology, Royal Victoria Hospital/Cedars Cancer Centre, 1001 Decarie Boulevard, Montreal, Quebec, H4A 3J1, Canada; [b] Dept of Radiation Oncology, University of Mississippi Medical Center, 2500 North State street, Jackson, MS, 39216, USA
* Corresponding author.
E-mail address: andreanne.leblanc@mail.mcgill.ca

Otolaryngol Clin N Am 56 (2023) 285–293
https://doi.org/10.1016/j.otc.2022.12.004
0030-6665/23/© 2022 Elsevier Inc. All rights reserved.

with poor functional status who are not eligible for definitive treatments. For patients who are not candidates for laryngeal preservation therapy, laryngectomy with adjuvant radiotherapy therapy is recommended with or without chemotherapy.

Functional organ-sparing treatments do not provide survival benefits over total laryngectomy. Some patients with extensive T3 or large T4a lesions with vocal cord destruction and poor pretreatment laryngeal function may derive better survival benefits and quality of life with primary surgical management.[1]

This article describes the evidence for therapeutic approaches for functional organ preservation and indications for adjuvant therapy in treating locoregionally advanced laryngeal cancer. Other treatments currently under investigation will also be discussed.

COMBINED MODALITY THERAPY FOR LOCOREGIONALLY ADVANCED LARYNGEAL CANCER

For patients with good functional status, combined modality therapy has replaced total laryngectomy as the standard of care.[2] The decision to proceed with this treatment approach requires the patient to tolerate the prolonged course of treatment (often 6–7 weeks) and associated toxicities and to participate in swallowing therapy after treatment.[3]

Concurrent Chemoradiation

Concurrent chemoradiation is the administration of systemic chemotherapy simultaneously with RT. The goal is to achieve disease control and laryngeal function preservation and is the first-line recommended for medically fit patients. Chemotherapy is used at a lower dose to act as a radiosensitizer to increase the cytotoxic effect of RT. The radiosensitivity of a cell depends on its current cell cycle phase. Cells in the S phase are more radioresistant, whereas cells in the G2–M phase are most radiosensitive.[4] Radiosensitizers arrest the cell cycle at the G2–M phase, thereby increasing radiotherapy's cytotoxic effect on tumor cells. Cisplatin, 5-FU, and taxanes are the most commonly used radiosensitizers and have cytotoxic activity.

A meta-analysis assessing the benefit of concurrent chemoradiation by tumor site demonstrated a 20% risk reduction of death (hazard ratio [HR] 0.80, 95% CI 0.71–0.90) with the addition of chemotherapy to locoregional treatment, with a 5-year overall survival (OS) of 47%.[5] Another meta-analysis showed an OS benefit with an HR 0.83 (0.79:0.86) ($P < 0.0001$) at 9.2 years in favor of CCRT when compared with induction and adjuvant chemotherapy and an absolute benefit of 6.5% and 3.6% at 5 and 10 years, respectively.

A platinum-based chemotherapy regimen with high-dose cisplatin (100 mg/m^2 every 3 weeks)[6,7] or weekly carboplatin and infusional 5-FU[8,9] is recommended as first-line treatments with category 1 evidence. However, the ConCERT trial has recently shown that weekly cisplatin (40 mg/m^2) concurrently with RT resulted in a non-inferior 2-year locoregional disease control and OS as well as an improved toxicity profile when compared with q3 weeks bolus cisplatin.[10] Weekly carboplatin with paclitaxel is an alternative for cis-ineligible patients.[11] More recently, docetaxel has also been shown to be appropriate for a CCRT approach for cis-ineligible patients and showed progression-free survival (PFS) and OS benefit over RTx alone.[12]

Patients are deemed ineligible for cisplatin-based treatment if they have any of the following criteria: Eastern Cooperative Oncology Group (ECOG) performance status of 2 or less, creatinine clearance of less than 60 mL/min, grade 2 or more hearing loss as evaluated by the Common Terminology Criteria for Adverse Events (CTCAE), grade 2 or above neuropathy as per CTCAE, heart failure with New York Heart Association class 3.[13]

A phase III trial has also looked at weekly cetuximab, a monoclonal antibody targeting epidermal growth factor receptor (EGFR), compared with weekly cisplatin for CCRT and showed inferior locoregional disease control at 3 years with cetuximab (23% cetuximab vs. 9% cisplatin, $P = 0.0036$).[14]

Sequential Chemoradiation

Sequential chemoradiation involves IC followed by CCRT. In theory, IC decreases the incidence of distant metastases and increases local disease control, whereas CCRT provides additional robust locoregional disease control. The literature on sequential chemotherapy is conflicting. Data supporting sequential therapy come from a phase III trial in which patients were randomly assigned to docetaxel, cisplatin, and fluorouracil, followed by chemoradiation versus chemoradiation alone.[15] Patients who received IC followed by CCRT had improved locoregional control, PFS, and OS (HR 0.74, 95% CI 0.56–0.97). However, there was no difference in distant metastasis in both arms. Two other phase III trials have not shown statistically significant improvement in 3-year survival or PFS, though one trial showed a decreased cumulative incidence of distance metastases in the sequential therapy arm when using docetaxel, cisplatin, and 5-FU (TPF) ×2 cycles followed by CCRT with docetaxel, fluorouracil, and hydroxyurea (10% vs. 19% for CCRT, $P = 0.025$).[16] Other trials have shown similar laryngeal preservation, function, and survival benefit but with an increased risk of severe toxicity.[17] If a sequential therapy approach is chosen, IC with TPF followed by CCRT with weekly cisplatin or carboplatin is recommended.[18]

Sequential chemotherapy is not the standard of care. Still, patients with large primary tumors (bulky T3 or T4) might benefit the most from sequential therapy. Patients with the advanced nodal disease at increased risk for distant metastases might also benefit.[16]

Induction Chemotherapy

IC followed by definitive radiotherapy is not the standard of care but remains an alternative organ-preserving treatment of patients with locally advanced laryngeal cancers. Treatment with TPF is recommended as first line.[18,19] Two trials have looked at IC with TPF versus cisplatin and fluorouracil (PF), and both trials showed a statistically significant survival benefit and improved locoregional disease control with TPF.[18,20] However, a recent meta-analysis demonstrated a survival benefit with PF with HR 0.90 (95% CI, 0.82–0.99) but did not show a survival benefit with TPF IC.[21] Although IC followed by definite radiotherapy has been shown to be an effective and safe option, there remains controversy regarding the overall benefit of IC and RT over CCRT. Laryngectomy-free survival (LFS) and locoregional disease control in patients with stage III and IV laryngeal cancer treated with either concurrent chemoradiation, IC followed by RT, or definitive RT alone were studied in the RTOG 91-11 trial.[7] Cisplatin was used for the CCRT arm, and PF was used in the IC arm. LFS was significantly increased with both combined modality approaches compared with RT alone, but locoregional disease control was significantly increased with concurrent chemoradiation compared with IC or RT alone. The actively accruing GORTEC SALTORL trial comparing IC with TPF followed by RT versus CCRT with TPF will help determine which treatment is preferred for this patient population (ClinicalTrials.gov Identifier: NCT03340896).

OLDER PATIENTS AND PATIENTS WITH POOR PERFORMANCE STATUS

It is often more appropriate for older patients and those with poor functional status to offer definitive RT alone to avoid treatment-related morbidity and mortality, such as aspiration pneumonia, severe mucositis, and weight loss. Although this approach may result in decreased locoregional disease control and functional organ preservation, risks and benefits must be considered to preserve the quality of life and prevent serious complications.

ADJUVANT TREATMENT

For patients undergoing larynx preservation surgery and total laryngectomy, adjuvant radiotherapy is indicated for all T3 and T4 tumors. The addition of concurrent chemotherapy is indicated for patients with high-risk features, such as positive resection margins or lymph nodes with extracapsular extension.[22] Radiotherapy with or without chemotherapy should be initiated within 6 weeks of surgery.

For cisplatin-eligible patients, concurrent weekly cisplatin (40 mg/m^2) with RT has shown non-inferior survival benefit and an improved toxicity profile compared with bolus 3 weekly high-dose (100 mg/m^2) cisplatin.[23] Bolus cisplatin is associated with significant acute and late toxicities.[24] For cisplatin-ineligible patients due to age, comorbidities, or poor functional status, adjuvant RT alone is recommended rather than concurrent RT with carboplatin. No significant improvement in locoregional disease control or OS has been shown with concurrent carboplatin and RT for adjuvant treatment.[25]

Alternatively, docetaxel and cetuximab have category 2B evidence for use with RT for cisplatin-ineligible patients who have a high-risk disease.[26]

RADIATION DOSE, FRACTIONATION, AND TECHNIQUES
Radiation Dose, Fractionation, and Techniques for Definitive Chemoradiation and Adjuvant Chemoradiation

Since the early 2000s, intensity-modulated radiation therapy (IMRT) technique has been used for head and neck radiation treatment planning given the improved toxicity profile, especially xerostomia.[27] The gross tumor, high-risk subclinical areas, and low-risk subclinical areas can be treated simultaneously at different doses using a dose-painting approach.[28] Depending on the radiation oncologist's experience and preference, a three-dose or two-dose plan can be used. If a three-dose regimen is used, the gross primary tumor and the nodes with a margin can be treated to 70 Gy in 35 fractions at 2 Gy daily, simultaneously with high-risk areas (remaining larynx, involved and adjacent nodal levels, indeterminate nodes, tracheostomy site) which can be treated to 59.4 Gy to 63 Gy in 35 fractions along with the low-risk elective nodal areas which can be treated to 56 Gy in 35 fractions. If a two-dose approach is used, the whole larynx and involved nodes with a margin will be treated to 70 Gy in 35 fractions, whereas elective nodal areas are treated to 56 Gy in 35 fractions. In the adjuvant setting, patients are treated with 60 to 66 Gy in 30 to 33 fractions, using the IMRT technique.

Definitive Radiation Dose, Fractionation, and Techniques for Chemotherapy Non-ineligible Patients

Patients ineligible for concurrent systemic therapy with cisplatin or cetuximab but eligible for definitive treatment can be treated with definitive radiation treatment using altered fractionation schemes. There are multiple altered fractionation schemes available, and they are listed below. The Meta-Analysis of Radiotherapy in squamous cell Carcinoma of Head and neck showed that the altered fractionation radiotherapy is associated with improved OS and PFS compared with conventional radiotherapy, with hyper fractionated radiotherapy showing the greatest benefit.[29]

1. Hyper fractionation technique: The primary tumor and the involved nodes should be treated to a dose as high as 79.2 Gy in 1.2 Gy twice daily. There should be at least 6 hours gap between daily fractions to limit toxicity.
2. Concomitant boost technique: Low- and high-risk areas are treated with 54 Gy in 30 fractions at 1.8 Gy daily, along with an afternoon boost (with >6-hour gap) using 1.5 Gy is given to the high-risk areas during the last 12 days of treatment, to a total of 72 Gy.
3. DAHANCA regimen: Patients are treated to 70 Gy in 35 fractions, using six fractions per week. The second fraction is given once weekly, with a 6-hour gap from the morning dose.

Palliative Radiation Treatment

Patients who are not eligible for definitive treatment, either due to poor performance status or the presence of metastatic disease, may benefit from palliative radiation treatment. An ideal radiation regimen should improve cancer symptoms with minimal treatment-related toxicity while improving the quality of life.[30] Various doses ranging from 30 Gy to 70 Gy and techniques (3D or IMRT) can be used depending on the patient's performance status and life expectancy.[30]

TREATMENT-ASSOCIATED TOXICITIES

Mucositis is a common side effect and is increased with concurrent chemoradiation with cisplatin, where 70% of patients will develop grade 3 or 4 oral mucositis.[31] These patients have visible ulcers and only tolerate a liquid diet (grade 3 mucositis) or cannot tolerate an oral diet and require enteral feeding (grade 4). Grade 4 occurs in about 20%–25% of patients.[32] Grade 3 and 4 mucositis significantly affects patients' quality of life and results in morbidity, hospitalizations, and often requires treatment interruptions. Other common radiotherapy-associated complications include vocal and swallowing difficulties, loss of taste and smell, fibrosis, and hypothyroidism.[33] Possible complications from cisplatin include fatigue, renal impairment, hearing impairment, neuropathy, and cytopenia. These complications and their management are outside the scope of this article. Vocal and swallowing rehabilitation are discussed in Cecelia E. Schmalbach and Jessica Anne Tang's article, "Vocal Rehabilitation and Quality of Life"; and Maude Brisson-McKenna's article, "Swallowing Function After Treatment of Laryngeal Cancer," in this issue.

FUTURE DIRECTIONS
Immune-Checkpoint Inhibitors

Immune-checkpoint inhibitors are already approved for the treatment of recurrent or metastatic head and neck cancers. Pembrolizumab, combined with platinum-based chemotherapy and 5FU, is approved as first line based on the KEYNOTE-048 trial, which showed improved OS compared with cetuximab with platinum and 5FU. CHECKMATE-141 showed increased OS with monotherapy nivolumab and is now approved as second line.[34,35] However, to date, no phase III trials have shown a statistically significant improvement in event-free survival with the addition of immunotherapy to CCRT in the curative intent. The Javelin HN 100 and KEYNOTE 412 trials looked at concurrent and maintenance durvalumab and pembrolizumab, respectively, and failed to show a statistical difference in PFS or OS.[2,36] Other trials evaluating the addition of immune-checkpoint inhibitors in the adjuvant setting for high-risk patients are currently ongoing.[37,38]

Recently, a randomized phase II trial looked at the optimal sequencing of a PD-1 inhibitor with CCRT for previously untreated, locally advanced head and neck squamous cell carcinoma, including laryngeal cancer.[39] They used pembrolizumab with cisplatin and radiation, either concurrently or sequentially. Both arms met their composite primary endpoint of less than 60% 1-year failure rate and ≥60% 1-year PFS. Although the study was not designed to compare both arms, sequential use of pembrolizumab resulted in a numerically superior 1-year PFS at 89% versus 82%, continuing through years 2 and 3. A numerically superior OS at 1 year was also observed (95% vs. 82%) and continued through years 2 and 3. Concurrent therapy resulted in higher ≥ grade 3 toxicity than sequential therapy (95% vs. 87%). Data regarding correlation with PDL1 status and circulating tumor biomarkers are ongoing.

Reducing Treatment-Induced Mucositis

A recent phase III trial demonstrated a statistically significant and clinically meaningful reduction in severe oral mucositis incidence and duration with avasopasem manganese (GC 4419) when administered intravenously Monday to Friday, during the entire duration of radiotherapy, to patients undergoing CCRT with cisplatin.[40] Multiple other trials studying preventative agents are ongoing.

SUMMARY

The decision-making process for patients with locoregionally advanced laryngeal cancer requires a multidisciplinary approach. Treatment decisions depend on the patient's functional status, comorbidities, and preferences. Although the literature offers conflicting data on the benefits of induction and sequential chemotherapy, the evidence is clear for concurrent chemoradiation. For medically fit patients with locoregionally advanced laryngeal cancer, concurrent chemoradiation is the standard of care, with weekly cisplatin as a new standard option.[10,21]

Although immunotherapy has shown benefits in the recurrent and metastatic setting, the addition of immunotherapy to curative chemoradiation has failed to show a PFS and OS benefit so far. More phase III trials are needed to establish if immunotherapy has a place in the curative treatment of locoregionally advanced head and neck cancers.

CLINICS CARE POINTS

- Neoadjuvant chemotherapy may be more appropriate for rapidly progressing disease.
- Weekly low-dose cisplatin is given at 40 mg/m^2.
- Severe mucositis and weight loss may warrant a percutaneous endoscopic gastrostomy (PEG) feeding tube.

DISCLOSURE

The authors have nothing to disclose.

REFERENCES

1. Forastiere AA, Ismaila N, Lewin JS, et al. use of larynx-preservation strategies in the treatment of laryngeal cancer: American Society of Clinical Oncology clinical practice guideline update. J Clin Oncol 2018;36(11):1143–69.
2. Lee NY, Ferris RL, Psyrri A, et al. Avelumab plus standard-of-care chemoradiotherapy versus chemoradiotherapy alone in patients with locally advanced

squamous cell carcinoma of the head and neck: a randomised, double-blind, placebo-controlled, multicentre, phase 3 trial. Lancet Oncol 2021;22(4):450–62.

3. Silver CE, Beitler JJ, Shaha AR, et al. Current trends in initial management of laryngeal cancer: the declining use of open surgery. Eur Arch Otorhinolaryngol 2009;266(9):1333–52.

4. Sinclair W, Morton R. X-ray sensitivity during the cell generation cycle of cultured Chinese hamster cells. Radiat Res 1966;29(3):450–74.

5. Blanchard P, Baujat B, Holostenco V, et al. Meta-analysis of chemotherapy in head and neck cancer (MACH-NC): a comprehensive analysis by tumour site. Radiother Oncol 2011;100(1):33–40.

6. Adelstein DJ, Li Y, Adams GL, et al. An intergroup phase III comparison of standard radiation therapy and two schedules of concurrent chemoradiotherapy in patients with unresectable squamous cell head and neck cancer. J Clin Oncol 2003;21(1):92–8.

7. Forastiere AA, Zhang Q, Weber RS, et al. Long-term results of RTOG 91-11: a comparison of three nonsurgical treatment strategies to preserve the larynx in patients with locally advanced larynx cancer. J Clin Oncol 2013;31(7):845.

8. Bourhis J, Sire C, Graff P, et al. Concomitant chemoradiotherapy versus acceleration of radiotherapy with or without concomitant chemotherapy in locally advanced head and neck carcinoma (GORTEC 99-02): an open-label phase 3 randomised trial. Lancet Oncol 2012;13(2):145–53.

9. Denis F, Garaud P, Bardet E, et al. Final results of the 94–01 French Head and Neck Oncology and Radiotherapy Group randomized trial comparing radiotherapy alone with concomitant radiochemotherapy in advanced-stage oropharynx carcinoma. J Clin Oncol 2004;22(1):69–76.

10. Sharma A., Kumar M., Bhasker S., et al., An open-label, noninferiority phase III RCT of weekly versus three weekly cisplatin and radical radiotherapy in locally advanced head and neck squamous cell carcinoma (ConCERT trial), *Am Soc Clin Oncol*, 40 (16) 2022, 6004.

11. Suntharalingam M, Haas ML, Conley BA, et al. The use of carboplatin and paclitaxel with daily radiotherapy in patients with locally advanced squamous cell carcinomas of the head and neck. Int J Radiat Oncol Biol Phys 2000;47(1):49–56.

12. Patil V.M., Noronha V., Menon N.S., et al., Results of phase 3 randomized trial for use of docetaxel as a radiosensitizer in patients with head and neck cancer unsuitable for cisplatin-based chemoradiation, *Am Soc Clin Oncol*, 40 (17) 2022, LBA6003.

13. Galsky MD, Hahn NM, Rosenberg J, et al. A consensus definition of patients with metastatic urothelial carcinoma who are unfit for cisplatin-based chemotherapy. Lancet Oncol 2011;12(3):211–4.

14. Gebre-Medhin M, Brun E, Engström P, et al. ARTSCAN III: a randomized phase III study comparing chemoradiotherapy with cisplatin versus cetuximab in patients with locoregionally advanced head and neck squamous cell cancer. J Clin Oncol 2021;39(1):38.

15. Ghi MG, Paccagnella A, Ferrari D, et al. induction TPF followed by concomitant treatment versus concomitant treatment alone in locally advanced head and neck cancer. A phase II–III trial. Ann Oncol 2017;28(9):2206–12.

16. Cohen E.E., Karrison T., Kocherginsky M., et al., DeCIDE: A phase III randomized trial of docetaxel (D), cisplatin (P), 5-fluorouracil (F)(TPF) induction chemotherapy (IC) in patients with N2/N3 locally advanced squamous cell carcinoma of the head and neck (SCCHN), *Am Soc Clin Oncol*, 30 (15),2012, 5500.

17. Lefebvre JL, Pointreau Y, Rolland F, et al. Induction chemotherapy followed by either chemoradiotherapy or bioradiotherapy for larynx preservation: the TREMPLIN randomized phase II study. J Clin Oncol 2013;31(7):853–9.
18. Posner MR, Hershock DM, Blajman CR, et al. cisplatin and fluorouracil alone or with docetaxel in head and neck cancer. N Engl J Med 2007;357(17):1705–15.
19. Janoray G, Pointreau Y, Garaud P, et al. Long-term results of a multicenter randomized phase III trial of induction chemotherapy with cisplatin, 5-fluorouracil,±docetaxel for larynx preservation. J Natl Cancer Inst 2016;108(4):djv368.
20. Vermorken JB, Remenar E, Van Herpen C, et al. Cisplatin, fluorouracil, and docetaxel in unresectable head and neck cancer. N Engl J Med 2007;357(17):1695–704.
21. Lacas B, Carmel A, Landais C, et al. Meta-analysis of chemotherapy in head and neck cancer (MACH-NC): An update on 107 randomized trials and 19,805 patients, on behalf of MACH-NC Group. Radiother Oncol 2021;156:281–93.
22. Bernier J, Cooper JS, Pajak T, et al. Defining risk levels in locally advanced head and neck cancers: a comparative analysis of concurrent postoperative radiation plus chemotherapy trials of the EORTC (# 22931) and RTOG (# 9501). Head Neck: J Sci Specialties Head Neck 2005;27(10):843–50.
23. Kiyota N, Tahara M, Mizusawa J, et al. Weekly cisplatin plus radiation for postoperative head and neck cancer (JCOG1008): A multicenter, noninferiority, phase II/III randomized controlled trial. J Clin Oncol 2022;40(18):1980.
24. Bernier J, Domenge C, Ozsahin M, et al. Postoperative irradiation with or without concomitant chemotherapy for locally advanced head and neck cancer. N Engl J Med 2004;350(19):1945–52.
25. Racadot S, Mercier M, Dussart S, et al. Randomized clinical trial of post-operative radiotherapy versus concomitant carboplatin and radiotherapy for head and neck cancers with lymph node involvement. Radiother Oncol 2008;87(2):164–72.
26. Harari PM, Harris J, Kies MS, et al. Postoperative chemoradiotherapy and cetuximab for high-risk squamous cell carcinoma of the head and neck: Radiation Therapy Oncology Group RTOG-0234. J Clin Oncol 2014;32(23):2486.
27. Sher DJ, Neville BA, Chen AB, et al. Predictors of IMRT and conformal radiotherapy use in head and neck squamous cell carcinoma: a SEER-Medicare analysis. Int J Radiat Oncol Biol Phys 2011;81(4):e197–206.
28. Grégoire V, Evans M, Le QT, et al. Delineation of the primary tumour Clinical Target Volumes (CTV-P) in laryngeal, hypopharyngeal, oropharyngeal and oral cavity squamous cell carcinoma: AIRO, CACA, DAHANCA, EORTC, GEORCC, GORTEC, HKNPCSG, HNCIG, IAG-KHT, LPRHHT, NCIC CTG, NCRI, NRG Oncology, PHNS, SBRT, SOMERA, SRO, SSHNO, TROG consensus guidelines. Radiother Oncol 2018;126(1):3–24.
29. Lacas B, Bourhis J, Overgaard J, et al. Role of radiotherapy fractionation in head and neck cancers (MARCH): an updated meta-analysis. Lancet Oncol 2017; 18(9):1221–37.
30. Grewal AS, Jones J, Lin A. Palliative Radiation Therapy for Head and Neck Cancers. Int J Radiat Oncol Biol Phys 2019;105(2):254–66.
31. Rosenthal DI, Trotti A. Strategies for managing radiation-induced mucositis in head and neck cancer. Semin Radiat Oncol 2009;19(1):29–34.
32. Henke M, Alfonsi M, Foa P, et al. Palifermin decreases severe oral mucositis of patients undergoing postoperative radiochemotherapy for head and neck cancer: a randomized, placebo-controlled trial. J Clin Oncol 2011;29(20):2815–20.
33. Levendag PC, Teguh DN, Voet P, et al. Dysphagia disorders in patients with cancer of the oropharynx are significantly affected by the radiation therapy dose to

the superior and middle constrictor muscle: a dose-effect relationship. Radiother Oncol 2007;85(1):64–73.

34. Burtness B, Harrington KJ, Greil R, et al. Pembrolizumab alone or with chemotherapy versus cetuximab with chemotherapy for recurrent or metastatic squamous cell carcinoma of the head and neck (KEYNOTE-048): a randomised, open-label, phase 3 study. Lancet 2019;394(10212):1915–28.
35. Ferris RL, Blumenschein G Jr, Fayette J, et al. Nivolumab vs investigator's choice in recurrent or metastatic squamous cell carcinoma of the head and neck: 2-year long-term survival update of CheckMate 141 with analyses by tumor PD-L1 expression. Oral Oncol 2018;81:45–51.
36. Machiels J-P, Tao Y, Burtness B, et al. Pembrolizumab given concomitantly with chemoradiation and as maintenance therapy for locally advanced head and neck squamous cell carcinoma: KEYNOTE-412. Future Oncol 2020;16(18):1235–43.
37. Haddad R, Wong D, Guo Y, et al. IMvoke010: Randomized phase III study of atezolizumab (atezo) as adjuvant monotherapy after definitive therapy of squamous cell carcinoma of the head and neck (SCCHN). Ann Oncol 2018;29:viii397.
38. Specenier P. Immunotherapy for head and neck cancer: From recurrent/metastatic disease to (neo) adjuvant treatment in surgically resectable tumors. Curr Opin Otolaryngol Head Neck Surg 2021;29(2):168–77.
39. Clump D.A., Zandberg D.P., Skinner H.D., et al., A randomized phase II study evaluating concurrent or sequential fixed-dose immune therapy in combination with cisplatin and intensity-modulated radiotherapy in intermediate-or high-risk, previously untreated, locally advanced head and neck cancer (LA SCCHN), *Am Soc Clin Oncol*, 40 (16),2022, 6007.
40. Anderson C.M., Lee C.M., Kelley J.R., et al., ROMAN: Phase 3 trial of avasopasem manganese (GC4419) for severe oral mucositis (SOM) in patients receiving chemoradiotherapy (CRT) for locally advanced, nonmetastatic head and neck cancer (LAHNC), *Am Soc Clin Oncol*, 40 (16), 2022, 6005.

Surgery for Supraglottic Laryngeal Cancer

Rusha Patel, MD

KEYWORDS

- Supraglottic laryngectomy • Horizontal partial laryngectomy
- Supracricoid laryngectomy • Transoral robotic surgery • Transoral laser surgery

KEY POINTS

- Total and partial laryngectomies both have a role in the initial treatment of supraglottic laryngeal cancer, with the latter technique gaining prominence due to technologic advances and high rates of cure and function.
- The goals of supraglottic laryngeal surgery are disease eradication and functional preservation, both of which are dependent on appropriate patient selection and surgeon experience.
- Surgical treatment should consider treatment of the neck lymphatics.
- Advanced stage cases and salvage cases should be approached with caution by experienced surgeons and, in specific cases, can be performed with success.

INTRODUCTION

The management of supraglottic cancer has undergone a shift during the last several decades, from a historic reliance on radiation and chemoradiation to the consideration of open and transoral partial laryngectomy techniques. Earlier laryngeal preservation studies led to widespread use of radiation and chemoradiation as primary management for supraglottic tumors. As partial and transoral techniques developed, the term "laryngeal preservation" expanded to include partial laryngectomy procedures. With continued development of technology, transoral surgical techniques have now become increasingly prevalent in the treatment of early supraglottic laryngeal cancer. In this section, we will review surgical indications, techniques, and outcomes in the management of supraglottic laryngeal cancer, with a focus on laryngeal preservation surgery.

BACKGROUND

Supraglottic laryngeal cancer is a unique and separate subtype of laryngeal cancer in both presentation and disease course. Lesions of the supraglottis tend to be

Oklahoma University, 800 Stanton L Young Boulevard, Suite 1400, Oklahoma City, OK 73104, USA
E-mail address: Rusha-patel@ouhsc.edu

Otolaryngol Clin N Am 56 (2023) 295–303
https://doi.org/10.1016/j.otc.2023.01.002
0030-6665/23/© 2023 Elsevier Inc. All rights reserved.
oto.theclinics.com

asymptomatic in the early stages, leading to around 70% of patients presenting with stage III or stage IV disease. Contributing to advanced stage presentation are the abundant lymphatics from the supraglottis, which account for advanced stage presentation in up to 40% of patients.[1] Unlike glottic cancer, supraglottic cancer has comparatively worse treatment outcomes, with overall survival being about 54% at 5 years. About 15% of patients diagnosed with supraglottic laryngeal cancer in the United States are treated with surgery alone.[2]

Patients presenting with advanced stage tumors extending outside of the laryngeal framework, and for those who have significant baseline laryngeal incompetence and functional loss, surgical management with total laryngectomy remains a mainstay of treatment. However, for otherwise functional patients with limited tumor burden, there has long been interest in laryngeal preservation surgery in the management of supraglottic laryngeal cancer. These surgeries include both open techniques and transoral techniques, the latter of which include transoral laser surgery (TLS) and transoral robotic surgery.

Open partial laryngectomy procedures for the management of supraglottic laryngeal cancer have been in practice since the mid-1900s and continue to be used today with success.[3,4] Transoral techniques evolved during the same timeframe. In the late 1970s, the development of precision surgical laser instruments led to a concurrent rise in TLS for laryngeal tumors.[5] The study of Steiner and colleagues during subsequent years established TLS as safe and effective in the management of supraglottic laryngeal cancer.[6,7] As technology advanced in the early 2000s, transoral robotic surgery developed and gained traction. This platform was readily applied to the management of the supraglottic malignancies.[8–10] In more than 2 decades since its implementation, transoral robotic surgery (TORS) has been found to be safe and provide comparable surgical cure rates to other techniques.[11–13] This article will focus on the above-mentioned laryngeal preservation surgeries in the management of supraglottic cancer, and review indications, methods, applications, and outcomes.

DISCUSSION
Pre-Operative Evaluation

A comprehensive preoperative assessment should factor in the tumor, the patient, and the disease process. The surgeon must weigh the likelihood of disease eradication with that of preserving laryngeal function. Given that radiation/chemoradiation continue to provide high cure rates for early-stage laryngeal cancer, the decision to proceed with surgery should additionally consider the ability to provide similar cure and function and to avoid triple-modality treatment.[14,15] Appropriate patient selection is paramount for the success of laryngeal preservation in the surgical management of supraglottic laryngeal cancer.

Tumor Factors: A complete assessment of tumor stage and sites of laryngeal involvement is critical to ensure the ability to clear margins with conservation surgery. Negative margins at the supraglottis have been defined as 2 to 5 mm from the tumor edge.[16,17] At a patient's initial patient evaluation, one can gather valuable information about the status of the tumor and staging to predict resectability. This visit should include flexible laryngoscopy to assess tumor subsite involvement and vocal cord mobility. Staging imaging should be obtained and carefully reviewed for the involvement of the inner thyroid cartilage and the extent of disease in the preepiglottic and/or paraglottic spaces. The tongue base should also be evaluated on imaging and invasion into the deep tongue musculature should be assessed. Supraglottic laryngectomy has been most studied for early stage (T1/T2) tumors with high cure rates for both open and transoral techniques.[11,18–21]

T3 tumors should be approached with caution, and the decision to operate should consider surgeon experience and the ability to achieve complete resection. Conservation surgery for these cases can be successful, although patients with vocal cord fixation, extensive preepiglottic space or base of tongue involvement, and/or uncertainty about the ability to obtain a negative margin along the thyroid lamina may be poor surgical candidates.[22–24] Additional contraindications for transoral approaches include glottic extension, bilateral arytenoid involvement, and involvement of the posterior commissure. In patients being considered for open procedures, contraindications depend on surgery type. Horizontal partial laryngectomy (HPL) should be avoided in patients with involvement of the glottis, invasion of the thyroid or cricoid cartilage, or extensive preepiglottic/base of tongue involvement.[25] Contraindications for supracricoid laryngectomy (SCL) include arytenoid cartilage fixation, invasion of the cricoid or posterior commissure, or subglottic extension to the level of the cricoid.[26]

Neck Disease: Evaluation of neck disease is critical in planning treatment. The supraglottis has a rich lymphatic spread and a rate of occult neck disease reported to be 17% to 30%.[27–30] Surgical candidates with N0 disease are ideal because their disease has the potential to be managed with single modality treatment. For patients who present with adenopathy, clinical examination and workup should focus on identifying patients with clinical evidence of extranodal extension, who may be better served with concurrent chemoradiation to avoid the morbidity of triple-modality treatment.

Patient Factors: The importance of appropriate patient selection for partial laryngectomy procedures cannot be understated. On initial evaluation, patients should be assessed for their baseline ability to carry out the main functions of the laryngeal construct: deglutition and airway maintenance. Baseline dysfunction in swallow mechanisms will likely not improve and may worsen after surgery. This is particularly true for open techniques, which have a rate of temporary aspiration of 32% to 89%.[31] As such, adequate pulmonary reserve is important in the success of these surgeries. Pulmonary function testing can help with risk stratification, and a FEV1/FVC ratio of less than 50% may be predictive of postoperative aspiration.[32] An additional factor associated with aspiration includes increasing age older than 70 years, although age alone should not be an exclusion criterion.[31] In contrast to open approaches, transoral techniques require adequate exposure, which may be limited due to earlier spinal surgery or body habitus. In all cases, patients who undergo conservation surgery for supraglottic cancer should be assessed for their willingness and ability to participate in speech and swallow therapy, both of which are critical in achieving long-term functional success. Finally, patients with significant baseline laryngeal dysfunction, such as tracheostomy or gastrostomy tube dependence, may be better served with total laryngectomy.

Salvage cases

Specific mention should be given to approaching salvage cases after definitive radiation or chemoradiation. Conservatively, salvage surgery for supraglottic cancers is thought to be most beneficial for patients with prior early-stage disease and limited primary site recurrence.[33] However, advanced imaging techniques and transoral surgery have expanded surgical options for this subset of patients, with success being reported for salvage conservation laryngectomy in T1-T3 tumors.[34] A meta-analysis of salvage TLS demonstrated rates of laryngeal preservation of 73% with complication rates of 14%. Margin clearance is particularly important in salvage situations where radiation fibrosis and occult disease can complicate surgery. Earlier reports suggest a marginal cure rate of 38% to 50% after TLS for salvage cases, suggesting a high degree of caution should exist when assessing a patient for salvage partial laryngectomy.[35,36] Open techniques for recurrent disease are more controversial. Several authors have demonstrated success with supracricoid partial laryngectomy in salvage situations with high rates of local control and survival and organ preservation in about 66% of patients at 5 years.[37–40] Complication rates for open salvage surgery range from 20% to 28% with fistula rates of 8% to 14%.[41–43] Appropriate patients for salvage cases are those who meet the criteria as outlined above, and additionally understand the increased risk of prolonged functional loss.

Surgical Methods

Open techniques

Both HPL and SCL have been used in the treatment of qualifying supraglottic malignancies. A conventional supraglottic laryngectomy involves resection of the epiglottis, hyoid, thyrohyoid membrane, the upper half of the thyroid cartilage, and the supraglottic mucosa. The plane of resection is at the level of the laryngeal ventricles, thus making the inferior extent of the tumor margin an important consideration in patient selection. As initially described, the HPL technique involved preservation of both arytenoid cartilages to maintain function and cure.[44,45] Certain exceptions apply, including tumors with superficial spread along the posterior vestibular fold or aryepiglottic fold. In these cases, resection of one arytenoid can be considered.[46] Tumors with extensive involvement of the arytenoid cartilage or cricoarytenoid joint may be better served with total laryngectomy.

In contrast to HPL, SCL allows for resection of tumors with a small degree of inferior extension—usually defined as less than 10 mm of subglottic extension. In the case of supraglottic malignancies, resection margins during SCL include the epiglottis and the hyoid superiorly. Inferiorly, the plane of resection is through the cricothyroid membrane. Reconstruction is performed with cricohyoidopexy.

In both HPL and SCL, tracheostomy is usually performed to maintain the airway during wound healing. A feeding tube is placed until swallowing can be rehabilitated.

Transoral techniques

Transoral supraglottic laryngectomy is a broad term that encompasses endoscopic resection, microlaryngoscopy, and robotic techniques. Regardless of instrumentation, the technique for transoral procedures remains essentially the same as originally described by Steinbeck. The epiglottis is divided in the midline to gain access to the tumor and the vallecula mucosa is transected. Key anatomic structures are identified including the superior edge of the thyroid cartilage, and the superior laryngeal artery. Resection continues around the petiole of the epiglottis, which is divided, and laterally to dissect the paraglottic space from the inner aspect of the thyroid cartilage. The final cuts are made to separate the false fold from the arytenoid cartilage and the tumor is removed. The described resection procedure may differ based on tumor subsite involvement.[47] In contrast to open procedures, tracheostomy may be avoided in specific cases, although it should be considered for patients with extensive tumors.[48] Return to swallowing can occur sooner than both HPL and SCL, and is often begun in the immediate postoperative period.[49–51]

Neck management

Neck management should always be considered as part of the treatment plan for supraglottic malignancies. In addition to the ipsilateral neck, the contralateral neck nodes must be considered in the treatment plan. Rates of occult disease to the contralateral neck can be as high as 44%,[28,52] the incidence of which is increased for tumors with N+ ipsilateral disease and tumors approaching or crossing the midline. The routine performance of bilateral neck dissections during the surgical treatment of supraglottic cancers can be done safely and can reduce recurrent cervical disease.[53,54] Radiation of the contralateral neck for patients anticipated to need adjuvant treatment can be considered. Select cases—early stage (T1), well lateralized tumors with clinically N0 neck disease—may be adequately treated with ipsilateral neck dissection alone.[55,56]

Postoperative Complications

In the immediate postoperative period, patients undergoing partial laryngectomy can be subject to the routine complications of surgery, in addition to those of airway loss, dysphonia, and persistent dysphagia. HSL and SCL have been associated with fistula formation in 2.9% to 3%[19,57] of patients undergoing primary resection. Transoral techniques can be associated with airway hemorrhage, with rates reported between 2% and 16%.[11,58] As such, careful identification and control of the superior laryngeal vessels should be performed to prevent major hemorrhage after transoral procedures. Steroid administration is typically recommended to reduce laryngeal edema in the first 24 hours after surgery, and patients undergoing extensive resections should be counseled about prophylactic tracheostomy. For patients undergoing open procedures, nutrition should be optimized before surgery to allow for adequate wound healing. In all cases, preoperative counseling should include a discussion of the functional rehabilitation issues discussed above.

Outcomes

Oncologic outcomes

Open, organ-sparing approaches to supraglottic carcinoma have a historical track record of high cure rates, particularly for early-staged disease. Five-year overall survival rates range from 68% to 89% across all stages, with local control rates up to 90%.[19,20,59] Transoral techniques boast similar rates of overall survival, with 5-year OS ranging from 78.7% to 80.2%.[11,60]

In a recent publication that compared oncologic outcomes among TORS, TLS, and open surgery for early laryngeal cancer, there was no difference in margin status or the need for adjuvant radiation between the 3 surgical modalities. Similarly, there was no difference between TORS or open surgery in overall survival for patients with supraglottic carcinoma.[61] This is in keeping with prior studies showing comparable oncologic outcomes across modalities and speaks to surgeon experience with a given technique being paramount to obtaining high cure rates.

Functional Outcomes

Open approaches to organ preservation tend to be associated with at least temporary need of tracheostomy and feeding tube placement, with up to 14% of patients requiring long-term tracheostomy and up to 18% requiring long-term gastrostomy.[62,63] In contrast, transoral techniques can result in up to 100% of patients resuming an oral diet shortly after surgery and low rates of tracheostomy, with several authors reporting a 0% rate of tracheostomy in the right clinical scenario.[9,11,50] Functional outcomes of conservation surgery for supraglottic cancer depend heavily on patient selection. Swallowing outcomes may be affected by the degree of tongue base involvement, and patients with tumors who undergo a partial tongue base resection may require focused speech and swallow rehabilitation.[64]

SUMMARY

Surgical treatment of supraglottic laryngeal cancer has evolved during the last several decades. Total laryngectomy continues to be the treatment of choice for advanced disease. However, both open and transoral techniques can provide laryngeal preservation with high rates of cure and function. Outcomes from both open and transoral techniques are highly dependent on patient selection and surgeon experience. The ultimate choice of treatment modality depends heavily on surgeon training and experience. Advanced stage tumors and salvage cases represent a challenging subset of supraglottic laryngeal surgery and should be approached with caution. In all cases, the treatment plan should include the management of neck lymphatics, as well as assessment of the need for adjuvant therapy, with the ultimate treatment goals being disease eradication, functional preservation, and avoiding triple-modality treatment. Surgical treatment of supraglottic laryngeal cancer continues to evolve as transoral techniques gain popularity.

CLINICS CARE POINTS

- Total and partial laryngectomies both have a role in the initial treatment of supraglottic laryngeal cancer, with the latter technique gaining prominence due to technologic advances and high rates of cure and function.
- The goals of supraglottic laryngeal surgery are disease eradication and functional preservation, both of which are dependent on appropriate patient selection and surgeon experience.
- Surgical treatment should consider treatment of the neck lymphatics.
- Advanced stage cases and salvage cases should be approached with caution by experienced surgeons and in specific cases can be performed with success.

DISCLOSURE

R. Patel has no relevant financial relationships with ineligible companies to disclose.

REFERENCES

1. Karatzanis AD, Psychogios G, Waldfahrer F, et al. Management of locally advanced laryngeal cancer. J Otolaryngol Head Neck Surg 2014;43:4.
2. Patel TD, Echanique KA, Yip C, et al. Supraglottic Squamous Cell Carcinoma: A Population-Based Study of 22,675 Cases. Laryngoscope 2019;129(8):1822–7.
3. Alonso Regules JE. Horizontal Partial Laryngectomy. Historical Review and Personal Technique. In: Wigand ME, Steiner W, Stell PM, editors. Functional Partial Laryngectomy. Berlin, Heidelberg: Springer; 1984.
4. Sperry SM, Rassekh CH, Laccourreye O, et al. Supracricoid partial laryngectomy for primary and recurrent laryngeal cancer. JAMA Otolaryngol Head Neck Surg 2013;139(11):1226–35.
5. Eckel HE. Endoscopic laser resection of supraglottic carcinoma. Otolaryngol Head Neck Surg 1997;117(6):681–7.
6. Iro H, Waldfahrer F, Altendorf-Hofmann A, et al. Transoral laser surgery of supraglottic cancer: follow-up of 141 patients. Arch Otolaryngol Head Neck Surg 1998; 124(11):1245–50.
7. Ambrosch P, Kron M, Steiner W. Carbon dioxide laser microsurgery for early supraglottic carcinoma. Ann Otol Rhinol Laryngol 1998;107(8):680–8.
8. Smith RV. Transoral robotic surgery for larynx cancer. Otolaryngol Clin North Am 2014;47(3):379–95.

9. Mendelsohn AH, Remacle M. Transoral robotic surgery for laryngeal cancer. Curr Opin Otolaryngol Head Neck Surg 2015;23(2):148–52.

10. Mendelsohn AH, Remacle M, Van Der Vorst S, et al. Outcomes following transoral robotic surgery: supraglottic laryngectomy. Laryngoscope 2013;123(1):208–14.

11. Hans S, Chekkoury-Idrissi Y, Circiu MP, et al. Surgical, Oncological, and Functional Outcomes of Transoral Robotic Supraglottic Laryngectomy. Laryngoscope 2021;131(5):1060–5.

12. Ozer E, Alvarez B, Kakarala K, et al. Clinical outcomes of transoral robotic supraglottic laryngectomy. Head Neck 2013;35(8):1158–61.

13. Razafindranaly V, Lallemant B, Aubry K, et al. Clinical outcomes with transoral robotic surgery for supraglottic squamous cell carcinoma: Experience of a French evaluation cooperative subgroup of GETTEC. Head Neck 2016; 38(Suppl 1):E1097–101.

14. Patel KB, Nichols AC, Fung K, et al. Treatment of early stage Supraglottic squamous cell carcinoma: meta-analysis comparing primary surgery versus primary radiotherapy. J Otolaryngol Head Neck Surg 2018;47(1):19.

15. Woo JS, Baek SK, Kwon SY, et al. T3 supraglottic cancer: treatment results and prognostic factors. Acta Otolaryngol 2003;123(8):980–6.

16. Michel J, Fakhry N, Duflo S, et al. Prognostic value of the status of resection margins after endoscopic laser cordectomy for T1a glottic carcinoma. Eur Ann Otorhinolaryngol Head Neck Dis 2011;128(6):297–300.

17. Peretti G, Piazza C, Ansarin M, et al. Transoral CO2 laser microsurgery for Tis-T3 supraglottic squamous cell carcinomas. Eur Arch Otorhinolaryngol 2010;267(11): 1735–42.

18. Bocca E, Sixteenth Daniel C, Baker Jr. memorial lecture. Surgical management of supraglottic cancer and its lymph node metastases in a conservative perspective. Ann Otol Rhinol Laryngol 1991;100(4 Pt 1):261–7.

19. Bron L, Brossard E, Monnier P, et al. Supracricoid partial laryngectomy with cricohyoidoepiglottopexy and cricohyoidopexy for glottic and supraglottic carcinomas. Laryngoscope 2000;110(4):627–34.

20. Bron LP, Soldati D, Monod ML, et al. Horizontal partial laryngectomy for supraglottic squamous cell carcinoma. Eur Arch Otorhinolaryngol 2005;262(4):302–6.

21. Carta F, Mariani C, Sambiagio GB, et al. CO2 Transoral Microsurgery for Supraglottic Squamous Cell Carcinoma. Front Oncol 2018;8:321.

22. Canis M, Ihler F, Martin A, et al. Results of 226 patients with T3 laryngeal carcinoma after treatment with transoral laser microsurgery. Head Neck 2014;36(5): 652–9.

23. Peretti G, Piazza C, Penco S, et al. Transoral laser microsurgery as primary treatment for selected T3 glottic and supraglottic cancers. Head Neck 2016;38(7): 1107–12.

24. Vilaseca I, Blanch JL, Berenguer J, et al. Transoral laser microsurgery for locally advanced (T3-T4a) supraglottic squamous cell carcinoma: Sixteen years of experience. Head Neck 2016;38(7):1050–7.

25. Daly JF, Kwok FN. Laryngofissure and cordectomy. Laryngoscope 1975;85(8): 1290–7.

26. Tufano RP, Stafford EM. Organ preservation surgery for laryngeal cancer. Otolaryngol Clin North Am 2008;41(4):741–55, vi.

27. Birkeland AC, Rosko AJ, Issa MR, et al. Occult Nodal Disease Prevalence and Distribution in Recurrent Laryngeal Cancer Requiring Salvage Laryngectomy. Otolaryngol Head Neck Surg 2016;154(3):473–9.

28. Hicks WL Jr, Kollmorgen DR, Kuriakose MA, et al. Patterns of nodal metastasis and surgical management of the neck in supraglottic laryngeal carcinoma. Otolaryngol Head Neck Surg 1999;121(1):57–61.
29. Sharbel DD, Abkemeier M, Groves MW, et al. Occult Metastasis in Laryngeal Squamous Cell Carcinoma: A Systematic Review and Meta-Analysis. Ann Otol Rhinol Laryngol 2021;130(1):67–77.
30. Wang SX, Ning WJ, Zhang XW, et al. Predictors of Occult Lymph Node Metastasis and Prognosis in Patients with cN0 T1-T2 Supraglottic Laryngeal Carcinoma: A Retrospective Study. ORL J Otorhinolaryngol Relat Spec 2019; 81(5–6):317–26.
31. Benito J, Holsinger FC, Perez-Martin A, et al. Aspiration after supracricoid partial laryngectomy: Incidence, risk factors, management, and outcomes. Head Neck 2011;33(5):679–85.
32. Beckhardt RN, Murray JG, Ford CN, et al. Factors influencing functional outcome in supraglottic laryngectomy. Head Neck 1994;16(3):232–9.
33. Shaw HJ. Role of partial laryngectomy after irradiation in the treatment of laryngeal cancer: a view from the United Kingdom. Ann Otol Rhinol Laryngol 1991; 100(4 Pt 1):268–73.
34. Hong JC, Kim SW, Lee HS, et al. Salvage transoral laser supraglottic laryngectomy after radiation failure: a report of seven cases. Ann Otol Rhinol Laryngol 2013;122(2):85–90.
35. de Gier HH, Knegt PP, de Boer MF, et al. CO2-laser treatment of recurrent glottic carcinoma. Head Neck 2001;23(3):177–80.
36. Steiner W, Vogt P, Ambrosch P, et al. Transoral carbon dioxide laser microsurgery for recurrent glottic carcinoma after radiotherapy. Head Neck 2004;26(6):477–84.
37. Laccourreye O, Weinstein G, Naudo P, et al. Supracricoid partial laryngectomy after failed laryngeal radiation therapy. Laryngoscope 1996;106(4):495–8.
38. Makeieff M, Venegoni D, Mercante G, et al. Supracricoid partial laryngectomies after failure of radiation therapy. Laryngoscope 2005;115(2):353–7.
39. Pellini R, Pichi B, Ruscito P, et al. Supracricoid partial laryngectomies after radiation failure: a multi-institutional series. Head Neck 2008;30(3):372–9.
40. Spriano G, Pellini R, Romano G, et al. Supracricoid partial laryngectomy as salvage surgery after radiation failure. Head Neck 2002;24(8):759–65.
41. Ganly I, Patel SG, Matsuo J, et al. Analysis of postoperative complications of open partial laryngectomy. Head Neck 2009;31(3):338–45.
42. Nibu K, Kamata S, Kawabata K, et al. Partial laryngectomy in the treatment of radiation-failure of early glottic carcinoma. Head Neck 1997;19(2):116–20.
43. Watters GW, Patel SG, Rhys-Evans PH. Partial laryngectomy for recurrent laryngeal carcinoma. Clin Otolaryngol Allied Sci 2000;25(2):146–52.
44. Ogura JH. Supraglottic subtotal laryngectomy and radical neck dissection for carcinoma of the epiglottis. Laryngoscope 1958;68(6):983–1003.
45. Som ML. Surgical treatment of carcinoma of the epiglottis by lateral pharyngotomy. Trans Am Acad Ophthalmol Otolaryngol 1959;63(1):28–48, discussion -9.
46. Ogura JH, Sessions DG, Ciralsky RH. Supraglottic carcinoma with extension to the arytenoid. Laryngoscope 1975;85(8):1327–31.
47. Rodrigo JP, Suarez C, Silver CE, et al. Transoral laser surgery for supraglottic cancer. Head Neck 2008;30(5):658–66.
48. Stubbs VC, Rajasekaran K, Gigliotti AR, et al. Management of the Airway for Transoral Robotic Supraglottic Partial Laryngectomy. Front Oncol 2018;8:312.
49. Chiesa Estomba CM, Betances Reinoso FA, Lorenzo Lorenzo AI, et al. Functional outcomes of supraglottic squamous cell carcinoma treated by transoral laser

microsurgery compared with horizontal supraglottic laryngectomy in patients younger and older than 65 years. Acta Otorhinolaryngol Ital 2016;36(6):450–8.

50. Karabulut B, Deveci I, Surmeli M, et al. Comparison of functional and oncological treatment outcomes after transoral robotic surgery and open surgery for supraglottic laryngeal cancer. J Laryngol Otol 2018;132(9):832–6.

51. Kaya KH, Karaman Koc A, Kayhan FT. Health-Related Quality-of-Life Outcomes after Transoral Robotic Surgery for T1 and T2 Supraglottic Laryngeal Carcinoma Compared to the Transcervical Open Supraglottic Approach. ORL J Otorhinolaryngol Relat Spec 2022;84(5):378–86.

52. Ozturkcan S, Katilmis H, Ozdemir I, et al. Occult contralateral nodal metastases in supraglottic laryngeal cancer crossing the midline. Eur Arch Otorhinolaryngol 2009;266(1):117–20.

53. Chiu RJ, Myers EN, Johnson JT. Efficacy of routine bilateral neck dissection in the management of supraglottic cancer. Otolaryngol Head Neck Surg 2004;131(4):485–8.

54. Weber PC, Johnson JT, Myers EN. The impact of bilateral neck dissection on pattern of recurrence and survival in supraglottic carcinoma. Arch Otolaryngol Head Neck Surg 1994;120(7):703–6.

55. Kurten CHL, Zioga E, Gauler T, et al. Patterns of cervical lymph node metastasis in supraglottic laryngeal cancer and therapeutic implications of surgical staging of the neck. Eur Arch Otorhinolaryngol 2021;278(12):5021–7.

56. Rodrigo JP, Cabanillas R, Franco V, et al. Efficacy of routine bilateral neck dissection in the management of the N0 neck in T1-T2 unilateral supraglottic cancer. Head Neck 2006;28(6):534–9.

57. Mercante G, Grammatica A, Battaglia P, et al. Supracricoid partial laryngectomy in the management of t3 laryngeal cancer. Otolaryngol Head Neck Surg 2013;149(5):714–20.

58. Turner MT, Stokes WA, Stokes CM, et al. Airway and bleeding complications of transoral robotic supraglottic laryngectomy (TORS-SGL): A systematic review and meta-analysis. Oral Oncol 2021;118:105301.

59. Damiani M, Mercante G, Abdellaoui M, et al. Prognostic Features in Intermediate-Size Supraglottic Tumors Treated With Open Supraglottic Laryngectomy. Laryngoscope 2021;131(6):E1980–6.

60. Doazan M, Hans S, Moriniere S, et al. Oncologic outcomes with transoral robotic surgery for supraglottic squamous cell carcinoma: Results of the French Robotic Surgery Group of GETTEC. Head Neck 2018;40(9):2050–9.

61. Hanna J, Brauer PR, Morse E, et al. Is robotic surgery an option for early T-stage laryngeal cancer? Early nationwide results. Laryngoscope 2020;130(5):1195–201.

62. de Vincentiis M, Greco A, Campo F, et al. Open partial horizontal laryngectomy for T2-T3-T4a laryngeal cancer: oncological outcomes and prognostic factors of two Italian hospitals. Eur Arch Otorhinolaryngol 2022;279(6):2997–3004.

63. Muscatello L, Piazza C, Peretti G, et al. Open partial horizontal laryngectomy and adjuvant (chemo)radiotherapy for laryngeal squamous cell carcinoma: results from a multicenter Italian experience. Eur Arch Otorhinolaryngol 2021;278(10):4059–65.

64. Breunig C, Benter P, Seidl RO, et al. Predictable swallowing function after open horizontal supraglottic partial laryngectomy. Auris Nasus Larynx 2016;43(6):658–65.

Management of Subglottic Cancer

Hayley Mann, MD[a], Kristen Seligman, MD[a], Nicholas Colwell, MD[a],
Adam Burr, MD, PhD[b], Tiffany A. Glazer, MD[a],*

KEYWORDS

- Squamous cell carcinoma • Subglottic cancer • Management • Surgery
- Laryngectomy • Partial laryngectomy • Radiation

KEY POINTS

- Management of subglottic cancer requires a multidisciplinary approach.
- Most patients with subglottic carcinoma present at an advanced stage due to a relative lack of early signs and symptoms.
- Primary radiation therapy offers similar 5-year overall and disease-specific survival rates compared with surgery in early-stage subglottic carcinoma.
- Patients with advanced stage subglottic carcinoma are typically treated with total laryngectomy and adjuvant radiation therapy.
- Paratracheal nodal metastases are found in about 20% of patients.

INTRODUCTION

Primary subglottic cancer is a rare entity comprising less than 5% of all laryngeal malignancies, most of which is histologically defined as squamous cell carcinoma (SCCa).[1,2] Management of primary subglottic carcinoma requires a multidisciplinary approach to consider disease stage, functional status, comorbidities, and other patient factors. The focus of this article is to provide evidence-based management strategies for carcinoma originating from the subglottic laryngeal subsite.

Although primary subglottic SCCa is known to represent a low percentage of laryngeal cancers, exact incidence is difficult to establish given that the subglottis does not have a standardized anatomic definition. The general consensus in the literature places the inferior boundary at the inferior border of the cricoid cartilage. However, the superior border has no clear embryologic or anatomic boundary and can be

[a] Department of Surgery, Division of Otolaryngology-Head & Neck Surgery, University of Wisconsin Hospital & Clinics, 600 Highland Avenue, K4/723, Madison, WI 53792, USA;
[b] Department of Human Oncology, University of Wisconsin Hospital & Clinics, 600 Highland Avenue, Madison, WI 53792, USA
* Corresponding author.
E-mail address: glazer@surgery.wisc.edu

Otolaryngol Clin N Am 56 (2023) 305–312
https://doi.org/10.1016/j.otc.2022.11.001
0030-6665/23/Published by Elsevier Inc.
oto.theclinics.com

considered as fused with the glottis. Definitions of the superior boundary have included an imaginary line passing 5 mm below the vocal cords, 0 to 1 cm below the vocal cords, or 1 cm below the apex of the laryngeal ventricle.[3] Additionally, the literature frequently conflates primary subglottic lesions with subglottic extension from glottic primaries.[3,4] Consequently, understanding of subglottic SCCa and reporting on treatment outcomes is inconsistent and can be difficult to interpret. Survival outcomes for primary subglottic SCCa are reported to be worse than in other laryngeal subsites, because patients more commonly present with locally advanced disease due to a lack of early symptoms such as dysphonia or dysphagia.[2] Subglottic SCCa tends to spread submucosally and through the intercartilaginous infrastructure of the subglottis, rather than within the cartilaginous boundaries of the larynx, which allows for growth of the tumor with minimal symptom development. The lymphatic drainage of the subglottis passes bilaterally through the prelaryngeal (Delphian), pretracheal, and paratracheal nodes, with nodal metastasis occurring in 2% to 21.5% of patients.[3,5] Given these characteristics, there is no consensus on treatment of primary subglottic carcinoma and much of clinical practice is guided by studies that do not differentiate by cancer subtype. This article seeks to inform and provide practical clinical guidance for the management of primary subglottic SCCa.

DISCUSSION
Management of Early-Stage Subglottic Squamous Cell Carcinoma

Treatment of subglottic SCCa varies based on tumor stage. The American Joint Committee on Cancer (AJCC) Staging Manual defines early-stage subglottic cancers as stage I tumors limited to the subglottis, and stage II tumors that extend to vocal cord(s) with normal or impaired mobility. Patients with early-stage disease have significantly better 5-year overall survival (55.5%) compared with those with advanced-stage disease (43.4%; $P < .01$).[5] Studies have shown that most early-stage tumors can be treated with a *single modality*, either surgical excision or primary radiation.[4,6,7] Surgery varies depending on the location of the primary tumor, and often entails a total laryngectomy versus a partial supratracheal laryngectomy. One study demonstrated that a supratracheal laryngectomy could be performed in cases with a fixed arytenoid but without cricoarytenoid joint invasion, with contraindications defined as tumors with cricoid invasion or extension to the first tracheal ring.[8] Primary radiotherapy has been shown in retrospective studies to be effective for early stage subglottic carcinoma.[2,5] Marchiano and colleagues represents the largest study to date using patient data from the SEER database (889 cases) and demonstrates no difference in 5-year overall survival or 5-year disease-specific survival between patients treated with curative-intent radiation and surgery.[2] However, due to the rarity of primary subglottic carcinoma, many of these studies are underpowered and do not report long-term laryngectomy-free survival.[2,9]

Management of Advanced-Stage Subglottic Squamous Cell Carcinoma

Advanced-stage lesions, including stages III and IV, are defined by vocal cord fixation, the presence of nodal disease, and locally or distally invasive disease (AJCC). These tumors have been shown to be most effectively treated with *multimodal therapy*, historically entailing a total laryngectomy with thyroidectomy; pretracheal, bilateral paratracheal, and possible lateral neck lymph node dissection; and adjuvant radiotherapy.[2,9] Jumaily and colleagues retrospectively examined 549 patients with subglottic SCCa and found that patients with stage III and IV disease who received surgery-based treatment as compared with nonsurgical treatment had significantly higher 5-year overall survival.[5] On multivariate analysis, factors associated with worse overall survival included patients with older age, higher comorbidities (Charlson-Deyo comorbidity score of >2), positive nodal status, clinical stage T4, and those who received chemoradiation.

PRIMARY THERAPIES
Surgical Therapy

Surgical therapy for subglottic carcinoma is the standard of care in most locally advanced disease, although data is limited and split on the overall and disease-specific outcome measures of radiation versus surgery as primary treatments in early stage disease.[2,5] Given the paucity of randomized controlled trials and reliance on mixed evidence from retrospective, institution-specific data, surgical management of laryngeal cancer requires a multidisciplinary approach with consideration for patient factors such as age, comorbidities, disease stage, and functional status. Depending on the stage, bulk, and patient tolerance of surgical therapy, various surgical strategies can be considered as primary, adjuvant, or salvage therapies. The anatomic specificity and associated advanced presentation of subglottic carcinoma limits the operative techniques that can be used; these techniques are described below.

Total laryngectomy

With an increased emphasis on organ-preservation surgery, total laryngectomy is reserved for locally advanced T3 and T4 subglottic SCCa. Criteria for T3 disease include vocal cord fixation, invasion of paraglottic space and/or the inner cortex of the thyroid cartilage, whereas T4 disease is defined by the invasion of cricoid or thyroid cartilage or neck soft tissues beyond the larynx (AJCC). Total laryngectomy may also be used as salvage therapy for patients who have failed radiation therapy (either by residual or recurrent disease). Additional absolute indications for total laryngectomy include invasion of the thyroid cartilage and extension of tumor to soft tissues of the neck.[10]

Although total laryngectomy is the mainstay of treatment of locally advanced subglottic cancer, it comes with the cost of significant morbidity and decrease in quality of life due to the loss of native voice and swallow function. Management of subglottic carcinoma with total laryngectomy requires patients to be healthy enough to undergo surgery but also requires a significant amount of postoperative follow-up for swallow and speech therapy, social and home health support, and physical rehabilitation.[11] When used as a salvage procedure, the rate of complication increases, with the most commonly reported being pharyngocutaneous fistula in 28% of patients, followed by wound complications, dysphagia, and stomal stenosis.[12]

Thyroidectomy

Although thyroidectomy is not routinely indicated for all total laryngectomy patients, those requiring total laryngectomy for T3 or T4 subglottic carcinoma should undergo thyroidectomy due to the high incidence of direct spread through the cricothyroid membrane and lymphatic invasion into the gland.[3,13]

Stomal spread

Typically, if a patient requires a tracheostomy for airway protection before definitive treatment, the tracheotomy is performed as proximal along the trachea as possible, often between tracheal rings 1 and 2. Caution must be taken if a patient is to require a tracheostomy in the setting of subglottic SCCa; due to its predilection for lymphatic spread to the prelaryngeal (Delphian) and paratracheal nodes, subglottic carcinoma has a high frequency of stomal spread of disease. Even after definitive total laryngectomy surgery, stomal relapses can be frequent.[6]

Partial laryngectomy
Typically, subglottic spread of disease is a contraindication for partial laryngectomies (ie, supracricoid partial laryngectomy). However, supratracheal partial laryngectomies (STPLs), also referred to as type III open partial horizontal laryngectomies, may allow select patients with early stage subglottic carcinoma to avoid total laryngectomy.[8,14] STPL involves resection of the entire glottis and subglottis with the inferior limit of resection reaching the first tracheal ring. Resection may include the thyroid cartilage but must spare one functioning cricoarytenoid unit.[8] Patients must have minimal anterior extralaryngeal extension. Typically, adjuvant radiation should be avoided in this population. This surgical option limits some of the morbidity associated with total laryngectomy, allowing preservation of some speech and swallow function.[8] Contraindications to the use of this technique are largely related to disease extension and include lesions originating from the epilarynx; lesions with major invasion of the preepiglottic space involving the hyoid bone, the interarytenoid space, the posterior commissure and both arytenoid cartilages; and lesions reaching the first tracheal ring.[8] The technique and intraoperative photos are described in detail elsewhere.[8]

Selective lymph node dissection
The lymphatic drainage pathway of the subglottis includes the pretracheal, prelaryngeal (Delphian), paratracheal, and mediastinal lymph nodes in a pattern that crosses midline. Up to 21.5% of patients with subglottic carcinoma will have lymph node involvement in these basins.[2,3] The paratracheal lymph nodes represent a more clinically occult group of nodes, with pretreatment imaging demonstrating poor ability to identify nodal disease.[15] Laryngeal tumors with subglottic involvement, including both those originating from the subglottis as well as those originating from other subsites with subglottic extension, are reported to have a statistically significant increase in paratracheal nodal disease compared with tumors involving only the supraglottic and glottic subsites.[15,16] Involvement of prelaryngeal (Delphian) nodes is associated with decreased overall survival, increased nodal metastasis in lateral neck levels, and increased tumor recurrence.[2,5,17] Although subglottic carcinomas have been demonstrated to have a significantly higher stomal recurrence rate, central neck dissection has been shown to reduce stomal recurrence.[6] As such, routine central neck dissection for subglottic SCCa is recommended to improve prognosis.[3,6,17]

PRIMARY RADIATION THERAPY

Due to the typical locally advanced stage of presentation, most patients with primary subglottic carcinoma are treated with laryngectomy followed by postoperative radiation. In the SEER analysis by Marchiano, 38.8% underwent combined surgery and radiation, whereas 33.9% underwent radiation alone.[2]

Early-Stage Disease

Early stage, T1 and T2 disease is equally managed with surgery or radiation in terms of survival. Because the embryonic origin of the subglottic and glottic larynx are identical, it follows that a similar approach to treatment would be effective. Cassidy and colleagues demonstrated 100% local control with 63 Gy for T1 lesions and 65.25 Gy for T2 lesions in 2.25 Gy per fraction using small larynx-directed fields with a 1 to 2-cm margin.[7] Paisley and colleagues treated slightly larger larynx-directed fields measuring 8 × 12 cm to a dose of 50 to 52 Gy in 20 fractions, treating more cervical and paratracheal lymphatics.[18] They demonstrated local control in 63.6% of T1 tumors and 66.7% of T2 tumors. This lower rate of local control suggests that biological effective dose (BED), accounting for total time is an important factor in this disease, similar to glottic larynx cancers.[19]

The study of Hata took a different approach incorporating chemoradiation and elective nodal treatment of early-stage disease.[20] The rationale for elective nodal coverage in early stage disease is analogous to supraglottic cancers given the increased nodal risk. They achieved local control in 7 of 8 patients. The failure occurred in a patient treated with 70 Gy in conventional fractionation without chemotherapy, again potentially due to the lower BED of this regimen. Chemoradiation therapy has also been suggested as primary treatment of stage II disease by others, with some studies demonstrating survival benefit over radiation treatment alone.[21–23] Thus both chemoradiation and radiation alone with altered fractionation seem effective with avoidance of chemotherapy-related toxicities, an expected advantage of radiation alone.

Cassidy and colleagues recommended adding nodal coverage with accelerated or hyperfractionated radiation for disease extending 1 cm below the vocal folds.[7] A unifying theory of why larynx directed radiation seems effective in a disease with high-nodal risk could be due to the highest risk Delphian node being included in the larynx-directed fields. Thus, our overall recommended approach would be radiation alone with altered fractionation, and to include elective nodal coverage for bulkier tumors or disease that extends more than 1 cm below the cords. Chemoradiation also seems effective and could be considered for bulkier or more invasive stage II tumors.

Advanced Disease

Advanced stage disease can be treated either with surgery followed by adjuvant radiation or with chemoradiation therapy. Radiation alone should likely be reserved for patients with poor performance status although subglottic cancers were not well represented in trials that established chemoradiation as standard of care.[21] Despite this, it seems prudent to offer chemoradiation to patients with good performance status for whom larynx preservation is selected given the large improvement in larynx preservation demonstrated on RTOG 9111. Patients should receive concurrent cisplatin if possible. Cetuximab or carboplatin and paclitaxel are reasonable alternatives for those who are cisplatin ineligible.[24,25] The criteria for initial surgery versus chemoradiation derive from the treatment of glottic and supraglottic larynx cancers. Local control in T4 subglottic larynx cancer was achieved in 5 of 7 patients by Cassidy and colleagues; however, similar to glottic cancers, T4 subglottic disease should likely be treated with initial laryngectomy followed by adjuvant radiation.[7]

Stage III (T3) tumors have been managed effectively by surgery followed by adjuvant radiation, radiation alone, and chemoradiation. The University of Florida uses a criterion of primary tumor volume less than 3.5 cm^3 to select patients for larynx preservation.[7] Patient swallow function, laryngeal function, and eligibility for concurrent chemotherapy all enter into the patient-centered discussion of larynx preservation versus laryngectomy. In a population study performed by Hill-Madsen and colleagues, the disease-specific mortality for patients treated with curative intent was not significantly different between treatment modalities but was significantly influenced by disease stage, which aligns with the findings of Marchiano.[1,2] This further supports a patient-centered discussion and multidisciplinary evaluation to arrive at individualized treatment of advanced stage disease.

Adjuvant Radiation

In general, adjuvant radiation therapy should generally be delivered to advanced stage patients, due to National Comprehensive Cancer Network guidance toward radiation in T3 and T4 disease in addition to the increased risk of a stomal recurrence in subglottic cancers. Subglottic extension or subglottic tumor location is an indication for stomal boost to 63 to 66 Gy. In addition to the stoma and postoperative BED, the radiation field for adjuvant therapy should encompass levels II to IV and VI in these patients given the level VI risk incurred by subglottic extension. Additional attention should be paid to anterior extension of tumor into strap musculature. Here, multidisciplinary interaction with the head and neck surgeon can give great insight into the local areas at greatest risk. Additionally, although base of tongue is included in most postlaryngectomy fields, this can likely be omitted or truncated if no extension to the supraglottic larynx is observed. The addition of concurrent chemoradiation should be included for patients with extranodal extension or positive margin.

RECURRENT OR METASTATIC SUBGLOTTIC SQUAMOUS CELL CARCINOMA

For patients with recurrent or metastatic subglottic SCCa, immunotherapy with checkpoint inhibitors can be used. Nivolumab and pembrolizumab, which are monoclonal antibodies to the PD-1 receptor, were Food and Drug Administration approved for use in patients in platinum-refractory recurrent and metastatic head and neck SCCa in 2016.[26]

SUMMARY

Subglottic SCCa is a rare subtype of laryngeal SCCa and typically presents at an advanced stage. Up to 21% of these patients will have nodal disease, primarily in the prelaryngeal, pretracheal, and paratracheal basins. Early-stage patients can be treated with a single modality treatment, with surgery and radiation therapy having equivalent overall survival rates. Elective nodal treatment in early-stage patients remains controversial. Advanced-stage patients require multimodal therapy, typically in the form of total laryngectomy followed by adjuvant radiation or chemoradiation therapy. Patients with recurrent or metastatic disease can be given checkpoint inhibitors. Due to the rare nature of subglottic SCCa, management requires a multidisciplinary approach at a tertiary care institution.

CLINICS CARE POINTS

- Subglottic carcinoma often presents in advanced stages.
- Early-stage disease (T1, T2) can be treated with either partial laryngectomy or radiation.
- Advanced-stage disease (T3, T4) can be treated with either total laryngectomy followed by adjuvant radiation or chemoradiation therapy.
- Pretracheal, paratracheal, and mediastinal nodal basins and the thyroid gland are common sites of spread and must be considered in the treatment plan.
- Because of the rarity of subglottic carcinoma, a multidisciplinary approach is recommended.

DISCLOSURES

Dr A. Burr receives salary support from Siemens and GE.

REFERENCES

1. Hill-Madsen L, Kristensen CA, Andersen E, et al. Subglottic squamous cell carcinoma in Denmark 1971-2015 - a national population-based cohort study from

DAHANCA, the Danish Head and Neck Cancer group. Acta Oncol 2019;58(10): 1509–13. Epub 2019 Jul 31. PMID: 31364888.

2. Marchiano E, Patel DM, Patel TD, et al. Subglottic Squamous Cell Carcinoma: A Population-Based Study of 889 Cases. Otolaryngol Head Neck Surg 2016;154(2): 315–21. Epub 2015 Nov 25. PMID: 26607281.

3. Coskun H, Mendenhall WM, Rinaldo A, et al. Prognosis of subglottic carcinoma: is it really worse? Head Neck 2019;41(2):511–21. Epub 2018 Jun 26. PMID: 29947111.

4. Garas J, McGuirt WF Sr. Squamous cell carcinoma of the subglottis. Am J Otolaryngol 2006;27(1):1–4. PMID: 16360814.

5. Jumaily M, Gallogly JA, Gropler MC, et al. Does Subglottic Squamous Cell Carcinoma Warrant a Different Strategy Than Other Laryngeal Subsites? Laryngoscope 2021;131(4):E1117–24. Epub 2020 Aug 26. PMID: 32846040.

6. Chiesa F, Tradati N, Calabrese L, et al. Surgical treatment of laryngeal carcinoma with subglottis involvement. Oncol Rep 2001;8(1):137–40. PMID: 11115585.

7. Cassidy R, Morris C, Kirwan J, et al. Radiation therapy for squamous cell carcinoma of the subglottic larynx. J Radiat Oncol 2012;1:333–6.

8. Succo G, Peretti G, Piazza C, et al. Open partial horizontal laryngectomies: a proposal for classification by the working committee on nomenclature of the European Laryngological Society. Eur Arch Otorhinolaryngol 2014;271(9):2489–96. Epub 2014 Apr 2. PMID: 24691854.

9. MacNeil SD, Patel K, Liu K, et al. Survival of patients with subglottic squamous cell carcinoma. Curr Oncol 2018;25(6):e569–75. Epub 2018 Dec 1. PMID: 30607125; PMCID: PMC6291284.

10. Pou A. "Total Laryngectomy." In Oper Otolaryngol Head Neck Surg, 16, 118-123. E1.

11. LoTempio MM, Wang KH, Sadeghi A, et al. Comparison of quality of life outcomes in laryngeal cancer patients following chemoradiation vs. total laryngectomy. Otolaryngol Head Neck Surg 2005;132(6):948–53.

12. Hasan Z, Dwivedi RC, Gunaratne DA, et al. Systematic review and meta-analysis of the complications of salvage total laryngectomy. Eur J Surg Oncol 2017;43(1): 42–51. Epub 2016 May 27. PMID: 27265037.

13. Xie J, Wu P, Liu H, et al. Thyroid gland invasion in total laryngectomy: A systematic review and meta-analysis. Int J Surg 2022;99:106262. Epub 2022 Feb 13. PMID: 35172203.

14. Crosetti E, Fantini M, Maldi E, et al. Open partial horizontal laryngectomy using CO_2 fiber laser. Head Neck 2019;41(8):2830–4. Epub 2019 May 8. PMID: 31066480.

15. Lucioni M, D'Ascanio L, De Nardi E, et al. Management of paratracheal lymph nodes in laryngeal cancer with subglottic involvement. Head Neck 2018;40(1): 24–33. Epub 2017 Sep 27. PMID: 28960661.

16. Chabrillac E, Jackson R, Mattei P, et al. Paratracheal lymph node dissection during total (pharyngo-)laryngectomy: A systematic review and meta-analysis. Oral Oncol 2022;132:106017. Epub 2022 Jul 10. PMID: 35830760.

17. Medina JE, Ferlito A, Robbins KT, et al. Central compartment dissection in laryngeal cancer. Head Neck 2011;33(5):746–52. Epub 2010 Jul 22. PMID: 20652888.

18. Paisley S, Warde PR, O'Sullivan B, et al. Results of radiotherapy for primary subglottic squamous cell carcinoma. Int J Radiat Oncol Biol Phys 2002;52(5): 1245–50.

19. Dixon LM, Douglas CM, Shaukat SI, et al. Conventional fractionation should not be the standard of care for T2 glottic cancer. Radiat Oncol 2017;12(1):178. PMID: 29137654; PMCID: PMC5686811.
20. Hata M, Taguchi T, Koike I, et al. Efficacy and toxicity of (chemo)radiotherapy for primary subglottic cancer. Strahlenther Onkol 2013;189(1):26–32. Epub 2012 Nov 18. PMID: 23161117.
21. Yang F, He L, Rao Y, et al. Survival analysis of patients with subglottic squamous cell carcinoma based on the SEER database. Braz J Otorhinolaryngol 2021; S1808-S8694(21):00167–71. Epub ahead of print. PMID: 34716102.
22. Komatsubara Y, Tachibana T, Orita Y, et al. Clinical characteristics of subglottic cancer: emphasis on therapeutic management strategies for stage II subglottic cancer. Acta Otolaryngol 2020;140(9):773–8. Epub 2020 Jun 3. PMID: 32491952.
23. Hirasawa N, Itoh Y, Ishihara S, et al. Radiotherapy with or without chemotherapy for patients with T1-T2 glottic carcinoma: retrospective analysis. Head Neck Oncol 2010;2:20. PMID: 20673360; PMCID: PMC2919535.
24. Jhawar SR, Bonomi M, Harari PM. Treating Advanced Head and Neck Cancer When Cisplatin Is Not an Option. J Clin Oncol 2021;39(1):7–12.
25. Bonomi MR, Blakaj A, Blakaj D. Organ preservation for advanced larynx cancer: A review of chemotherapy and radiation combination strategies. Oral Oncol 2018; 86:301–6.
26. Campbell G, Glazer TA, Kimple RJ, et al. Advances in Organ Preservation for Laryngeal Cancer. Curr Treat Options Oncol 2022;23(4):594–608. Epub 2022 Mar 18. PMID: 35303749; PMCID: PMC9405127.

The Role of Robotic Surgery in Laryngeal Cancer

Wei Jia, MBchB, BSC, MRCS (ENT), PGcert*, Emma King, FRCS, PhD

KEYWORDS

- Larynx • Laryngectomy • TORS • Robotic surgery • Cordectomy
- Supraglottic laryngectomy

KEY POINTS

- Transoral robotic surgery (TORS) is a minimally invasive technique that offers many technical advantages over transoral laser microsurgery (TLM).
- The feasibility of TORS supraglottic laryngectomy, cordectomy, and laryngectomy has been proven; more research is required to determine the long-term oncological and functional outcomes.
- TORS cordectomy has a higher complication rate than TLM; better technology or techniques are required to justify replacing TLM.

INTRODUCTION

Transoral robotic surgery (TORS) is a growing field in the treatment of head and neck cancers. Its use for the treatment of early oropharyngeal cancer is well established in the literature.[1] For early HPV-positive squamous cell carcinomas (SCCs) of the oropharynx, the application of TORS can potentially replace the need for chemoradiation or reduce the dosage required, thus leading to decreased late sequelae of chemoradiation for patients. For oropharynx cancers, TORS has helped to usher primary surgery back to the forefront of early-stage oropharyngeal cancer treatment. Treatment of larynx cancers has historically been open approaches or chemoradiation. The introduction of transoral laser microsurgery (TLM) in the larynx has changed the management of larynx cancers. This minimally invasive technique has allowed organ preservation and improved quality of life for patients. Oncological outcomes for TLM, open surgery, and chemoradiation are similar,[2] which makes the transoral minimal approach very appealing for the treatment of larynx cancers. Driven by the good TLM outcomes in the treatment of larynx cancer, institutions have sought to apply the same concept with TORS. Although the current evidence is not extensive, institutions are increasingly exploring its role in the management of laryngeal cancers and

ENT Department, Poole Hospital, Longfleet Road, Poole BH15 2JB, UK
* Corresponding author.
E-mail address: wei.jia@nhs.net

Otolaryngol Clin N Am 56 (2023) 313–322
https://doi.org/10.1016/j.otc.2022.12.010
0030-6665/23/© 2023 Elsevier Inc. All rights reserved.

using this technology for its apparent advantages. Specifically, in the larynx, TORS can be used to resect supraglottic and glottic tumors. Specific TORS procedures in the larynx include transoral robotic supraglottic laryngectomy, TOR cordectomy, and TOR laryngectomy.

Treatment Goals of Transoral Robotic Surgery

- To achieve cure via good oncological resection with negative margins.
- To aim for single modality treatment if possible, for example, TOR-SGL with negative margins and neck dissections.
- To reduce morbidity as associated with open procedures or chemoradiation.
- To preserve the anatomical and neurophysiological functions of the larynx (voice, breathing, and swallowing).
- To achieve long-term cure rates.
- To reduce complications and hospital stay.

Comparisons with Transoral Laser Microsurgery

TORS shares many of the principles as TLM as a technique. There are advantages that TORS offers over TLM. TORS provides superior visualization of the operative field via a wide field view while still also magnifying the area of interest. This is especially appreciated in large tumors where the boundaries extend beyond the margins of the laryngoscope. The ability to replicate three dimensional (3D) vision is also beneficial to the surgeon. Adjusting the endoscopic view of the robot is much more ergonomic compared with the microscope adjustments required in TLM surgery.

Greater degrees of movement and rotation of the robotic wrists provide increased dexterity thus allowing a greater degree of maneuverability that is not possible with TLM. TORS also eliminates the tremor sometimes noted under the microscope in TLM cases requiring the use of long instruments. For larger lesions, TORS allows the possibility of en-bloc resection as well as suturing to close defects. Suturing is also a possibility in the larynx to close defects. The two arms of the robot also mimic the two-handed surgical experience compared with TLM.

However, TORS is more expensive and not readily available at all centers. It can be associated with increased procedure time due to set up time. Working in the distal larynx (glottis) requires optimum access. Current robotic systems with two robotic arms and a camera may crowd the operative field and limited visibility. Newer single port systems may overcome this problem.

Education and Training

TORS also provides an improved learning experience. Robots have two modules where the trainee surgeon can observe a first person's view of the primary operative field in 3D. Some of the newer machines also allow the transfer of control between primary surgeon and trainee surgeon, allowing a controlled environment for learning, this surgical technique. Training modules on the robotic systems allow simulation training which allows a standardized training program.

TRANSORAL ROBOTIC SUPRAGLOTTIC LARYNGECTOMY

Outside of oropharyngeal cancers, transoral robotic supraglottic laryngectomy (TOR-SGL) is the most common indication. Most TORS performed in the larynx are done for early (T1–T2) supraglottic lesions and some T3 tumors, to allow for complete en-bloc resection with negative margins, while at the same time preserving the anatomical and neurophysiological functions of the glottic larynx. TOR-SGL shares the same principles as TLM. Depending on the location and the size of the tumor, the technique should be adapted to the particular needs of the patient. The European Laryngological Society (ELS) classification for SGL can be used as a frame work for surgical resection (**Fig. 1**).[3]

A review by LeChien and colleagues[4] pooled 422 patients with SCC treated with TOR-SGL. The tumor location mainly consisted of epiglottis (55.4%), aryepiglottic fold (31.2%), and ventricular band (5.1%). TOR-SGL was performed mainly for T1 (35.8%) and T2 (48.6%), with some T3 (13.9%) and no T4 tumors. Commonest ELS procedure performed includes type I (13.4%), type II (21.7%), type III (19.3%), and type IV classification for endoscopic supraglottic laryngectomy (45.7%). Lechien and colleagues[4] concluded the survival outcomes of supraglottic laryngectomies performed on patients with scc of the supraglottis, outlined **Table 1**.[4] A review by Turner and colleagues[5] identified 503 patients who underwent TOR-SGL for SCC of the larynx. Two hundred ninety-five patients (58.65%) underwent concurrent neck dissection, whereas 131 patients (26.04%) underwent delayed neck dissections. Two hundred twenty-three patients (44.33%) required bilateral neck dissections, whereas 174 (29.22%) were treated with unilateral, ipsilateral neck dissection. Many patients also required adjuvant chemoradiation or radiation. 1.7% of cases were for recurrent SCC of supraglottis as a salvage procedure. The mean hospital stay was 9.53 days (3.9–15.1 days). Positive margin rate was identified in 5.4% of patients. Intraoperative blood loss was estimated to be between 9.4 and 200 mL. The mean operative time for tumor resection varied from 25.3 to 124.0 minutes. The mean setup time ranged from 5.0 to 40.0 minutes. The 24 month local and regional control rates ranged from 94.3 to 100% and 87.5% to 94.0%, respectively. The 2- year and 5- year overall survival rates ranged from 66.7% to 88.0% and 78.7% to 80.2%, respectively.

Functional Outcomes

Functional outcomes after TOR-SGL are limited in the literature and available studies are heterogeneous in nature. The resumption of oral intake varies between day 1 and 5.3 weeks. Feeding tube and percutaneous endoscopic gastrostomy are used in 62.5% and 8.82% of patients, respectively.[4]

Complications

Bleeding following TOR-SGL can be catastrophic due to hemorrhage or airway obstruction. A review by Turner and colleagues[5] identified a bleed rate of 3.74% in 503 patients. Two-thirds of this group required surgical intervention. This was most often managed by transoral clipping or cautery of the internal branch of the superior laryngeal artery. On average, this happened around day 10 (range of 2–14 days). Three patients' deaths related to massive hemorrhage. Two patients had surgical tracheostomies to secure the airway. No use of interventional radiological embolization of bleeding vessels was reported 103 of 303 patients (33.9%) were treated with elective intraoperative tracheostomy.

There is heterogeneity in the reasoning for the placement of tracheostomy tubes in different centers. Some centers routinely performed tracheostomy for all patients (Park and colleagues[16]). Other groups did so for selected patients only. Concurrent bilateral neck dissection has been identified as a risk factor for tracheostomy due to an increased risk of post-op airway edema. The other reasons for a prophylactic tracheostomy were to anticipate for airway compromise or postoperative hemorrhage, surgeon's discretion for large resections, and difficult intubation due to trismus and patients with a high risk for aspiration. Decannulation rate was around 12 days. In this review, there were also centers that do not routinely use planned tracheostomy.

T1	For excision of small superficial tumours of the supraglottis (any part of the supraglottis including free border of the epiglottis, the aryepiglottic fold, the arytenoid or the ventricular fold). Wide local excision around the lesion with a margin.	
T2a	Partial epiglottectomy: For small T1 tumours on the laryngeal surface of the epiglottis located above the hyoid bone. Excise the superior portion of the epiglottis above the hyoid bone with a margin.	
T2b	Total epiglottectomy: For tumours extending below the hyoid bone, a total epiglottectomy is performed. The section line goes through the pre-epiglottic space without its complete excision. The pharyngo-epiglottic, ary-epiglottic and ventricular folds are preserved	
T3a	The resection of T1–T2 tumors extending to the petiole of the epiglottis must include the pre-epiglottic space with the steps mentioned above.	
T3b	T1–T2 tumors of the infrahyoid epiglottis extending to the ventricular fold can be resected with the same technique (Type 3a). The ventricular folds can be completely dissected from the thyroid cartilage along the inner surface towards the ventricle of Morgagni	
Type 4 a	Tumours of the threefolds' region (lateral free edge of the epiglottis, the ary-epiglottic fold and the pharyngo-epiglottic fold) with possible extension to the ventricular folds, the resection includes the free edge of the epiglottis, the threefolds' region and the ventricular fold	
Type 4b	Type 4a resection including arytenoid excision with medial or anterior piriform fossa mucosa if necessary	

Table 1 Survival outcomes of transoral robotic surgery supraglottic laryngectomy for supraglottic squamous cell carcinoma[4]			
Disease outcomes		Disease outcomes	Disease outcomes
12-month local control	92.3%–98.0%	2-y Overall Survival	66.7%–88.0%
24-month local control	94.3%–100%	2-y Disease free survival	91.0%–95.1%
24-month regional control	87.5%–94.0%	5-y Overall Survival	78.7%–80.2%
5-y local control	90.2%–93.2%	5-y Disease free survival	94.3%
5-y regional control	87.7%–89.2%	2-y rate of distant metastasis	<9%

Instead, some use prolonged intubation for 24 to 36 hours or immediate intubation following surgery. The conclusion was that prophylactic perioperative tracheotomy largely depends on surgeon experience and/or preference. Other complications included aspiration pneumonia (6.56%, the commonest), temporary emergency tracheostomy (3.38%), tracheostomy dependence (1.39%), laryngeal stenosis (0.99%), and reports of bilateral temporary vocal fold immobility.

The evidence for TOR-SGL is encouraging to support its use. It is not possible to make direct comparisons for different staging groups. Multicentered comparative studies are needed to evaluate the oncological and functional role of TOR-SGL.

Transoral Robotic Cordectomy

There has been an evolution of treatment over the last century for treatment of early larynx SCC, moving from open procedures such as the transcervical partial laryngectomy to chemoradiotherapy, with the hope for organ preservation, back to minimally invasive and organ preservation techniques such as TLM. The introduction of TLM has revolutionized the management of early glottic cancer. It can provide similar oncological outcomes as open surgery and radiotherapy +/- chemotherapy.[6] It is organ preserving and mitigates the long-term sequelae of radiation therapy. TOR cordectomy is a new arm under the umbrella of minimally invasive surgery introduced over the last decade. However, TLM remains the gold-standard surgical approach for the treatment of early glottic carcinoma. Nonetheless, different institutions have sought to demonstrate the use of TORS for the treatment of glottic cancers. Unlike supraglottic cancers, glottic cancers require more exposure as it is more distal in the larynx compared with the more capacious supraglottis. The use of TORS shares many of the similar principles as TLM. Patient selection is the key, and the right exposure is required.

The evidence in the literature for transoral robotic cordectomy is limited to a handful of retrospective or prospective case series only. The only review to date by Lechien and colleagues[7] looked at the current evidence for TOR cordectomy; 114 patients in total were included. The type of cordectomy performed was classified using the ELS classification (Fig. 2).[8,17] Types 2 to 6 were carried out for T1–T2 lesions. Conversion to transoral laser surgery was 4%. This was due to access either the length of the robotic arms was insufficient or a prominent tongue base impeded surgical access.

Fig. 1. ELS classification for supraglottic laryngectomy. (*Adapted from* Remacle, M., Hantzakos, A., Eckel, H. et al. Endoscopic supraglottic laryngectomy: a proposal for a classification by the working committee on nomenclature, European Laryngological Society. Eur Arch Otorhinolaryngol 266, 993–998 (2009). https://doi.org/10.1007/s00405-008-0901-8.)

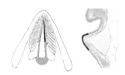 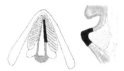 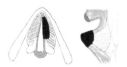

| Subepithelial cordectomy (type I) | Subligamental cordectomy (type II) | Transmuscular cordectomy (type III). In order to expose the entire vocal fold, partial resection of the ventricular fold may be necessary (grey area) to improve access |

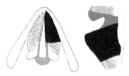

Total or complete cordectomy (type IV). The ipsilateral ventricular fold can be removed partially or totally to ensure complete resection of the vocal fold (grey area)

Extended cordectomy encompassing the contralateral vocal fold (type Va). The extent of the resected contralateral vocal fold depends on the extent of the tumour

Extended cordectomy encompassing the arytenoid (type Vb)

Extended cordectomy encompassing the ventricular fold (type Vc). The inferior resection of the vocal fold is maximum

Extended cordectomy encompassing the subglottis to a distance of 1 cm (type Vd). Partial resection of the ventricular fold may be necessary (grey area) to improve access

Resection of the anterior commissure (Type VI)

Fig. 2. ELS classification for cordectomy. (*Adapted from* Remacle M, Eckel HE, et.al. Endoscopic cordectomy. A proposal for a classification by the Working Committee, European Laryngological Society. Eur Arch Otorhinolaryngol. 2000;257(4):227-31. https://doi.org/10.1007/s004050050228. PMID: 10867840 and Remacle M, Van Haverbeke C, Eckel H, Bradley P, Chevalier D, Djukic V, de Vicentiis M, Friedrich G, Olofsson J, Peretti G, Quer M, Werner J et.al. Proposal for revision of the European Laryngological Society classification of endoscopic cordectomies. Eur Arch Otorhinolaryngol. 2007 May;264(5):499-504. doi: 10.1007/s00405-007-0279-z. Epub 2007 Mar 22. Erratum in: Eur Arch Otorhinolaryngol. 2007 Jun;264(6):709. PMID: 17377801.)

The robot installation and vocal fold exposure time ranged from 26 to 42 minutes, and the procedure time ranged from10 to 40 minutes. Blood loss was noted to be 10 to 20 mL.

There was a great deal of heterogeneity in the pooled outcome measures in the review paper by Lechien and colleagues.[7] Positive margins were identified in 4.5% (three cases out of the reported cases on this measure). Local recurrence occurred in 10.7% ($N = 8/75$). The mean hospital stay was 3.25 days (range 2–7 days). Tracheotomy was required in 22.3% of patients ($N = 25$, out of the cases that reported this measure) and removed after a mean of 7.1 days. Feeding tube was required in 15.8% (15 patients out of the cases that reported this measure) and was removed after a mean of 9.3 days. Gastrostomy was used in one patient. The complication rate was 12.6% which included granuloma, postoperative bleeding, dyspnea, synechia, tongue hematoma, and dysesthesia. Overall, local recurrence occurred in 10.7% ($N = 8/75$). No conclusions about the overall survival were available.

The higher tracheostomy and feeding tube rates reported after using Da Vinci S, Si, Xi, or Medrobotics robot systems are an important limiting factor to support the routine use of TORS in glottic cancers. Owing to the heterogeneity of outcome measures and few numbers of patients in the studies, it is not possible to draw any concrete conclusions. The low positive margin rate and local reoccurrence rate compared with TLM are encouraging. More research in terms of direct comparisons with controlled measures is required to gain further insight into this. One theory of higher complication rate is the high thermal injury to surrounding tissue via the cautery techniques, leading to more tissue swelling, trauma, and scarring therefore more tracheostomy rates. Newer robotic systems such as the single-port robots may allow better exposure.[9] The combined use of TORS and lasers may further reduce the prementioned morbidity and access problem. More research is needed on this area to truly determine the short-term and long-term outcomes.

Transoral Robotic Laryngectomy

Similar to the use of TORS in the treatment of early glottic cancers, the place of TORS for total laryngectomy is not yet well-defined. There is only a five-case series demonstrating the feasibility of transoral robotic laryngectomy (TOR-LG).[10–14] The aim of the robotic laryngectomy is to reduce the treatment-related morbidities of the open procedures and improve the quality of life of patients. The theoretic treatment goals specific to TOR-LG are to reduce the pharyngocutaneous fistula rate, via smaller pharyngotomy incisions. By sparing more mucosa, this can potentially lead to a shorter healing time. Having maximum mucosa preserved allows for more of a horizontal closure, leading to a more capacious neopharynx, thus less likely to develop strictures. Second, a saliva leak laterally from a fistula into the vascular compartment can lead to complications such as pseudoaneurysms and carotid blowout. The TORS approach can lead to more natural barriers such as the fascia being left intact, thus reducing the likelihood of this.

Most of the patients requiring a laryngectomy are for locally advanced SCC of the larynx with or without neck disease. Bilateral neck dissections are often required. The benefits of a minimally invasive approach are therefore questionable in this setting. The precise indications for TOR-LG are yet to be well-defined. For specific situations where neck dissections can be avoided, TOR-LG may have a role.[15] Firstly, in the setting of salvage surgery for recurrent SCC following the local failure of radiotherapy or chemoradiotherapy, where there is no radiological or clinical neck disease. In this setting, primary closure without the need for a flap reconstruction is possible. There must be no invasion of the thyroid cartilage, so that of the infrahyoid muscles can be preserved. Secondly, in rare benign or malignant cancers of the larynx, where there is a limited local extension potential. Some examples include adenoid cystic carcinoma and low-grade chondrosarcoma or chondroma. Thirdly, laryngeal failure with recurrent aspirations, long-term tracheostomies, and enteral feeding. The pathologies involved in these cases include neurodegenerative disease, severe chemoradiotherapy toxicity, with or without chondronecrosis, and patients with laryngeal stenosis who have had multiple procedures, including tracheostomy.

A combined total of 25 cases of TOR-LG cases have been reported in five series.[10–14] The procedure could not be completed in four additional cases due to inadequate exposure: one was converted to the open approach and the other was presumed to be converted to open, as the authors completed the superior resection transorally, but did not explicitly state if open conversion was used. Two cases were excluded by the Hans and colleagues[14] group due to inadequate exposure. They advise preprocedure assessment with the Feyh-Kastenbauer retractors for all cases in order to adequately assess the larynx.

Fistula rates were reported in 25% of the cases (5/25). Three patients had prior radiotherapy, one had laryngeal stenosis, and one had a dysfunctional larynx. Two patients had post-op bleeding, with one reported occurrence at day 9, which required return to theater for cauterization; 18 patients had swallow outcomes reported. In the largest series of 10 patients by Hans and colleagues, all had their nasogastric tubes removed within a mean of 9.3 days (6–24 days), without gastrostomy insertion. The other series reported oral feeding outcomes between 7 to 21 days and 10 to 12 days. Two patients in the Krishnan and colleagues group were gastrostomy dependent before TOR-LG due to neurological conditions. Out of the reported outcomes, 14 patients reported tracheoesophageal voice use and 2 reported esophageal voice use. Two had nonfunctional voice capability due to neurological disease. There were mixtures of primary and secondary punctures. The rest did not have outcomes reported.

The mean length of stay in three series was 9.6, 13.9, and 21 days. The average total operative times from the three groups were 4 hours 58 minutes, 4 hours 32 minutes, and 4 hours 22 minutes. Hans and colleagues had the largest series ($n = 10$) for oncological outcomes. There were no reported local recurrences at 5 years for the recurrent larynx SCC group ($n = 5$). One patient had distant metastasis and died at 5 years. One had local typo-recurrence of chondrosarcoma at 3 years. All patients had adequate pathological margins as reported at the time of surgery. Krishnan and colleagues reported free margins for the three patients operated on due to cancer in their series. The first patient had an rT2N0M0 SCC, the second patient had an adenoid cystic carcinoma, and the third patient had a low-grade chondrosarcoma. They were still alive and disease-free 54, 54, and 18 months, respectively, after the surgery.

Early reports have demonstrated the feasibility and safety of TOR-LG for a selected group of patients. This includes the salvage laryngectomy for recurrent SCC, rare low-grade tumors of the larynx, and nonfunctional larynx. A simultaneous neck dissection should not be required in TOR-LG. To date, the number of cases is far too few to draw any meaningful conclusions about the long-term outcomes and its benefits compared with the open approaches. Future multicenter-controlled studies are needed to determine the strengths and weaknesses of TOR-LG over open LG.

DISCUSSION

TORS as a minimally invasive procedure for the treatment of laryngeal cancer has been shown to be feasible for selected patients. TORS for supraglottic cancers has the most amount of evidence to support its role as primary treatment. The data are very heterogeneous and concrete conclusions cannot be drawn given the low-level evidence available. This is applicable to TORS cordectomy and laryngectomy. It has the potential to play a much bigger role in the treatment of laryngeal cancers, if more robust and randomized data can prove this. With glottic cancer, perhaps with better technological improvements, the associated complication rates can be reduced, making it comparable with TLM. As a minimally invasive surgical tool, it offers many operator advantages compared with TLM, thus making it a very effective tool for surgeons.

CLINICS CARE POINTS

- Transoral supraglottic laryngectomy is the commonest robotic procedure for SCC of the larynx. ELS classification for supraglottic laryngectomy can be used as a guide for excision.

- Transoral cordectomy shares the same principles as transoral laser microsurgery. ELS classification for cordectomy can be used as a guide for tumour excision.

- Indications for transoral robotic laryngectomy include recurrent SCC of the larynx without cervical node metastasis, non-functioning larynx causing aspiration and or rare benign and malignant cancers of the larynx with limited local extension potential.

DISCLOSURE

No funding was required.

REFERENCES

1. Garas G, Tolley N. Robotics in otorhinolaryngology - head and neck surgery. Ann R Coll Surg Engl 2018;100(Suppl 7):34–41.
2. Hartl DM, Ferlito A, Brasnu DF, et al. Evidence-based review of treatment options for patients with glottic cancer. Head Neck 2011;33:1638–48.
3. Remacle M, Hantzakos A, Eckel H, et al. Endoscopic supraglottic laryngectomy: a proposal for a classification by the working committee on nomenclature, European Laryngological Society. Eur Arch Otorhinolaryngol 2009;266:993–8.
4. Lechien JR, Fakhry N, Saussez S, et al. Surgical, clinical and functional outcomes of transoral robotic surgery for supraglottic laryngeal cancers: a systematic review. Oral Oncol 2020;109:104848.
5. Turner MT, Stokes WA, Stokes CM, et al. Airway and bleeding complications of transoral robotic supraglottic laryngectomy (TORS-SGL): a systematic review and meta-analysis. Oral Oncol 2021;118:105301.
6. Hans S, Baudouin R, Circiu MP, et al. Laryngeal cancer surgery: history and current indications of transoral laser microsurgery and transoral robotic surgery. J Clin Med 2022;11(19):5769.
7. Lechien JR, Baudoin R, Circiu MP, et al. Transoral robotic cordectomy for glottic carcinoma: a rapid review. Eur Arch Otorhinolaryngol 2022;279(11):5449–56.
8. Remacle M, Eckel HE, Antonelli A, et al. Endoscopic cordectomy. a proposal for a classification by the Working Committee, European Laryngological Society. Eur Arch Otorhinolaryngol 2000;257(4):227–31.
9. Remacle M, Prasad VMN, Lawson G, et al. Transoral robotic surgery (TORS) with the Medrobotics Flex™ System: first surgical application on humans. Eur Arch Otorhinolaryngol 2015;272(6):1451–5.
10. Smith RV, Schiff BA, Sarta C, et al. Transoral robotic total laryngectomy. Laryngoscope 2013;123:678–82.
11. Dowthwaite S, Nichols AC, Yoo J, et al. Transoral robotic total laryngectomy: report of 3 cases. Head Neck 2013;35:E338–42.
12. Krishnan G, Krishnan S. Transoral robotic surgery total laryngectomy: evaluation of functional and survival outcomes in a retrospective case series at a single institution. ORL J Otorhinolaryngol Relat Spec 2017;79:191–201.
13. Lawson G, Mendelsohn A, Fakhoury R, et al. Transoral robotic surgery total laryngectomy. ORL J Otorhinolaryngol Relat Spec 2018;80:171–7.

14. Hans S, Chebib E, Chekkoury-Idrissi Y, et al. Surgical and oncological outcomes of transoral robotic total laryngectomy: a case series. Oral Oncol 2021;121: 105511.

15. Gorphe P. A contemporary review of evidence for transoral robotic surgery in laryngeal cancer. Front Oncol 2018;8:121.

16. Park YM, Kim WS, Byeon HK, et al. Surgical techniques and treatment outcomes of transoral robotic supraglottic partial laryngectomy. Laryngoscope 2013;123(3): 670–7.

17. Remacle M, Van Haverbeke C, Eckel H, et al. Proposal for revision of the European Laryngological Society classification of endoscopic cordectomies. Eur Arch Otorhinolaryngol 2007;264(5):499–504.

Salvage Surgery

Somtochi Okafor, MD[a], Oluwaseyi O. Awaonusi[b],
Tammara L. Watts, MD, PhD[a], Trinitia Y. Cannon, MD[a,c],*

KEYWORDS

- Laryngeal cancer • Chemoradiation therapy • Tracheal esophageal puncture
- Elective neck dissection • Pectoralis major myocutaneous/myofascial flap

INTRODUCTION

During the last several decades, the primary treatment of advanced laryngeal cancers has been in the favor of organ preservation therapy.[1,2] This has included primary radiation therapy, concurrent chemoradiation therapy, and/or surgery with endoscopic microsurgical approaches. The risk of persistent or recurrent disease after such preservation approaches ranges from 25% to 50%.[3] In patients with recurrent or residual squamous cell carcinoma of the larynx, salvage total laryngectomy remains one of the few viable options for management.

BACKGROUND

Laryngeal cancer is one of the most common sites of malignancy presenting in the head and neck, affecting more than 175,000 patients worldwide.[4] It has an age-standardized incidence rate of 5.0/100,000 among men and 0.7/100,000 among women.[4] In 1873, in Vienna, Austria, Theodor Billroth performed the first successful laryngectomy. Before this novel procedure, laryngeal cancer was deemed a fatal disease with a palliative tracheostomy as its only treatment option. During the early developments of the procedure, mortality rates were as high as 39% to 54%.[5,6] Although minimally invasive techniques and advancements in radiation therapy have changed the scope of practice for some patients, surgical management of laryngeal cancer remains the only viable option for patients with contraindications for standard of care chemoradiation.

Surgical approaches such as total laryngopharyngectomy remained the mainstay of treatment until the landmark Veterans Administration (VA) Laryngeal Cancer Study Group trial in 1993[1] and the Radiation Therapy Oncology Group 91-11 (RTOG 91–

[a] Department of Head and Neck Surgery & Communication Sciences, Duke University Health System, 2301 Erwin Road, Durham, NC 27710, USA; [b] Indian University, School of Medicine, 340 West 10th Street, Indianapolis, IN 46202, USA; [c] Department of Head and Neck Surgery & Communication Sciences, Duke Raleigh Hospital, 3404 Wake Forest Road Suite 202, Raleigh, NC 27609, USA
* Corresponding author. Department of Head and Neck Surgery & Communication Sciences, Duke Raleigh Hospital, 3404 Wake Forest Road Suite 202, Raleigh, NC 27609.
E-mail address: trinitia.cannon@duke.edu

Otolaryngol Clin N Am 56 (2023) 323–331
https://doi.org/10.1016/j.otc.2022.12.002
0030-6665/23/© 2022 Elsevier Inc. All rights reserved.

11) trial in 2003.[2,7] Novel data from both studies supported the use of nonsurgical organ preservation therapies as adequate treatment in selected patients with advanced laryngeal disease.[8] New research and advancements have permitted combination and choice of treatment modalities to expand beyond surgery to include radiation with or without chemotherapy as viable treatment options based on the presenting stage. Since the publication of this data, standard treatment of primary disease has shifted toward nonsurgical organ-preserving modalities with chemotherapy and radiation therapy.[4] Surgery with partial or total laryngectomy is reserved for persistent or recurrent disease following organ preservation approaches and is considered salvage. Given laryngeal cancer recurrence rates ranging from 16% to 50%, salvage laryngectomy remains one of the most common definitive treatment options following failed primary nonsurgical organ preserving treatment.[9,10]

Surgical Technique

A u-shaped incision is made from mastoid tip to mastoid tip. Often the incision is made approximately 1 cm above the planned stoma or current surgical tracheostomy site to have some skin separating the stoma from the incision. Others will incorporate the incision into the stoma to avoid the possibility of skin loss. Subplatysmal flaps are elevated superiorly above the hyoid bone and the skin is folded. Inferiorly, skin flaps are dissected to the clavicles and retracted.

Next, the inferior aspect of the infrahyoid muscles is divided. The decision to perform a hemithyroidectomy or total thyroidectomy is determined based on the perioperative imaging. If staging imaging shows no invasion of the thyroid gland and/or no subglottic extension, the thyroid gland is divided at the isthmus and moved laterally to access the trachea. Preservation of the inferior thyroid vessels allows for adequate blood supply to the thyroid and parathyroid glands. For direct thyroid invasion and/or subglottic extension, a hemithyroidectomy or total thyroidectomy is performed depending on the extent of the spread. The trachea is transected between the second and the third tracheal rings. The decision to make the tracheal cuts lower will be based on any subglottic extension. The distal end is brought forward to create the stoma. The proximal end is bluntly dissected free of the esophagus. The posterior cricoid mucosa is dissected off the posterior cricoarytenoid muscle.

If a neck dissection was performed first, the fibrofatty tissue is now brought in bloc over the lateral aspects of the thyroid cartilage. The pharyngeal constrictors are dissected off the thyroid cartilage. The laryngeal vessels are ligated. The pyriform sinus mucosa is separated from the laryngeal framework.

Superiorly, the suprahyoid musculature is divided. Placement of a small Deever into the mouth aids in identification of the pre-epiglottic space. The pre-epiglottic space is opened transversely at the level of the hyoid. The epiglottis is grasped and retracted inferiorly to allow for direct visualization of the supraglottic larynx. Dissection is carried out laterally from the point of entry to allow for macroscopic removal of the tumor with a minimum of 0.5-cm margins. Using curved heavy Mayo scissors, the pharyngeal incisions are extended inferiorly on either side of the thyroid cartilage to the level of the cricoid.

The aforementioned technique describes entering the larynx through a transverse pharyngotomy at the level of the hyoid; however, the location of the primary tumor and involvement of adjacent structures ultimately determines the entry point. For example, laryngeal tumors with involvement of the vallecula may require the surgeon to enter the larynx inferiorly at the level of the trachea or laterally at the level of the pyriform sinuses.

The larynx is removed and sent for pathological inspection of the margins. A cricopharyngeal myotomy may be performed and the stoma is created. If the patient is a candidate for a primary tracheal esophageal puncture (TEP), this is usually performed along with placement of a prosthesis, after the stoma is created. However, some patients, especially those with wound healing concerns, may not be ideal candidates for a TEP at the time of total laryngectomy, and this can be performed as a secondary procedure at any time in the future.

Neck Dissection in Salvage Laryngectomy

The decision to perform an elective neck dissection (END), levels II-IV, at the time of surgical salvage remains controversial. The controversy is understandable because the risk of postsurgical complications remain high. According to Lin C and colleagues, (2019),[11] the relative risk (RR) of postoperative complication with END compared with observation was 1.72 (95% CI = 0.96–3.10, P = .07). However, because the rate of nodal metastasis in patients undergoing neck dissection in the salvage setting ranges from 0% to 31% in clinically N0 (cN0) patients, some authors elect to proceed with an END.[12–20]

In a retrospective review of 98 patients with neither clinical nor radiologic evidence of disease, positive nodal disease was identified on final pathology in ~10 of these patients.[21] The presence of microscopic nodal disease was associated with worse overall survival without an increased risk of complications.[21] The highest rates of occult nodal metastasis were seen in patients with advanced T-stage (T3/T4) and those with supraglottic cancers.[11] Moreover, Birkeland and colleagues, retrospectively reviewed 203 cN0 patients undergoing salvage total laryngectomy, and the risk of nodal metastasis was associated with advanced staged supraglottic. In this series, 50% of patients with T4 supraglottic disease had microscopic metastasis to regional lymph nodes compared with 21% of early stage T1/T2 tumors.[20] Therefore, it is our opinion that patients undergoing salvage laryngectomy should be considered for END.

Repair and Reconstruction

A total laryngectomy will result in some degree of pharyngeal mucosal loss, either partial or total. The remaining pharyngeal defect can then be closed primarily, for those with enough residual pharyngeal mucosa. However, vascularized flap reconstruction of the pharynx may be necessary to augment mucosa after extensive resection and/or to mitigate complications following radiation exposure. In cases where primary pharyngeal closure is possible, flaps may also be used to reinforce the closure or as an onlay to decrease fistula formation. The type of flap, either locoregional pedicled flaps or microvascular fee tissue transfer, is usually dependent on the degree of mucosal involvement, body habitus, and patient comorbidities.

In 1996, Hui Y and colleagues[22] measured the pharyngeal remnants of 52 patients following a total laryngectomy with partial pharyngectomy to determine how much residual tissue is needed for a primary closure free from dysphagia. They concluded that a minimum of 1.5 cm of relaxed or 2.5 cm of stretched mucosa was needed for primary closure. The same authors also reviewed each type of rotational and free flap available to aid in pharyngeal closure and their outcomes. For patients with significant comorbidities either a pectoralis major myocutaneous/myofascial flap or a supraclavicular artery island flap could be used to reinforce the primary pharyngeal closure. However, no one flap demonstrated superiority over the others.[22] Gonzalez-Orús Álvarez-Morujo R. concluded that prophylactic pectoris major flaps reduced the incidence, severity, and duration of fistula and should be considered during salvage cases.[23] In ongoing efforts to decreased pharyngeal fistula rates, several closure techniques have been devised. Chen DW and colleagues[24] harvested additional fascia from the quadriceps muscle from the anterolateral thigh flap and used it in a multilayered underlay technique as a second layer of closure. This reinforced primary epithelial-mucosal reconstruction reduced to fistula rate to 3% compared with 20% in those who received a single-layered closure.[24]

Postoperative Care and Complications

Following surgery, patients remain hospitalized receiving routine postlaryngectomy care with close monitoring of respiratory status, airway humidification, drain output, surgical site complications, and/or flap assessment.[25] Primary laryngectomy is often associated with postoperative complications such as surgical site infection, drain failure, hematoma, and pharyngocutaneous fistula (PCF).[9] Given prior treatment with chemotherapy and/or radiation therapy and the associated effects on wound healing, patients who undergo salvage laryngectomy are at greater risk of postoperative complications. The pathophysiologic effects of chemoradiation include decreased vascularity, hypoxia, and poorer nutritional and immune status, thus providing a poor foundation for wound healing.[26] In a systematic review by Hasan and colleagues,[27] the overall complication rates for patients who underwent salvage laryngectomy rate was 42% to 67.5%.

Surgical Site Infections

Surgical site infections occur as frequently as 40% to 61% in patients who have undergone salvage laryngectomy.[28] Susceptibility to wound breakdown associated with prior nonsurgical treatment places patients at an increased risk for infection due to subsequent toxicities of chemoradiation therapy. However, in a retrospective study by Scotton and colleagues,[25,28] higher rates of postoperative infection were observed in patients of advanced age, low BMI and albumin levels, who also had a history of tobacco and alcohol use. The majority of surgical site infections are managed with intravenous antibiotics with de-escalation to enteral antibiotics pending culture sensitivities and clinical improvement.

Hematoma

Rates of hematoma range from 5.4% to 11% among patients who have recently undergone salvage laryngectomy.[17,29,30] Patients presenting with hematoma must return to the operating room for surgical exploration and control of bleeding.

Pharyngocutaneous Fistula

For patients undergoing salvage laryngectomy, PCF is one of the most common complications seen with incidence rates similar to those observed for wound infection, bleeding, pharyngeal stenosis/stricture, and dysphagia.[4,5,7] Monitoring drain output is critical for the early identification of PCF, which typically presents with high volume output, turbid fluid, erythema, and edema of the wound closure.[9] Thus, most allow drains to remain in place until output is less than 30 mL over at least 48 hours. In retrospective review of 259 patients who underwent total laryngectomy at the University of Alabama at Birmingham, 56.4% of whom underwent salvage laryngectomy, hypothyroidism and a history of previous radiation treatment were significant risk factors associated with the development of PCF.[31]

Morbidity that arises with PCF consists of delayed initiation of oral diet, prolonged dysphagia, delay in discharge and financial constraints associated with prolonged lengths of stay, and fatal sequela such as carotid blowout.[8,26] Treatment of PCF includes conservative management with daily fistula packing dressings, antibiotics, strict nothing by mouth (NPO) status as well as keeping drains in place to help divert saliva and prevent saliva accumulation.[9] White and colleagues[31] noted 55% of patients who underwent salvage laryngectomy healed with conservative measures over an average of 54 days. Although such patients do not experience additional morbidity associated with another surgical procedure, the protracted hospital course further adds to the financial costs associated with initial surgical treatment as well as further delays clearance to start a diet, which inevitably affects quality of life.

If conservative management proves futile, surgical intervention includes salivary bypass tube placement to divert saliva from accumulating near critical structures (ie, carotid artery) and/or placement of a flap to definitively close such defects. Flap placement offers the benefit of establishing a protective barrier around vital structures such as the great vessels as well as providing well-vascularized tissue and antibacterial properties to an avascular, infected area.[9,23,32] Ultimately, close clinical monitoring following salvage laryngectomy is warranted to monitor for the development of PCF, which can lead to life-threatening consequences if appropriate treatment is not initiated promptly.

Stomal Stenosis and Pharyngoesophageal Stenosis

Late complications following salvage laryngectomy include the development of tracheostomal and pharyngoesophageal stenosis, both of which are a challenge to manage in the salvage setting. Tracheostomal stenosis causes significant distress to patients due to respiratory insufficiency secondary to reduced airflow, subsequent turbulence, and poor secretion clearance.[33] Rates of stoma stenosis following total laryngectomy range from 4% to 42% based on varying definitions of stomal stenosis.[34] Stomal stents may provide temporizing relief of airflow impedance; however, symptomatic patients and those requiring stenting for more than 3 months require surgical revision.[17,29]

Pharyngoesophageal stenosis causes dysphagia, which is known to negatively affect patients' quality of life.[5,35] However, concern for recurrence remains of the utmost priority when a patient status after total laryngectomy presents with pharyngoesophageal stenosis.[9] Once recurrence has been ruled out by panendoscopy and biopsy, further evaluation and treatment of stenosis with dilation may proceed. Various retrospective reviews have associated higher rates of pharyngeal stricture necessitating dilation procedures with patients who underwent salvage total laryngectomy with flap reconstruction.[30,36] Ziegler and colleagues[35] noted patients who underwent salvage laryngectomy with primary closure and an onlay flap fared better with postoperative swallowing results compared with those who underwent procedures with incorporated musculocutaneous flaps. Ziegler and colleagues[35] attributed differences in stricture presentation to additional scarring associated with added suture lines and relative narrowing of the pharynx secondary to added bulky layer of incorporated flap to the neopharynx. Fung and colleagues[36] reported similar findings with higher rates of pharyngeal stricture requiring dilation interventions in their treatment arm that involved flap reconstruction. However, Schuman and colleagues performed a retrospective analysis involving 233 patients who underwent salvage total laryngectomy and reported approximately one-third of patients underwent dilation procedures for pharyngeal stricture. Noted associated factors for the development of stricture postsalvage laryngectomy included the formation of PCF and smoking status before salvage surgery.[37] Ultimately, close follow-up of patients in the postoperative period remains critical for evaluating both stomal and pharyngoesophageal stricture, which present with airway and recurrence concerns, respectively.

Hypothyroidism

Prior radiation therapy as well as hemithyroidectomy place patients at greater risk for hypothyroidism due to toxicity to the thyroid gland and surgical removal, respectively.[9] One study retrospectively reviewed a cohort of 128 patients noting hypothyroidism developed in 84% of patients who underwent salvage laryngectomy and hemithyroidectomy and 38% who underwent salvage laryngectomy without thyroid gland surgery.[38] White and colleagues[26] identified an association between hypothyroidism and postlaryngectomy PCF formation. Thus, thyroid function laboratories must be monitored postoperatively and appropriately treated with thyroid supplementation.

Rehabilitation

Swallowing

Surgical resection of the hyoid and larynx as well as the disruption of the anatomical position between the trachea and esophagus alter the swallowing mechanism and passage of food bolus, thus resulting in dysphagia.[8,39] Given the high risk of developing PCF, oral intake is delayed up to 3 weeks after salvage laryngectomy.[40] However, Eustaquio and colleagues[41] document initiating oral feeds as early as postoperative day 5 following salvage laryngectomy, reporting a fistula rate of 10%. During the initial hospital stay, patients receive enteral nutrition through either nasogastric tube feeding or gastrostomy tube feeding. Once patients have not exhibited evidence of a fistula, they are trialed on liquid PO and gradually diet is advanced accordingly.

Voice

Tracheoesophageal puncture (TEP) with placement of a prosthesis is the most common method of restoring voice after primary and salvage laryngectomies with successful outcomes. Other forms of voice rehabilitation are electrolarynx, esophageal speech, and writing as a means of communication. TEP with voice prosthesis placement can be primary, at the time of total laryngectomy, or secondary, delayed for a few months after wound healing.[42] The timing of the TEP and voice prosthesis placement varies widely among institutions.[10] There is no robust evidence that shows a statistically significant difference in voice outcome based on timing; however, placement of the prosthesis at the time of laryngectomy is associated with increased rates of complications such as leakage and displacement. Some known complications that can affect the success of tracheoesophageal speech are dislocation of the prosthesis and leakage of saliva around the prosthesis.[43] Studies by Starmer and colleagues,[44] show an increased risk of these complications in salvage laryngectomy compared with primary laryngectomy possibly due to the effect of previous radiotherapy exposure on poor wound healing. Early speech and language therapy intervention has been shown to improve a patient's long-term voice outcomes.[43]

SUMMARY

The Department of Veterans Affairs (VA) Laryngeal Cancer Study propelled the combination of chemotherapy and radiation therapy to the forefront of strategies used for management of locally advanced laryngeal cancer. Organ preservation approaches gained further validation as the Intergroup RTOG 91–11 demonstrated that primary concurrent chemoradiation had better outcomes when compared with induction chemotherapy and radiation therapy or primary radiation therapy alone. The organ preservation rate was 84%. However, during the past 30 years that these approaches have been in place, there have been concerns regarding long-term survival and high failure rates requiring salvage. Furthermore, salvage laryngectomy, if feasible when considering increased morbidity after CRT, is fraught with a higher risk of wound complications including fistula, longer hospitalization, and reduced quality of life.

CLINICS CARE POINTS

- Salvage total laryngectomy is a viable treatment option in surgically resectable patients who failed organ preservation approaches.

- The rate of occult nodal metastasis ranges from 0% to 30% with the highest rates seen in those with advanced T-stage and supraglotticcancer. Consider an END in these patients.

- Flap reconstruction is necessary to replace tissue loss, to reinforce mucosal closure, or to prevent complications such as fistula formation.[1]

- The overall complication rate for surgical salvage is as high as 67%.

- Complications for salvage laryngectomy include PCF (most common), wound infection, hematoma, stomal and pharyngoesophageal stenosis, and hypothyroidism.

- Rehabilitation of speech and swallow following salvage surgery is important for good quality of life.

DISCLOSURE

The authors have nothing to disclose.

REFERENCES

1. Department of Veterans Affairs Laryngeal Cancer Study Group, Wolf GT, Fisher SG, Hong WK, et al. Induction chemotherapy plus radiation compared with surgery plus radiation in patients with advanced laryngeal cancer. N Engl J Med 1991;324(24):1685–90.
2. Forastiere AA, Goepfert H, Maor M, et al. Concurrent chemotherapy and radiotherapy for organ preservation in advanced laryngeal cancer. N Engl J Med 2003;349(22):2091–8.
3. Goodwin WJ Jr. Salvage surgery for patients with recurrent squamous cell carcinoma of the upper aerodigestive tract: when do the ends justify the means? Laryngoscope 2000;110(3 Pt 2 Suppl 93):1–18.
4. Deng Y, Wang M, Zhou L, et al. Global burden of larynx cancer, 1990-2017: estimates from the global burden of disease 2017 study. Aging (Albany NY) 2020; 12(3):2545–83.
5. Holinger PH. Panel discussion: the historical development of laryngectomy. V. A century of progress of laryngectomies in the northern hemisphere. Laryngoscope 1975;85(2):322–32.
6. Weir NF. Theodore Billroth: the first laryngectomy for cancer. J Laryngol Otol 1973;87(12):1161–9.
7. Tsetsos N, Poutoglidis A, Vlachtsis K, et al. Twenty-year experience with salvage total laryngectomy: lessons learned. J Laryngol Otol 2021;135(8):729–36.
8. Silverman DA, Puram SV, Rocco JW, et al. Salvage laryngectomy following organ-preservation therapy - An evidence-based review. Oral Oncol 2019;88:137–44.
9. Sievert M, Goncalves M, Binder B, et al. Salvage laryngectomy after primary radio- and radiochemotherapy : a retrospective study. Salvage-Laryngektomie nach primärer Radio- und Radiochemotherapie : eine retrospektive Fallzusammenfassung. HNO 2021;69(Suppl 2):47–52.
10. Sullivan CB, Ostedgaard KL, Al-Qurayshi Z, et al. Primary Laryngectomy Versus Salvage Laryngectomy: a Comparison of Outcomes in the Chemoradiation Era. Laryngoscope 2020;130(9):2179–85.

11. Lin C, Puram SV, Bulbul MG, et al. Elective neck dissection for salvage laryngectomy: a systematic review and meta-analysis. Oral Oncol 2019;96:97–104.
12. Kligerman J, Olivatto LO, Lima RA, et al. Elective neck dissection in the treatment of T3/T4 N0 squamous cell carcinoma of the larynx. Am J Surg 1995;170(5): 436–9.
13. Petrović Z, Krejović B, Janosević S. Occult metastases from supraglottic laryngeal carcinoma. Clin Otolaryngol Allied Sci 1997;22(6):522–4.
14. Wax MK, Touma BJ. Management of the N0 neck during salvage laryngectomy. Laryngoscope 1999;109(1):4–7.
15. Farrag TY, Lin FR, Cummings CW, et al. Neck management in patients undergoing postradiotherapy salvage laryngeal surgery for recurrent/persistent laryngeal cancer. Laryngoscope 2006;116(10):1864–6.
16. Yao M, Roebuck JC, Holsinger FC, et al. Elective neck dissection during salvage laryngectomy. Am J Otolaryngol 2005;26(6):388–92.
17. Basheeth N, O'Leary G, Sheahan P. Elective neck dissection for no neck during salvage total laryngectomy: findings, complications, and oncological outcome. JAMA Otolaryngol Head Neck Surg 2013;139(8):790–6.
18. Deganello A, Meccariello G, Bini B, et al. Is elective neck dissection necessary in cases of laryngeal recurrence after previous radiotherapy for early glottic cancer? J Laryngol Otol 2014;128(12):1089–94.
19. Koss SL, Russell MD, Leem TH, et al. Occult nodal disease in patients with failed laryngeal preservation undergoing surgical salvage. Laryngoscope 2014;124(2): 421–8.
20. Birkeland AC, Rosko AJ, Issa MR, et al. occult nodal disease prevalence and distribution in recurrent laryngeal cancer requiring salvage laryngectomy. Otolaryngol Head Neck Surg 2016;154(3):473–9.
21. Freiser ME, Ojo RB, Lo K, et al. Complications and oncologic outcomes following elective neck dissection with salvage laryngectomy for the N0 neck. Am J Otolaryngol 2016 May-Jun;37(3):186–94. https://doi.org/10.1016/j.amjoto.2016.01.004. Epub 2016 Jan 22. PMID: 27178505.
22. Hui Y, Wei WI, Yuen PW, et al. Primary closure of pharyngeal remnant after total laryngectomy and partial pharyngectomy: how much residual mucosa is sufficient? Laryngoscope 1996;106:490–4.
23. Gonzalez-Orús Álvarez-Morujo R, Martinez Pascual P, Tucciarone M, et al. Salvage total laryngectomy: is a flap necessary? Braz J Otorhinolaryngol 2020; 86(2):228–36, 30683565.
24. Chen DW, Ellis MA, Horwich P, et al. Free flap inset techniques in salvage laryngopharyngectomy repair: impact on fistula formation and function. Laryngoscope 2021;131(3):E875–81.
25. Rassekh CH, Haughey BH. Total Laryngectomy and Laryngopharyngectomy. In: Cummings otolaryngology: head and neck surgery. 7th ed. Philadephia, PA: Elsevier Inc; 2021. p. 1660–976.
26. Ganly I, Patel S, Matsuo J, et al. Postoperative complications of salvage total laryngectomy. Cancer 2005;103(10):2073–81.
27. Hasan Z, Dwivedi RC, Gunaratne DA, et al. Systematic review and meta-analysis of the complications of salvage total laryngectomy. Eur J Surg Oncol 2017;43(1): 42–51.
28. Scotton W, Cobb R, Pang L, et al. Post-operative wound infection in salvage laryngectomy: does antibiotic prophylaxis have an impact? Eur Arch Otorhinolaryngol 2012;269(11):2415–22.

29. Furuta Y, Homma A, Oridate N, et al. Surgical complications of salvage total laryngectomy following concurrent chemoradiotherapy. Int J Clin Oncol 2008;13(6): 521–7.
30. Meulemans J, Demarsin H, Debacker J, et al. Functional outcomes and complications after salvage total laryngectomy for residual, recurrent, and second primary squamous cell carcinoma of the larynx and hypopharynx: a multicenter retrospective cohort study. Front Oncol 2020;10:1390.
31. White HN, Golden B, Sweeny L, et al. Assessment and incidence of salivary leak following laryngectomy. Laryngoscope 2012;122(8):1796–9.
32. Gosain A, Chang N, Mathes S, et al. A study of the relationship between blood flow and bacterial inoculation in musculocutaneous and fasciocutaneous flaps. Plast Reconstr Surg 1990;86:1152.
33. Karonidis A, Tsoutsos D. The inverted V-shaped fasciocutaneous advancement flap effectively solves the complication of tracheostomal stenosis. Ann Plast Surg 2021;86(3):298–301.
34. Seo GT, Wein LE, Dowling EM, et al. A novel technique for management of stenosis of the postlaryngectomy stoma with preservation of a functional tracheoesophageal puncture following tracheal resection. Head & Neck 2022;44(7): 1737–41.
35. Ziegler A, Pittman A, Thorpe E. Salvage total laryngectomy swallowing outcomes based on flap reconstruction: onlay vs incorporated technique. Otolaryngol Head Neck Surg 2021;165(6):827–9.
36. Fung K, Lyden TH, Lee J, et al. Voice and swallowing outcomes of an organ-preservation trial for advanced laryngeal cancer. Int J Radiat Oncol Biol Phys 2005;63(5):1395–9.
37. Schuman AD, Birkeland AC, Farlow JL, et al. Predictors of Stricture and Swallowing Function Following Salvage Laryngectomy. Laryngoscope 2021;131(6): 1229–34.
38. Plaat RE, van Dijk BAC, Muller Kobold AC, et al. Onset of hypothyroidism after total laryngectomy: Effects of thyroid gland surgery and preoperative and postoperative radiotherapy. Head Neck 2020;42(4):636–44.
39. Paleri V, Winter S, Fox H, et al. Tumours of the Larynx. In: Scott-Brown's otorhinolaryngology: head and neck surgery. 8th ed. Boca Raton, FL: Taylor & Francis Group; 2019. p. 237–62.
40. Boyce S, Meyers A. Oral feeding after total laryngectomy. Head Neck 1989;11: 269–73.
41. Eustaquio M, Medina JE, Krempl GA, et al. Early oral feeding after salvage laryngectomy. Head Neck 2009;31(10):1341–5.
42. Bertolin A, Lionello M, Zanotti C, et al. Oncological and functional outcomes of primary and salvage total laryngectomy. Laryngoscope 2021;131(2):E569–75.
43. van der Putten L, de Bree R, Kuik DJ, et al. Salvage laryngectomy: oncological and functional outcome. Oral Oncol 2011;47(4):296–301.
44. Starmer HM, Ishman SL, Flint PW, et al. Complications that affect postlaryngectomy voice restoration: primary surgery vs salvage surgery. Arch Otolaryngol Head Neck Surg 2009;135(11):1165–9.

Larynx Cancer
Reconstructive Options

Russel Kahmke, MD, MMCi[a], Mirabelle Sajisevi, MD[b],*

KEYWORDS

- Laryngeal cancer • Laryngectomy • Laryngeal reconstruction • Functional results
- Outcomes • Salvage surgery • Pedicled flap • Microvascular reconstruction

KEY POINTS

- Reconstruction for laryngeal cancer will depend on the defect left by surgical resection, patient-related factors, and surgeon preference.
- Vascularized tissue placed over the neopharynx closure in an onlay fashion may reduce pharyngocutaneous fistula in salvage laryngectomy.
- Multiple pedicled and free tissue flaps are available for the reconstruction of partial/total pharyngectomy or skin defects associated with total laryngectomy each with their advantages and disadvantages.

INTRODUCTION/HISTORY

Surgical resection of tumors involving the larynx often impair the primary functions of the organ, namely respiration, airway protection, phonation. The defect and resulting deficits will vary depending on the size and location of the tumor. Smaller lesions in accessible subsites of the larynx may be removed transorally and allowed to heal by secondary intention with good outcomes. Larger tumors may necessitate partial or total removal of the larynx and require reconstruction to preserve or restore function.

The first recorded total laryngectomy was performed by Theodor Billroth, in 1873, which was a success; however, later attempts demonstrated a 50% mortality rate.[1] Subsequently, there were major advances with a steep decline in mortality by the early 1900s.[1] The midtwentieth century was characterized as a period of partial laryngectomies.[2] Although nonoperative larynx preservation therapy resulted in a paradigm shift in the 1990s, surgery is still a mainstay of treatment. With the majority of patients surviving surgery, it is critical to preserve quality of life by maintaining the basic human functions of breathing, talking, and swallowing. This article discusses reconstruction

[a] Department of Head and Neck Surgery & Communication Sciences, Duke University Medical Center, DUMC 3805, Durham, NC 27710, USA; [b] Department of Surgery, Division of Otolaryngology, University of Vermont Medical Center, 89 Beaumont Avenue, Given B110L, Burlington, VT 05401, USA
* Corresponding author.
E-mail address: mirabelle.sajisevi@uvmhealth.org

Otolaryngol Clin N Am 56 (2023) 333–343
https://doi.org/10.1016/j.otc.2022.11.002
oto.theclinics.com

options for various types of open laryngectomy defects that can help optimize patient outcomes.

APPROACH

Reconstruction for laryngeal cancer will depend on the defect left by surgical resection and patient-related factors such as medical comorbidities and history of previous radiation therapy. Options include primary closure, locoregional flaps, and microvascular reconstruction. The approach to reconstruction outlined in this article is organized by type of laryngectomy: partial laryngectomy, total laryngectomy, and extended laryngectomy (**Fig. 1**).

Partial Laryngectomy

Vertical partial laryngectomies are typically performed for select T1–T2 glottic cancers and involve resection of one vocal fold with the underlying thyroid cartilage and can include resection of the anterior commissure and ipsilateral arytenoid depending on the extent of the tumor. Several reconstruction methods have been described including both local and free flap options. Local flaps that have been reported include the hyoid osteomuscular flap and pedicled stenothyroid or sternohyoid strap muscles.[3–5] Free flap reconstruction can also be performed with fascia lata (**Fig. 2**) or temporoparietal fascia. The fascia can be used as a lining or carrier for a free buccal mucosa graft and ear cartilage as described by Gilbert and colleagues.[6] The outcomes reported for each of these techniques are overall favorable for decannulation, voice, and swallow.[3–6] The benefits of a local flap include less technically challenging and time consuming; however, an extended vertical partial laryngectomy defect and/or radiated patient may benefit from free tissue transfer and structural support offered by a vascularized carrier.

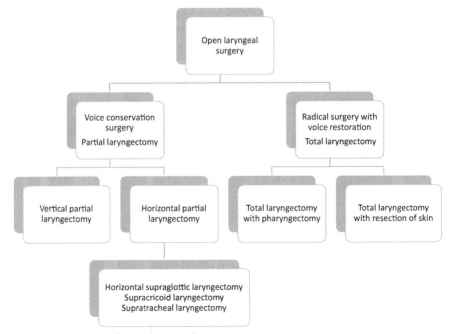

Fig. 1. Classification of open laryngeal surgeries.

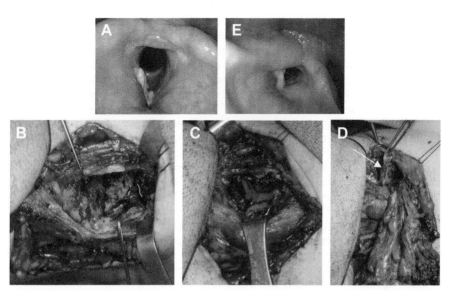

Fig. 2. Vertical partial laryngectomy with reconstruction. (*A*) Right true vocal fold squamous cell carcinoma seen on flexible laryngoscopy. (*B*) Intraoperative view of tumor after laryngofissure (*asterisk*). (*C*) Defect after resection. (*D*) Reconstruction using free tissue transfer with fascia lata to create neo cord (*arrow*) and laryngeal lining. (*E*) Early postoperative result.

Horizontal laryngectomy is typically performed for select early and intermediate stage tumors (T1–T3), particularly for those with inadequate transoral exposure or radiation failure. It involves resection of the laryngeal segment affected by disease including the mucosal layer, membranous layer, submucosal visceral spaces, muscles, and corresponding cartilage.[2,7] The extent of open partial laryngectomy is classified as types 1 to 3 with type 1 involving preservation of some of the thyroid cartilage (horizontal supraglottic laryngectomy), type 2 involving resection of the entire thyroid cartilage (supracricoid laryngectomy), and type 3 involving resection of the thyroid and cricoid cartilage (supratracheal laryngectomy). Reconstruction of these defects involves impaction between the residual cartilaginous and bony structures, that is, crico-hyoidopexy, crico-hyoido-epiglottopexy, tracheo-hyoidopexy, and tracheo-hyoido-epiglottopexy.[2] The reported functional outcomes for open partial laryngectomy vary widely depending on extent of surgery and prior treatment status, however, in a systematic review of 251 patients who underwent salvage supracricoid laryngectomy, the laryngeal preservation rate was 85.2% and the decannulation and swallowing recovery rates were 85.2% and 96.5%, respectively.[2,7,8]

Total Laryngectomy

Total laryngectomy involves complete resection of all laryngeal structures and a section of the upper trachea, which leads to disconnection of the airway and a permanent stoma. Removal of the larynx results in pharyngeal defect, which must be reconstructed. If there is sufficient pharyngeal mucosa, the edges can be bought together and closed primarily. A study by Hui and colleagues[9] showed that a residual strip of mucosa 1.5 cm relaxed, 2.5 cm stretched was sufficient in restoring swallowing function. The pharyngeal mucosal layer may be closed in a vertical, horizontal or T-shaped line. Studies suggest inferior swallowing outcomes with a vertical closure, likely due increased development of a pseudodiverticulum.[10,11] Use of laser-assisted indocyanine green dye angiography, commonly used to assess perfusion of reconstructive tissues, can be used to evaluate areas of decreased native pharyngeal mucosa perfusion to aid in closure decisions.[12] A modified continuous Connell suture to close the mucosal layer is recommended over an interrupted submucosal suture.[13] Stapler suture of the pharynx has also been described with reported advantages of fast application and no increased rate of complications.[14] If there is not adequate residual mucosa for primary closure, then a patch reconstruction is required (see "Total Laryngectomy with Pharyngectomy" section for further discussion).

One of the major complications associated with total laryngectomy includes pharyngocutaneous fistula (PCF), and the rates are significantly increased in the salvage setting. PCF after concurrent chemoradiation has been reported to occur in 30% to 75% of patients.[15] Several studies have attempted to evaluate the utility of incorporating vascularized tissue either as an onlay or patch closure to decrease PCF rates. Multiple systematic reviews demonstrate that prophylactic flaps used in an onlay technique reduce fistula incidence in salvage total laryngectomy.[16–18] The vast majority of the onlay reconstructions in these analyses was a pectoralis major muscle flap although the systematic reviews by Sayles and colleagues[17] and Paleri and colleagues[18] included publications with free tissue transfer.

Incorporating vascularized tissue in the closure as an interposition graft when there is enough mucosa for primary closure has shown conflicting results. A multi-institutional study by Patel and colleagues[15] showed an interposed free flap improved incidence of fistula compared with primary closure (25% vs 34%, $P = .07$) but not to the same degree as pectoralis onlay (15% vs 34%, $P = .02$). Similarly, Cabrera and colleagues[16] found lower rates of fistula with pectoralis onlay compared with interposition reconstruction. Furthermore, Harris and colleagues[19] showed primary closure to be associated with oral diet success and faster pharyngeal transit times compared with patch closure with a pedicled or free flap. However, Withrow and colleagues conversely showed free tissue patch to decreased PCF from 50% in primary closure to 18% with decrease in rate of stricture and feeding tube dependence. Comparable alaryngeal tracheoesophageal prosthesis speech outcomes are reported for free flap reconstruction and primary closure.[20,21]

In summary, primary closure of the pharynx is preferred when there is adequate, healthy mucosa remaining after total laryngectomy. The data suggest that an onlay flap reduces incidence and severity of PCF in salvage laryngectomy. The decision for pedicled versus free flap is dependent on multiple factors including prior treatment, patient health and body habitus, status of neck vessels and surgeon preference.

Total Laryngectomy with Pharyngectomy

Partial pharyngectomy may be needed as part of total laryngectomy when the tumor extends beyond the endolarynx to involve a portion of the hypopharyngeal wall or pyriform sinus. Typically, there is not enough mucosa for primary closure and the defect requires patch reconstruction. Multiple regional and free flap options are available each with their advantages and disadvantages (**Table 1**). Regional options include pectoralis major myocutaneous, supraclavicular artery island, and deltopectoral flaps based on the pectoral branch of thoracoacromial, supraclavicular, and internal mammary arteries, respectively. Commonly used free flaps include the radial forearm free flap and anterolateral thigh (ALT) based on the radial artery and descending branch of the lateral circumflex femoral system, respectively.

Subtotal or circumferential resection of pharyngeal and/or cervical esophageal mucosa can be reconstructed with the flaps outlined above either in a tubed fashioned or

Table 1
Pros and cons of reconstructive options for total laryngectomy with pharyngectomy

	Advantages	Disadvantages	Relative Contraindications	Surgical Tips	Complication/Success Rates
Pectoralis major	• Short operative time/ ease of harvest • Large amount of well-vascularized tissue • Low donor site morbidity	• Skin is not 100% reliable • Flap may have excessive bulk preventing tubulization • Long-term fibrotic muscle retraction	• Obese/muscular patients	• Avoid small skin paddle • Center skin flap over muscle	• Flap loss 2.4%–4%, partial necrosis 12%[26] • PCF 0%–57% (mean 27%)[22] • Stenosis 0%–43% (mean 17%)[22]
Supraclavicular	• Short operative time/ ease of harvest • Pliable • Low donor site morbidity	• Limited by arc of rotation • Potential for distal tip necrosis	• Prior radical neck dissection or shoulder surgery (resulting in ligation/injury of pedicle)	• Avoid flap longer than 22 cm due to increased risk of flap necrosis	• Flap loss rate 0%–5.6%, Partial necrosis 4.2%–14.9%[27] • PCF: 11%[28] • Stenosis 11%[22]
Deltopectoral	• Short operative time/ ease of harvest	• Need for skin grafting donor site • Potential for distal tip necrosis	• Prior cardiac surgery (compromise to internal mammary artery)	• Can stage/delay flap to improve reliability	• Overall flap survival rate 96.3%[29]
RFFF	• Thin, pliable tissue • Long pedicle	• Need for skin grafting and splinting of donor site • Limited flap size • Microvascular expertise required	• Prior forearm injury/ surgery • Inadequate collateral flow to hand via ulnar artery	• Preserve paratenon to increase graft survival at donor site • Edge deepithelialization with 2-layered sutures to reduce PCF • z-plasty technique at distal esophageal anastomosis to reduce stenosis	• Flap failure 0%–5%[22] • PCF 2%–53% (mean 20%) • Stenosis 0%–36% (mean 11%) • Superior voicing compared with PMMC and visceral flaps

(continued on next page)

Table 1
(continued)

	Advantages	Disadvantages	Relative Contraindications	Surgical Tips	Complication/Success Rates
ALT	• Low donor site morbidity • Large amount of tissue available	• May have excessive bulk • Variable perforator anatomy • Microvascular expertise required	• Severe peripheral vascular disease • Previous surgery or trauma of thigh • Obesity	• Flap can be primarily thinned above level of fascia • Wrap first layer suture with fascia lata for tubed reconstruction	• Flap failure 0%–9%[22] • PCF 0%–25% (mean 15%) • Stenosis 0%–30% (mean 9%) • Superior voicing compared with PMMC and visceral flaps
Jejunum	• Naturally tubed • Peristalsis allowing active food transport	• Morbidity of open abdominal surgery • Limited ischemic tolerance • Short pedicle	• Prior abdominal surgery	• Laparoscopic harvest	• Flap failure 0%–17%[22] • PCF 0–32% (mean 12%) • Stenosis 0%–40% (mean 11%) • Suboptimal voicing compared with fasciocutaneous FF
Gastro-omental	• Naturally tubed • Long length and mobility of flap	• Morbidity of open abdominal surgery	• Prior abdominal surgery	• Highly vascularized omentum can be used to drape soft tissues	• Flap failure 0%[22] • PCF 0–27% (mean 16%) • Stricture 0%–60% (mean 13%)

Abbreviation: RFFF, radial forearm free flap.

designed in a U-shape and sutured to the prevertebral fascia. Additionally, free visceral flaps including jejunum and gastro-omentum are options for circumferential defects with the appeal of already being naturally tubed (see **Table 1**). However, these carry the risks associated with open abdominal surgery and higher perioperative morbidity. For subtotal/total pharyngeal defects, the ALT free flap has a favorable profile with respect to morbidity from the donor site and outcomes related to PCF and stenosis rates.[22] The ALT allows for ample tissue that can be tubed to maintain a circumference of 3 cm and still allow for primary closure of the thigh. The flap can be sutured over a salivary bypass tube and be designed to include an external monitoring segment that is incorporated into the stoma (**Fig. 3**).

Total Laryngectomy with Skin Resection

Advanced laryngeal cancer with skin involvement or fibrotic cervical soft tissues may result in a skin defect that cannot be closed primarily. The same regional and nonvisceral free flap options discussed for *total laryngectomy with pharyngectomy* reconstruction are available for skin defects each with their advantages and disadvantages (see **Table 1**). Regional flaps such as the supraclavicular artery island flap can provide thin pliable tissue with good skin contour and match, avoiding need for microvascular reconstruction (**Fig. 4**). In situations where both external skin and pharyngeal reconstruction is required, a chimeric ALT flap can provide ample soft tissue.[23] Alternatively, a dual pedicled flap using a deltopectoral flap for posterior wall reconstruction and pectoralis major to construct the anterior pharyngeal wall and external skin can be used in patients who are not candidates for free flap reconstruction.[24,25]

COMPLICATIONS

The most feared complication related to reconstructive surgery is flap loss, which for laryngeal defects can result in PCF, prolonged hospitalization, and need for additional

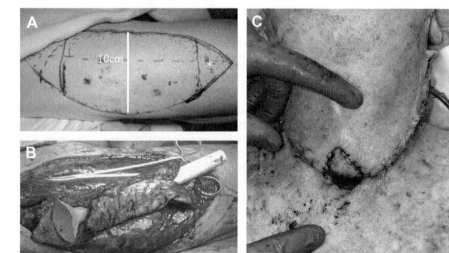

Fig. 3. Tubed anterolateral thigh free flap. (*A*) Flap designed to include external monitoring segment (*asterisk*), (*B*) skin edges sutured over salivary bypass tube, and (*C*) monitoring segment flipped outward and incorporated into stoma for flap monitoring.

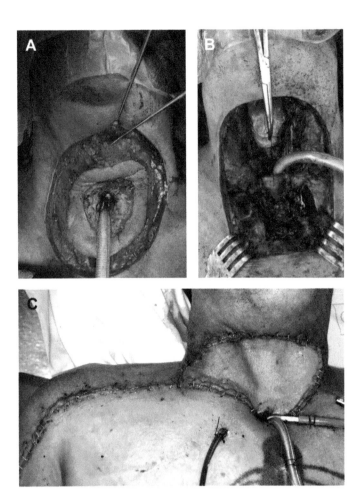

Fig. 4. Reconstruction of skin defect with supraclavicular artery island flap. (*A*) Laryngeal squamous cell carcinoma eroding though skin at tracheostomy site. (*B*) Defect after total laryngectomy with resection of involved skin. (*C*) Supraclavicular artery island flap inset into defect with primary closure of donor site.

surgeries including a second flap. Several risk factors for free flap failure have been reported in the literature including tobacco use, diabetes mellitus, peripheral vascular disease, renal failure, prior (chemo) radiation, ischemia time, alcohol withdrawal, and length of anesthesia. Patients who have several nonmodifiable risks factors may be better candidates for regional tissue transfer. Ultimately, after oncologic resection, the reconstructive surgeon is tasked to prevent life-threatening perioperative complications (infection), to allow the patient to return to activities of daily living (swallowing, breathing, communicating), and to provide an acceptable cosmetic state.

SUMMARY

Reconstruction for laryngeal cancer will depend on the defect left by surgical resection and patient-related factors such as medical comorbidities and history of previous radiation treatment. The goals of reconstruction are to preserve and/or restore the primary functions of the larynx (breathing, swallowing, voicing). Options include primary closure, locoregional flaps, and microvascular free tissue each with their advantages and disadvantages, which should be considered when planning reconstruction.

CLINICS CARE POINTS

- Reconstruction for laryngeal cancer will depend on the defect left by surgical resection, patient-related factors, and surgeon preference
- Vascularized tissue placed over the neopharynx closure in an onlay fashion may reduce PCF in salvage laryngectomy
- For subtotal/total pharyngectomy defects, ALT free flaps have a favorable donor site morbidity profile and outcomes related to PCF and stenosis rates
- The supraclavicular artery island flap can supply a large area of thin pliable tissue for reconstruction of pharyngeal or skin defects associated with laryngectomy while still allowing for primary closure at the donor site

DISCLOSURE

The authors have no conflict of interests.

REFERENCES

1. Matev B, Asenov A, Stoyanov G, et al. Losing one's voice to save one's life: a brief history of laryngectomy. Cureus J Med Sci 2020;12:e8804.
2. Hans S, Baudouin R, Circiu M, et al. Open partial laryngectomies: history of laryngeal cancer surgery. J Clin Med 2022;11:5352.
3. Jurek-Matusiak O, Wójtowicz P, Szafarowski T, et al. Vertical partial frontolateral laryngectomy with simultaneous pedunculated sternothyroid muscle flap reconstruction of the vocal fold – surgical procedure and treatment outcomes. Otolaryngologia Polska 2018;72:23–9.
4. Yagudin RK, Yagudin KF. Reconstruction of the larynx with unipedicled sternohyoid myofascial flap following open extended vertical partial laryngectomy. Int J Otorhinolaryngol Head Neck Surg 2018;5:231–5.
5. WEI B, SHEN H, XIE H. Laryngeal function reconstruction with hyoid osteomuscular flap in partial laryngectomy for laryngeal cancer. Oncol Lett 2015;10:637–40.
6. Gilbert R, Goldstein D, Guillemaud J, et al. Vertical Partial Laryngectomy With Temporoparietal Free Flap Reconstruction for Recurrent Laryngeal Squamous Cell Carcinoma: Technique and Long-term Outcomes. Arch Otolaryngol Head Neck Surg 2012;138:484–91.
7. Succo G, Crosetti E. Limitations and opportunities in open laryngeal organ preservation surgery: current role of OPHLs. Front Oncol 2019;9:408.
8. DeVirgilio A, Pellini R, Mercante G, et al. Supracricoid partial laryngectomy for radiorecurrent laryngeal cancer: a systematic review of the literature and meta-analysis. Eur Arch Otorhinolaryngol 2018. https://doi.org/10.1007/s00405-018-4986-4.
9. Hui Y, Wei WI, Yuen PW, et al. Primary closure of pharyngeal remnant after total laryngectomy and partial pharyngectomy: how much residual mucosa is sufficient? Laryngoscope 1996. https://doi.org/10.1097/00005537-199604000-00018.
10. Chotipanich A. Total laryngectomy: a review of surgical techniques. Cureus 2021; 13:e18181.

11. van der Kamp MF, Rinkel RNPM, Eerenstein SEJ. The influence of closure technique in total laryngectomy on the development of a pseudo-diverticulum and dysphagia. Eur Arch Oto-rhino-l 2017;274:1967–73.

12. Partington E, Moore L, Kahmke R, et al. Laser-assisted indocyanine green dye angiography for postoperative fistulas after salvage laryngectomy. JAMA Otolaryngol Head Neck Surg 2017. https://doi.org/10.1001/jamaoto.2017.0187.

13. Avci H, Karabulut B. Is It important which suturing technique used for pharyngeal mucosal closure in total laryngectomy? modified continuous connell suture may decrease pharyngocutaneous fistula. Ear Nose Throat J 2020;99:664–70.

14. Dedivitis RA, Aires FT, Pfuetzenreiter EG, et al. Stapler suture of the pharynx after total laryngectomy. Acta Otorhinolaryngologica Italica Organo Ufficiale Della Soc Italiana Di Otorinolaringologia E Chir Cervico-facciale 2012;34:94–8.

15. Patel U, Moore B, Wax M, et al. Impact of pharyngeal closure technique on fistula after salvage laryngectomy. Jama Otolaryngol Head Neck Surg 2013;139: 1156–62.

16. Cabrera CI, Jones AJ, Parker NP, et al. Pectoralis major onlay vs interpositional reconstruction fistulation after salvage total laryngectomy: systematic review and meta-analysis. Otolaryngol Head Neck Surg 2020;164:972–83.

17. Sayles M, Grant DG. Preventing pharyngo-cutaneous fistula in total laryngectomy: a systematic review and meta-analysis. Laryngoscope 2014;124:1150–63.

18. Paleri V, Drinnan M, Brekel M, et al. Vascularized tissue to reduce fistula following salvage total laryngectomy: a systematic review. Laryngoscope 2014;124: 1848–53.

19. Harris BN, Hoshal SG, Evangelista L, et al. Reconstruction technique following total laryngectomy affects swallowing outcomes. Laryngoscope Invest Otolaryngol 2020;5:703–7.

20. Revenaugh PC, Knott PD, Alam DS, et al. Voice outcomes following reconstruction of laryngopharyngectomy defects using the radial forearm free flap and the anterolateral thigh free flap. Laryngoscope 2014. https://doi.org/10.1002/lary.23785.

21. Alam DS, Vivek PP, Kmiecik J. Comparison of voice outcomes after radial forearm free flap reconstruction versus primary closure after laryngectomy. Otolaryngology–Head Neck Surg 2008. https://doi.org/10.1016/j.otohns.2008.03.024.

22. Piazza C, Taglietti V, Nicolai P. Reconstructive options after total laryngectomy with subtotal or circumferential hypopharyngectomy and cervical esophagectomy. Curr Opin Otolaryngo 2012;20:77–88.

23. Liu J, Lv D, Deng D, et al. Free bipaddled anterolateral thigh flap for simultaneous reconstruction of large larynx and prelaryngeal skin defects after resection of the local recurrent laryngeal cancer invading the cricoid cartilage and prelaryngeal skin. Medicine 2019;98. e14199.

24. Ishimaru M, Ono S, Suzuki S, et al. Risk factors for free flap failure in 2,846 patients with head and neck cancer: a national database study in Japan. J Oral Maxillofac Surg 2016. https://doi.org/10.1016/j.joms.2016.01.009.

25. Crawley M, Sweeny L, Ravipati P, et al. Factors associated with free flap failures in head and neck reconstruction. Otolaryngology–Head Neck Surg 2019. https://doi.org/10.1177/0194599819860809.

26. Bussu F, Gallus R, Navach V, et al., Contemporary role of pectoralis major regional flaps in head and neck surgery. Acta Otorhinolaryngol Ital. 34 (5), 2014, 327-341.

27. Nikolaidou E, Pantazi G, Sovatzidis A, et al. The supraclavicular artery island flap for pharynx reconstruction. J Clin Med 2022;11:3126.

28. Reiter Maximilian. Baumeister & Philipp. Reconstruction of laryngopharyngectomy defects: Comparison between the supraclavicular artery island flap, the
radial forearm flap, and the anterolateral thigh flap. Microsurgery 2018. https://
doi.org/10.1002/micr.30406.

29. Chan RCL, Chan JYW. Deltopectoral Flap in the Era of Microsurgery. Surg Res
Pract 2014;2014:420892.

Non-squamous Laryngeal Cancer

Stephanie Danielle MacNeil, MD, MSc

KEYWORDS

- Non-squamous • Larynx • Laryngeal • Cancer • Malignancy • Chondrosarcoma
- Small-cell neuroendocrine carcinoma

KEY POINTS

- Non-squamous cancer of the larynx is a rare entity that usually presents with hoarseness and as a submucosal mass.
- Evaluation of patients with suspected non-squamous cancer of the larynx includes flexible endoscopy but may rely more heavily on imaging, in particular MRI.
- The most common non-squamous cancer of the larynx is chondrosarcoma, followed by small-cell neuroendocrine carcinoma.
- Treatment of non-squamous cancer of the larynx can be extrapolated for treatment based on the histology in nonlaryngeal sites.
- Organ preserving treatment is preferred but total laryngectomy may be required for some tumor types and locally advanced diseases.

INTRODUCTION

Non-squamous cell carcinoma (SCC) of the larynx represents approximately 5% of laryngeal malignancies.[1] These malignancies originate from minor salivary glands, bone, cartilage, muscles, fatty tissues, neuronal tissue and connective tissue. These cell types are seen throughout the upper aerodigestive tract including the larynx. Although the vast majority of new malignancies seen in the larynx are SCC, it is important to consider other histologic subtypes because these malignancies can present with submucosal spread resulting in delay of diagnosis. Further to this, the pathologic diagnosis, staging and treatment paradigms are not commonly accepted, therefore being aware of the most up to date data on this group of malignancies is important for appropriate treatment planning.

In this review, we adhere to the World Health Organization (WHO) classification of disease in our presentation.[2] We have excluded all benign tumors of the larynx with

Head and Neck Surgical Oncologist, Department of Otolaryngology-Head and Neck Surgery, Western University, Victoria Hospital, Room B3-439, 800 Commissioners Road East, London, Ontario, N6A 5W9, Canada
E-mail address: Danielle.Macneil@lhsc.on.ca

Otolaryngol Clin N Am 56 (2023) 345–359
https://doi.org/10.1016/j.otc.2023.01.003
0030-6665/23/© 2023 Elsevier Inc. All rights reserved.

oto.theclinics.com

Abbreviations	
MRI	Magnetic Resonance Imaging
WHO	World Health Organization
SCC	Squamous Cell Carcinoma
CT	Computed Tomography
MEC	Mucoepidermoid Carcinoma
DSS	Disease-specific Survival
NET	Neuroendocrine Tumor
SCNC	Small-cell Neuroendocrine Carcinoma
LCNC	Large-cell Neuroendocrine Carcinoma
OS	Overall Survival
SDHD	Succinate Dehydrogenase Complex Subunit D
SDHB	Succinate Dehydrogenase Complex Subunit B
SDHC	Succinate Dehydrogenase Complex Subunit C
NOS	Not Otherwise Specified
KS	Kaposi Sarcoma
HIV	Human Immunodeficiency Virus
RMS	Rhabdomyosarcoma
CS	Chondrosarcoma
MPNST	Malignant Peripheral Nerve Sheath Tumor
NF	Neurofibromatosis
MFH	Malignant Fibrous Histiocytoma
PNET	Peripheral Primitive Neuroectodermal Tumor
DLBCL	Diffuse Large B-Cell Lymphoma
MALT	Mucosa-associated Lymphoid Tumor

the exception of those that mimic malignant tumors in behavior. Although some previous articles have reported rare variants of SCC as non-squamous cell malignancies of the larynx, we have excluded these from the discussion here as they are considered variants of SCC by the WHO. We have excluded the following variants of SCC: verrucous, basaloid, papillary, spindle cell, adenosquamous, and lymphoepithelial.[2] Treatment of non-squamous cancer of the larynx is variable. Much of the evidence for optimal treatment relies on data extrapolated from treatment of SCC, similar histologies in non-laryngeal subsites or small case series.[3,4] As these tumors are relatively rare, the epidemiology and clinical behavior of non-SCC tumors of the larynx are not as well studied. Here we summarize the most up to date information on these histologic entities including treatment recommendations.

CLINICAL EVALUATION

The evaluation of patients with suspected non-squamous cancer of the larynx is the same as that for the SCC of the larynx. Direct visualization with flexible laryngoscopy and subsequent biopsy is required.[5] Although SCC usually presents as an area with obvious mucosal abnormality, non-squamous malignancies can present with submucosal lesions and are more challenging to identify.[6] Radiographic imaging in the form of computed tomography (CT) may help to establish a submucosal laryngeal lesion. However, MRI has good sensitivity and specificity for localization of tumor with respect to laryngeal subsites, submucosal infiltration into surrounding preepiglottic or paraglottic spaces, cartilage invasion, and metastasis to regional lymph nodes.[7–9] In the absence of a clear lesion on endoscopy in the presence of worsening or persistent symptoms, clinicians should be diligent in ordering imaging to rule out a submucosal tumor, potentially a non-squamous malignancy of the larynx.[6] Obtaining a definitive diagnosis on tissue sampling may also be challenging requiring deeper biopsies in the submucosal tissues. Review with an experienced head and neck pathologist and multidisciplinary tumor board of clinical presentation, imaging and pathology should be considered standard of care.

NON-SQUAMOUS CANCER OF THE LARYNX BY HISTOLOGY
Melanoma of the Larynx

Melanoma, commonly a cutaneous disease, presents rarely as a primary laryngeal mucosal tumor.[10] Malignant melanoma of the mucous membranes arises from melanocytes scattered in the mucosa, they represent 1.4% of all melanomas.[11,12] Primary laryngeal melanomas are estimated to represent the 3.6% to 7.4% of primary mucosal melanomas of the head and neck.[13] Males are more frequently affected with a mean age of 57.7 years (range 27 to 86).[11] Primary laryngeal melanoma tends to present with hoarseness, throat irritation or dyspnea, with spread to cervical lymph nodes and regional/distant metastasis in 66% and 79% of cases, respectively.[10,14] The most frequently affected laryngeal region is the supraglottis (60%) followed by the glottis (40%).[11] Radical surgery is generally recommended however no evidence of a better survival rate has been reported for total laryngectomy vs partial or endoscopic laser surgery.[11] Survival is in fact influenced primarily by distant metastases. Given that distant metastases highly impacts survival, appropriate preoperative work-up is essential to rule out metastatic disease.[11]

Malignant Salivary Gland Tumors

Malignant salivary gland tumors of the larynx are very rare neoplasms. They account for <1% of all laryngeal malignancies.[15] The most common malignant minor salivary gland tumors are adenoid cystic carcinoma (32% to 69%) and mucoepidermoid carcinomas (MECs) (15% to 35%).[16] Other salivary gland histology are much less common, including adenocarcinoma, acinic cell carcinoma, carcinoma ex pleomorphic adenoma, epithelial-myoepithelial cell carcinoma, and salivary duct carcinoma.[17] Malignant salivary gland tumors are not strongly associated with smoking and occur equally in males and females.[15,16,18] They are found most commonly in the subglottis and supraglottis, as they arise from subepithelial mucous glands which predominate in these locations.[19] Given that these tumors typically present in a subepithelial fashion, they can grow to a large size before they present with dysphonia or airway symptoms.

Adenoid cystic carcinoma

Laryngeal adenoid cystic carcinoma comprises less than 1% of all laryngeal carcinomas and is thought to arise from minor salivary glands or glandular elements in the larynx.[20] Most patients present with dyspnea or hoarseness; some present with nonspecific respiratory symptoms, which can delay diagnosis.[21,22] In the larynx, adenoid cystic carcinoma is found primarily in the subglottis (57%), supraglottis (30%), and glottis (5.8%).[23]

Laryngeal adenoid cystic carcinoma presents with local, regional, and distant involvement at rates of 60%, 26%, and 14%, respectively.[23] Surgery is the mainstay of treatment and has led to higher disease-specific survival at 5 years compared with nonsurgical treatment (73.7% disease specific survival (DSS) surgical group versus 44.4% DSS non-surgical group, $p = 0.02$).[20] Although not commonly used, chemotherapy (carboplatin/cisplatin +/- paclitaxel) has been used concurrently with radiation in the primary and adjuvant setting for the purpose of laryngeal preservation.[24,25] This indication for chemotherapy for the treatment of adenoid cystic carcinoma is based on case reports alone.[24,25]

Mucoepidermoid carcinoma

Mucoepidermoid carcinoma (MEC) of the larynx is uncommon.[26] It tends to present as a submucosal mass in the supraglottis with hoarseness or dyspnea.[27], Similar to other laryngeal tumors, MEC primarily presents in men in the 6th decade.[27]

The typical stage of presentation is unclear, but MEC of the larynx can have submucosal, perineural, and perivascular spread, which predisposes to locally advanced disease at presentation.[28] Primary treatment involves surgery.[26] A diagnosis of high-grade MEC or the presence of nodal metastases are indications for neck dissection.[29] Medium- and high-grade tumors are further treated with adjuvant radiotherapy, given the high incidence of local recurrence (approximately 50%).[30]

Acinic cell carcinoma

Acinic cell carcinoma, normally a parotid gland disease, has been documented occasionally in the larynx. The presentation tends to be a painless firm solitary mass in the supraglottis.[31] Treatment of this disease in the larynx has involved surgery with or without radical neck dissection, laser excision with radiotherapy, and radiotherapy alone.[32,33]

Neuroendocrine Neoplasms and Paraganglioma

Neuroendocrine neoplasms are divided into well-differentiated neuroendocrine tumors (NETs) and neuroendocrine carcinoma (small-cell neuroendocrine carcinoma [SCNC] and large-cell neuroendocrine carcinoma [LCNC]). Paraganglioma tumors are a separate classification in this group.

NETs include grades 1 to 3.[2] They are epithelial neuroendocrine neoplasms that arise from the cells of the dispersed neuroendocrine system in the upper aerodigestive tract and salivary gland.[2] Laryngeal tumors may cause hoarseness, dysphonia, sore throat and hemoptysis,[34] whereas some are asymptomatic and detected incidentally during laryngoscopy or intubation for unrelated reasons. Laryngeal NETs are more frequent in males in their sixth and seventh decades with a male-to-female ratio of 2.4:1.[35]

Well-differentiated neuroendocrine carcinoma, or Typical carcinoid tumor

Grade 1 NET, also known as a typical carcinoid tumor, is the least common NET.[36] Typical carcinoid tumor comprises less than 1% of all laryngeal carcinomas.[37] Treatment primarily involves surgical excision. Neck dissection is not indicated given the lack of lymph node metastasis.[38] Despite this cancer being less aggressive, approximately 35% of cases can recur locally, regionally or distally.[39] Low-grade NETs have a reported 5-year survival of approximately 80% after conservative surgical resection.[40]

Moderately differentiated neuroendocrine carcinoma, or Atypical carcinoid tumor

Atypical carcinoid tumor, Grade 2, is the most common laryngeal NET, and comprises less than 1% of all laryngeal carcinoma. It typically presents with hoarseness, dysphagia, and respiratory distress.[41] The tumor usually involved the supraglottis and occasionally the glottis and subglottis.[37] In contrast to other locations, laryngeal atypical carcinoid has particularly high rates of local and distant recurrence. Treatment of laryngeal atypical carcinoid primarily involves surgery with supraglottic or total laryngectomy, along with neck dissection, given the prevalence of early cervical metastasis.[42] Despite adequate treatment, most patients (62.5%) will experience disease recurrence, with 69.4% of these patients having distant metastasis.[39] In a meta-analysis of 436 reported cases published in 2015, the 5-year disease-free survival and overall survival (OS) were 52.8% and 46%, respectively.[39]

Small-cell neuroendocrine carcinoma

Small-cell neuroendocrine carcinoma (SCNC) is a poorly differentiated (high-grade) neuroendocrine carcinoma composed of epithelial cells with scant cytoplasm, hyperchromatic nuclei, finely granular chromatin, inconspicuous nucleoli, high mitotic count and frequent necrosis.[2,43] SCNC represents about 0.5% of all laryngeal cancers and commonly presents with hoarseness, stridor, dyspnea, and cough along with a neck mass.[42,44] Approximately 60% of head and neck small cell NETs arise in the larynx, the majority in the supraglottis.[45] SCNC comprises 40% to 50% of laryngeal neuroendocrine neoplasms,[39,46] it has a mean age of 59 to 62 years and a male-to-female ratio of 1.6 to 3.4:1. Approximately 67% to 76% of cases present with stage IV disease due to the propensity of distant metastasis.[39]

Chemoradiotherapy is the mainstay of treatment of SCNC, resulting in improved 5-year disease specific survival (31% vs 13%, $p = 0.001$) and median survival (19 vs 11 months, $p = 0.02$) compared with other treatment modalities.[39,44] Recommended chemotherapy regimen includes platinum/etoposide, similar to the small-cell lung carcinoma (SCLC) regimen.[47,48]

In the larynx, approximately 90% of SCNC develop distant metastases and 5-year survival is 5% to 20%.[39,49,50]

Large-cell neuroendocrine carcinoma

Large-cell neuroendocrine carcinoma (LCNC) of the larynx is a newly reclassified tumor and thus has an unknown incidence. It is a poorly differentiated neuroendocrine carcinoma composed of cells with abundant eosinophilic cytoplasm, vesicular chromatin and prominent nueleoli.[2] Previously grouped with atypical carcinoid, LCNC is currently considered a subtype of poorly differentiated neuroendocrine carcinoma, grade III, along with SCNC.[2] In the larynx, more than 80% arise in the supraglottis.[39] They are associated with tobacco use in more than 90% of cases. LCNC is aggressive, with 70% of patients presenting with stage IV disease.[39] The chance of recurrence is 81% and 5-year OS is 9%.[39] Surgery alone, radiotherapy alone, and varying combinations of multimodal therapy have been used in LCNC.[39,51]

Paraganglioma

Head and neck paraganglioma are well-differentiated non-epithelial neoplasms derived from paraganglion cells of the automatic nervous system.[2] The majority of paragangliomas of the larynx arise in the supraglottis.[2] They are associated with a hereditary predisposition in at least 40% of patients.[52] The most common germline mutation in patients with head and neck paragangliomas is succinate dehydrogenase complex subunit D (SDHD) (47%), followed by succinate dehydrogenase complex subunit B (SDHB) (30%) and succinate dehydrogenase complex subunit C (SDHC) (16%).[52] The clinical approach depends on several factors but may include clinical observation, secondary to the potential morbidity of surgery, placing cranial nerves at risk.[53]

Malignant Soft Tissue and Bone Tumors

The WHO Classification of soft tissue and bone tumors is based on tissue of origin. These tumors are classified based on whether they are benign, intermediate (locally aggressive) or malignant.

Malignant adipocytic tumors

Liposarcomas are included in this classification and are quite rare. They are a heterogenous group of malignant adipocytic neoplasms with features dependent on the type of liposarcoma. They generally occur in men aged 40 to 60 years.[54–56] The majority of laryngeal liposarcomas arise in the supraglottis (75%).[55] They are generally low grade, but they can behave aggressively and recur in up to 51% of cases.[55,57] The survival of patients with liposarcoma is significantly better for liposarcoma of the head and neck than other sites, this is thought to be because head and neck tumors are more likely to have a lower pathologic grade.58 However, prognosis depends on the subtype with pleomorphic liposarcomas demonstrating a significantly lower over-all survival than other histologies ($p = .001$) and well differentiated liposarcoma demonstrating the highest overall survival.[58]

Fibroblastic and myofibroblastic malignant tumors

Intermediate (rarely metastasizing) tumors in this group include Dermatofibrosarcoma protuberans NOS (not otherwise specified), and myofibroblastic sarcoma. Malignant tumors included in this group are fibrosarcoma NOS and solitary fibrous tumors, malignant.

Low-grade myofibroblastic sarcoma is an uncommon sarcoma. It usually affects middle aged patients, and there is a slight male predominance.[59,60] This tumor has a tendency to occur in the head and neck region, in particular the tongue, oral cavity, and rarely the larynx.[59,60] Although the prognosis is usually favorable,there is a high chance of recurrence, but they rarely metastasize. Surgical excision with negative margins is generally preferred.[60]

Fibrosarcoma is composed of fibroblasts arranged in fibrous fusiform bundles with an oval shape nucleus.[61] The primary treatment method is surgical resection with proper marginal tissue.[62] The role of chemotherapy and radiotherapy is not clear. The 5-year survival rates for highly differentiated and poorly differentiated fibrosar-coma are 50% and 5%, respectively.[63]

Malignant vascular tumors

Intermediate tumors in this category include Kaposi sarcoma (KS). More aggressive tumors in this group include epithelioid hemangioendothelioma NOS and angiosarcoma.

KS is an uncommon locally aggressive endothelial neoplasm and is also known as KS-associated herpesvirus 8. Human herpesvirus 8 associated diseases are most commonly diagnosed in individuals living with human immunodeficiency virus (HIV). KS represents 20% to 25% of all head and neck sarcomas.[64,65] It is estimated that 66% of mucosal KS involve head and neck sites, the hard palate is the most common location, followed by the gingiva and tongue.[66] KS rarely affects the larynx; however, it has been reported that patients with cutaneous and multiple oral cavity lesions have a higher risk of laryngeal involvement, and this should be excluded by direct laryngos-copy.[67] The recommended treatment of KS in patients with HIV is antiretroviral ther-apy and single -agent chemotherapy for advanced disease.[68,69]

Angiosarcoma originates from the endothelium, has a nodular appearance, is rich in blood vessels, or has unclear gross boundaries. The symptoms of angiosarcoma are non-specific. It demonstrates rapid progression and has a high metastatic rate via the hematogenous route. Surgery is the primary treatment and adjuvant radiotherapy may be beneficial.[70]

Pericytic (perivascular) tumors

Within this group of tumors are malignant glomus tumors. Glomus tumors are mostly benign and are derived from three components: glomus cells, vasculature, and smooth muscle cells.[71] Malignant glomus tumors are extremely rare. The features of malignant glomus tumors include the following: deep visceral location, large size (approximately 4 cm), and increased mitotic activity (20 mitoses/50 high-power field).[72] Malignant glomus tumors usually do not metastasize, and present a locally infiltrative malignancy.[73]

Smooth muscle tumors

Laryngeal leiomyosarcoma is mostly seen in adults, and there is a male predominance. It can occur in any part of the larynx.[74,75] Radiation exposure, immunosuppression, and tumor predisposition syndromes (Li-Fraumeni and retinoblastoma) are predisposing factors.[76,77]

Surgery is the primary treatment of laryngeal leiomyosarcoma.[78] Surgery should be performed with wide surgical margins, achieving tumor free margins affords the best prognosis.[79,80] For head and neck leiomyosarcomas as a group, prognosis is often poor (20% 5-year OS) due to late presentation and difficulties achieving tumor-free margins.[79]

Skeletal muscle tumors

Rhabdomyosarcoma (RMS) variants are included in this group. Variants of RMS include embryonal, alveolar, pleomorphic, and spindle cell/sclerosing. Although RMS is a malignancy that commonly presents in the head and neck, its presentation in the larynx has been rarely reported. Laryngeal RMS tends to present in the pediatric population with changes in voice, a lump sensation in the throat or in some cases dyspnea or stridor given its fast-growing nature.[81,82]

Given the rarity of laryngeal RMS, treatment has not been standardized and is often modeled after treatment of RMS in other sites. Various modalities have been implemented, including surgery, radiotherapy, and chemotherapy with varying success. Small series have suggested that laryngeal disease is less aggressive than other types of RMS, presenting as a localized disease with 5-year mean survival of 70% to 90%.[83] This may be due to the cartilaginous borders of the larynx restricting local tumor spread.[84] Given the presentation of RMS in the pediatric population, attempts have been made for organ preservation: in localized disease, local excision/partial laryngectomy in conjunction with chemotherapy has been considered. Similar chemotherapy regimens used for RMS in other sites can be used in laryngeal disease.[85]

Chondrosarcoma

Chondrosarcoma (CS) is the most common laryngeal sarcoma, whereas its benign counterpart, chondroma is exceedingly rare.[2,86] Both tumors arise in the laryngeal hyaline cartilages, the most common site is the cricoid cartilage, with more than 50% of cases presenting in the cricoid cartilage.[43,87] CS are most commonly found on the posterior lamina of the cricoid cartilage.[88] The other primary sites include the thyroid cartilage, arytenoid and epiglottis.[87] CS grows slowly as a submucosal, lobulated endolaryngeal mass.[43] The tumors are less invasive than in other areas and can remain localized for many years. Therefore, close attention should be paid to CT examination findings or vocal cord paralysis of unknown cause.[88] Clinically, laryngeal CS presents primarily with hoarseness or dyspnea.[87,89–91] It is more common in males (75%), with a mean age of presentation 62 years.[88,92] CT scan is the diagnostic imaging of choice, which reveals hypodense calcified lesions.[89,93,94] Nodal and distant metastasis are very rare.[92]

Despite most tumors presenting in the early stage (T1 or T2), treatment can remain challenging because the tumor has high local recurrence rates, with some studies reported rates as high as 50%.[90–92] Although there remains a lack of consensus regarding the optimal extent of initial surgery, a reasonable approach is preservation of organ function with the initial surgery, when appropriate. Based on SEER data in the United States, the mean survival for patients with CS of the larynx is 77.8 months (95%

confidence interval [CI]: 68.07 to 87.43 months).[88] Owing to its high recurrence rate, long-term monitoring and follow-up of patients is required. Posttreatment surveillance requires frequent office visits and imaging.

Osteosarcoma

Head and neck osteosarcomas are rare and account for ≤1% of all head and neck cancers. Histologic subtypes of head and neck osteosarcoma include osteoblastic, chondroblastic, fibroblastic, telangiectatic, and dedifferentiated. Osteosarcoma of the larynx is extremely rare and shows many differences from osteosarcomas of other head and neck sites. There are less than 30 reported cases in the literature. The median age at diagnosis is 64 years (range, 47 to 80 years) and there is a male predominance (92%).[95] The most common primary site is the true vocal cord, followed by the cricoid cartilage and thyroid cartilage. CT shows infiltrating and destructive lesions with calcifications. It can also be expansile. MRI is used to define the intramedullary and extramedullary extent of such tumors. Diagnosis of this tumor is difficult because of submucosal involvement, and several biopsies may be required. Laryngeal osteosarcoma is extremely rare with a poor prognosis. The 5-year survival rate is less than 50%.[96] Adequate surgical resection is likely the best predictor of prognosis.[96] The use of adjuvant therapy has not been established.

Peripheral nerve sheath tumors

Malignant peripheral nerve sheath tumors (MPNSTs) can arise in 50% of patients with neurofibromatosis type 1, sporadically from benign neurofibroma, or rarely following radiation treatment. MPNSTs typically present between 20 and 50 years of age, with younger ages for NF-1-associated tumors. Patients present with an enlarging mass that may be painful. MPNST show aggressive behavior with poor prognosis. For head and neck MPNST, 2- and 5-year disease-specific survivals are 50% and 30%, respectively,[97] NF-1 and radiation-induced MPNST are associated with 5-year survival of approximately 35% and 23% repsecitvely.[98,99]

Tumors of uncertain differentiation

Laryngeal synovial sarcoma is more common in young men mean age at diagnosis 32 years (range 11 to 79 years) (69.2% men).[100–102] Synovial sarcomas of the larynx typically present as a painless neck lump associated with airway symptoms in advanced cases. Although the imaging pathway for initial investigation remains undefined, final diagnosis is made based on tumor morphology, immunohistochemistry and molecular studies. The histological feature is bidirectional differentiation of the tumor; that has both spindle cell sarcoma-like and adenoid-like components lining epithelial cells.[103] The majority of cases of synovial sarcoma of the larynx are biphasic, however the significance of this for prognosis is unclear.[102,104] Radical surgical resection with a negative margin is the preferred treatment. Neck dissection is not recommended because the tumors do not involve the lymph nodes. The 2-, 5-, and 10-year DSS rates are 97%, 79%, and 68%, respectively.[105,106]

Malignant fibrous histiocytoma (MFH) or undifferentiated pleomorphic sarcoma is observed commonly in the extremities and retroperitoneum. Its presence in the larynx has been rarely described and is associated with prior radiotherapy. Hoarseness and voice changes are the most common presenting symptoms, which can be accompanied by difficulty swallowing and dyspnea.[107,108] Given that local recurrence of laryngeal MFH occurs in up to 85% of cases with close margins compared with 27% with radical resection, recommended treatment involves radical surgical excision with consideration of simultaneous neck dissection and radiotherapy for close or positive margins.[109] At 5 years, the relapse survival rate was 70.5% and OS rate was 75.0%.[110]

Malignant granular cell tumors of the larynx are rare, and at least four cases have been reported in the literature.[92,111–113] Patients with laryngeal tumors reportedly developed nodal and distant metastasis (lung and bone) and were alive after an average follow-up of 17 months.[92,111,113] The current recommended treatment is complete surgical resection with negative margins.[111]

Undifferentiated small round cell sarcomas of bone and soft tissue
Included in this group are Ewing's sarcomas. In some reviews, tumors have been separately classified as peripheral primitive neuroectodermal tumors (PNETs). These tumors are now considered the same entity as they have a similar phenotype and because they share an identical chromosome translocation.[114] Eighty-five to ninety percent of cases show t(11;22)(q24;q12) resulting in EWSR1::FLI1 fusion and 5-10% of cases show t(21;22)(q22;q12) resulting in EWSR1::ERG fusion.[2,114]

Hematolymphoid Tumors

A variety of non-Hodgkin's lymphomas have been described in the larynx, including diffuse large B-cell lymphoma (DLBCL), Burkitt lymphoma, extranodal NK/T-cell lymphoma, and mucosa-associated lymphoid tissue (MALT) lymphoma, although all in limited numbers.[115] Laryngeal lymphoma can present with dyspnea, dysphagia, voice changes, or hoarseness, along with fever and weight loss.[116] It often present in the supraglottis given the presence of lymphoid collections in the lamina propria and ventricles.[117] As laryngeal lymphoma is rare, treatment is modeled after management of these diseases in the lymph nodes and other extra-nodal sites.

Secondary Laryngeal malignancies

Metastatic spread of malignancy to the larynx is rare. The most common primary tumors metastasizing to the larynx are malignant melanoma and renal carcinoma.[118] Breast, lung, prostate, stomach, and colon metastases have also been reported.[119,120] The most common sites of metastatic are the supraglottis and subglottis because of the rich lymphatic and vascular supply.

SUMMARY

The pathology of non-squamous carcinoma of the larynx is broad and there is a wide differential diagnosis. The most common presenting symptoms for laryngeal malignancies, both squamous and non-squamous, are hoarseness and dyspnea. Presentation with persistent or worsening symptoms and a submucosal lesion should raise suspicion for a non-squamous malignancy of the larynx. Accurate histology determines the most appropriate treatment and has an impact on prognosis.

CLINICS CARE POINTS

- Although uncommon, not all malignancies of the larynx are squamous cell in origin. Clinicians should consider other histologies when the suspected malignancy is submucosal or the clinical presentation is unusual.

- MRI may be helpful for the diagnosis of non-squamous malignancies of the larynx. Biopsy is required at all times ot obtain a correct histologic diagnosis of malignancies of the larynx.

- Given the rarity of non-squamous cell cancer of the larynx, multidisciplinary tumor board presentation including pathology and radiology review at a high volume head and neck centre is imperative for appropriate management and treatment.

DISCLOSURE

The authors have nothing to disclose.

REFERENCES

1. Marioni G, Marchese-Ragona R, Cartei G, et al. Current opinion in diagnosis and treatment of laryngeal carcinoma. Cancer Treat Rev 2006;32(7):504–15.
2. El-Naggar AKJCG JR, Takata T, Slootweg PJ. 5th ed. WHO classification of head and neck tumors, 9. WHO classification of tumors series; 2017.
3. Haigentz M Jr, Silver CE, Hartl DM, et al. Chemotherapy regimens and treatment protocols for laryngeal cancer. Expert Opin Pharmacother 2010;11(8): 1305–16.
4. Tan E, Mody MD, Saba NF. Systemic therapy in non-conventional cancers of the larynx. Oral Oncol 2018;82:61–8.
5. Dogan S, Vural A, Kahriman G, et al. Non-squamous cell carcinoma diseases of the larynx: clinical and imaging findings. Braz J Otorhinolaryngol 2020;86(4): 468–82.
6. Rotsides JM, Patel E, Oliver JR, et al. Non-squamous cell malignancies of the larynx. Laryngoscope 2022;132(9):1771–7.
7. Banko B, Dukic V, Milovanovic J, et al. Diagnostic significance of magnetic resonance imaging in preoperative evaluation of patients with laryngeal tumors. Eur Arch Otorhinolaryngol 2011;268(11):1617–23.
8. Castelijns JA, Becker M, Hermans R. Impact of cartilage invasion on treatment and prognosis of laryngeal cancer. Eur Radiol 1996;6(2):156–69.
9. Blitz AM, Aygun N. Radiologic evaluation of larynx cancer. Otolaryngol Clin North Am 2008;41(4):697–713, vi.
10. Zaghi S, Pouldar D, Lai C, et al. Subglottic presentation of a rare tumor: primary or metastatic? Primary mucosal melanoma of the subglottic larynx. JAMA Otolaryngol Head Neck Surg 2013;139(7):739–40.
11. Fernandez IJ, Spagnolo F, Roncadi L, et al. Primary mucosal melanoma of the larynx: systematic review of the literature and qualitative synthesis. Eur Arch Otorhinolaryngol 2022;279(12):5535–45.
12. Chang AE, Karnell LH, Menck HR. The National Cancer Data Base report on cutaneous and noncutaneous melanoma: a summary of 84,836 cases from the past decade. The American College of Surgeons Commission on Cancer and the American Cancer Society. Cancer 1998;83(8):1664–78.
13. Wenig BM. Laryngeal mucosal malignant melanoma. A clinicopathologic, immunohistochemical, and ultrastructural study of four patients and a review of the literature. Cancer 1995;75(7):1568–77.
14. Cojocaru O, Aschie M, Mocanu L, et al. Laryngeal primary malignant melanoma: a case report. Rom J Morphol Embryol 2015;56(4):1513–6.
15. Batsakis JG, Luna MA, el-Naggar AK. Non-squamous carcinomas of the larynx. Ann Otol Rhinol Laryngol 1992;101(12):1024–6.
16. Ganly I, Patel SG, Coleman M, et al. Malignant minor salivary gland tumors of the larynx. Arch Otolaryngol Head Neck Surg 2006;132(7):767–70.
17. Moukarbel RV, Kwan K, Fung K. Laryngeal epithelial-myoepithelial carcinoma treated with partial laryngectomy. J Otolaryngol Head Neck Surg Oct 2010; 39(5):E39–41.
18. Karatayli-Ozgursoy S, Bishop JA, Hillel AT, et al. Malignant salivary gland tumors of the larynx: a single institution review. Acta Otorhinolaryngol Ital 2016;36(4):

289–94. Tumori maligni delle ghiandole salivari della laringe: un'unica review istituzionale.

19. Bak-Pedersen K, Nielsen KO. Subepithelial mucous glands in the adult human larynx. Studies on number, distribution and density. Acta Otolaryngol 1986; 102(3–4):341–52.

20. Dubal PM, Svider PF, Folbe AJ, et al. Laryngeal adenoid cystic carcinoma: a population-based perspective. Laryngoscope 2015;125(11):2485–90.

21. Liu W, Chen X. Adenoid cystic carcinoma of the larynx: a report of six cases with review of the literature. Acta Otolaryngol 2015;135(5):489–93.

22. Kashiwagi T, Kanaya H, Konno W, et al. Adenoid cystic carcinoma of the larynx presenting with unusual subglottic mass: Case report. Auris Nasus Larynx 2016; 43(5):562–5.

23. Marchiano E, Chin OY, Fang CH, et al. Laryngeal adenoid cystic carcinoma: a systematic review. Otolaryngol Head Neck Surg 2016;154(3):433–9.

24. Misiukiewicz KJ, Camille N, Tishler R, et al. Organ preservation for adenoid cystic carcinoma of the larynx. Oncologist 2013;18(5):579–83.

25. Subramaniam T, Lennon P, Kinsella J, et al. Laryngeal preservation in managing advanced tracheal adenoid cystic carcinoma. Case Rep Otolaryngol 2015; 2015:404586.

26. Ferlito A, Recher G, Bottin R. Mucoepidermoid carcinoma of the larynx. A clinicopathological study of 11 cases with review of the literature. ORL J Otorhinolaryngol Relat Spec 1981;43(5):280–99.

27. Mokhtari S, Mokhtari S. Clinical features and differential diagnoses in laryngeal mucoepidermoid carcinoma. Clin Med Insights Pathol 2012;5:1–6.

28. Zhang M, Li KN, Li C, et al. Malignant minor salivary gland carcinomas of the larynx. ORL J Otorhinolaryngol Relat Spec 2014;76(4):222–6.

29. Ferlito A, Rinaldo A, Devaney KO, et al. Management of the clinically negative cervical lymph nodes in patients with non-conventional squamous carcinoma of the larynx. J Laryngol Otol 1999;113(7):619–23.

30. Garden AS, el-Naggar AK, Morrison WH, et al. Postoperative radiotherapy for malignant tumors of the parotid gland. Int J Radiat Oncol Biol Phys 1997; 37(1):79–85.

31. Boscolo-Rizzo P, da Mosto MC, Marchiori C, et al. Transglottic acinic cell carcinoma. Case report and literature review. ORL J Otorhinolaryngol Relat Spec 2004;66(5):286–9.

32. Crissman JD, Rosenblatt A. Acinous cell carcinoma of the larynx. Arch Pathol Lab Med 1978;102(5):233–6.

33. Kallis S, Stevens DJ. Acinous cell carcinoma of the larynx. J Laryngol Otol 1989; 103(6):638–41.

34. Perez-Ordonez B. Neuroendocrine carcinomas of the larynx and head and neck: challenges in classification and grading. Head Neck Pathol 2018; 12(1):1–8.

35. Bal M, Sharma A, Rane SU, et al. Neuroendocrine neoplasms of the larynx: a clinicopathologic analysis of 27 neuroendocrine tumors and neuroendocrine carcinomas. Head Neck Pathol 2022;16(2):375–87.

36. Wang Q, Chen H, Zhou S. Typical laryngeal carcinoid tumor with recurrence and lymph node metastasis: a case report and review of the literature. Int J Clin Exp Pathol 2014;7(12):9028–31.

37. Ferlito A, Devaney KO, Rinaldo A. Neuroendocrine neoplasms of the larynx: advances in identification, understanding, and management. Oral Oncol 2006; 42(8):770–88.

38. Ferlito A, Silver CE, Bradford CR, et al. Neuroendocrine neoplasms of the larynx: an overview. Head Neck 2009;31(12):1634–46.
39. van der Laan TP, Plaat BE, van der Laan BF, et al. Clinical recommendations on the treatment of neuroendocrine carcinoma of the larynx: a meta-analysis of 436 reported cases. Head Neck 2015;37(5):707–15.
40. Soga J, Osaka M, Yakuwa Y. Laryngeal endocrinomas (carcinoids and relevant neoplasms): analysis of 278 reported cases. J Exp Clin Cancer Res 2002;21(1):5–13.
41. Kumar PD, Simha NV NS. Atypical carcinoid of larynx: a case study and a brief review. J Clin Diagn Res 2014;8(4):KD03–4.
42. Ferlito A, Rinaldo A. Primary and secondary small cell neuroendocrine carcinoma of the larynx: a review. Head Neck 2008;30(4):518–24.
43. Zidar N, Gale N. Update from the 5th edition of the World Health Organization classification of head and neck tumors: hypopharynx, larynx, trachea and parapharyngeal space. Head Neck Pathol 2022;16(1):31–9.
44. Baugh RF, Wolf GT, Beals TF, et al. Small cell carcinoma of the larynx: results of therapy. Laryngoscope 1986;96(11):1283–90.
45. Kuan EC, Alonso JE, Tajudeen BA, et al. Small cell carcinoma of the head and neck: a comparative study by primary site based on population data. Laryngoscope 2017;127(8):1785–90.
46. Ghosh R, Dutta R, Dubal PM, et al. Laryngeal neuroendocrine carcinoma: a population-based analysis of incidence and survival. Otolaryngol Head Neck Surg 2015;153(6):966–72.
47. Barker JL Jr, Glisson BS, Garden AS, et al. Management of nonsinonasal neuroendocrine carcinomas of the head and neck. Cancer 2003;98(11):2322–8.
48. Kalemkerian GP, Schneider BJ. Advances in small cell lung cancer. Hematol Oncol Clin North Am 2017;31(1):143–56.
49. Gnepp DR. Small cell neuroendocrine carcinoma of the larynx. A critical review of the literature. ORL J Otorhinolaryngol Relat Spec 1991;53(4):210–9.
50. Kao HL, Chang WC, Li WY, et al. Head and neck large cell neuroendocrine carcinoma should be separated from atypical carcinoid on the basis of different clinical features, overall survival, and pathogenesis. Am J Surg Pathol 2012;36(2):185–92.
51. Deep NL, Ekbom DC, Hinni ML, et al. High-grade neuroendocrine carcinoma of the larynx: the mayo clinic experience. Ann Otol Rhinol Laryngol 2016;125(6):464–9.
52. Smith JD, Harvey RN, Darr OA, et al. Head and neck paragangliomas: a two-decade institutional experience and algorithm for management. Laryngoscope Investig Otolaryngol 2017;2(6):380–9.
53. Williams MD. Paragangliomas of the head and neck: an overview from diagnosis to genetics. Head Neck Pathol Sep 2017;11(3):278–87.
54. Esclamado RM, Disher MJ, Ditto JL, et al. Laryngeal liposarcoma. Arch Otolaryngol Head Neck Surg 1994;120(4):422–6.
55. Han Y, Yang LH, Liu TT, et al. Liposarcoma of the larynx: report of a case and review of literature. Int J Clin Exp Pathol 2015;8(1):1068–72.
56. Pajaniappane A, Farzan J, Green DM, et al. Well-differentiated liposarcoma of the epiglottis. J Laryngol Otol 2014;128(3):296–8.
57. Kodiyan J, Rudman JR, Rosow DE, et al. Lipoma and liposarcoma of the larynx: case reports and literature review. Am J Otolaryngol 2015;36(4):611–5.
58. Gerry D, Fox NF, Spruill LS, et al. Liposarcoma of the head and neck: analysis of 318 cases with comparison to non-head and neck sites. Head Neck 2014;36(3):393–400.
59. Covello R, Licci S, Pichi B, et al. Low-grade myofibroblastic sarcoma of the larynx. Int J Surg Pathol 2011;19(6):822–6.

60. Kordac P, Nikolov DH, Smatanova K, et al. Low-grade myofibroblastic sarcoma of the larynx: case report and review of literature. Acta Med (Hradec Kralove) 2014;57(4):162–4.

61. Ferlito A. Laryngeal fibrosarcoma: an over-diagnosed tumor. ORL J Otorhinolaryngol Relat Spec 1990;52(3):194–5.

62. Cowan ML, Thompson LD, Leon ME, et al. Low-grade fibromyxoid sarcoma of the head and neck: a clinicopathologic series and review of the literature. Head Neck Pathol 2016;10(2):161–6.

63. Myssiorek D, Patel M, Wasserman P, et al. Osteosarcoma of the larynx. Ann Otol Rhinol Laryngol 1998;107(1):70–4.

64. Peng KA, Grogan T, Wang MB. Head and neck sarcomas: analysis of the SEER database. Otolaryngol Head Neck Surg 2014;151(4):627–33.

65. Stavrakas M, Nixon I, Andi K, et al. Head and neck sarcomas: clinical and histopathological presentation, treatment modalities, and outcomes. J Laryngol Otol 2016;130(9):850–9.

66. Thariat J, Kirova Y, Sio T, et al. Mucosal Kaposi sarcoma, a Rare Cancer Network study. Rare Tumors 2012;4(4):e49.

67. Mochloulis G, Irving RM, Grant HR, et al. Laryngeal Kaposi's sarcoma in patients with AIDS. J Laryngol Otol 1996;110(11):1034–7.

68. Dupont C, Vasseur E, Beauchet A, et al. Long-term efficacy on Kaposi's sarcoma of highly active antiretroviral therapy in a cohort of HIV-positive patients. CISIH 92. Centre d'information et de soins de l'immunodeficience humaine. AIDS 2000;14(8):987–93.

69. Bower M, Dalla Pria A, Coyle C, et al. Prospective stage-stratified approach to AIDS-related Kaposi's sarcoma. J Clin Oncol 2014;32(5):409–14.

70. Pisani P, Krengli M, Ramponi A, et al. Angiosarcoma of the hypopharynx. J Laryngol Otol 1994;108(10):905–8.

71. Aslam N, Qazi ZU, Ahmad AH, et al. Malignant glomus tumor of larynx: first case report and literature review. J Laryngol Otol 2012;126(7):743–6.

72. Folpe AL, Fanburg-Smith JC, Miettinen M, et al. Atypical and malignant glomus tumors: analysis of 52 cases, with a proposal for the reclassification of glomus tumors. Am J Surg Pathol 2001;25(1):1–12.

73. Oh SD, Stephenson D, Schnall S, et al. Malignant glomus tumor of the hand. Appl Immunohistochem Mol Morphol 2009;17(3):264–9.

74. Marioni G, Bertino G, Mariuzzi L, et al. Laryngeal leiomyosarcoma. J Laryngol Otol 2000;114(5):398–401.

75. Selcuk OT, Renda L, Erol B, et al. A case of laryngeal leiomyosarcoma and review of the literature. Ann Maxillofac Surg 2015;5(2):274–6.

76. Ognjanovic S, Olivier M, Bergemann TL, et al. Sarcomas in TP53 germline mutation carriers: a review of the IARC TP53 database. Cancer 2012;118(5):1387–96.

77. George S, Serrano C, Hensley ML, et al. Soft Tissue and Uterine Leiomyosarcoma. J Clin Oncol 2018;36(2):144–50.

78. Morera Serna E, Perez Fernandez CA, de la Fuente Jambrina C, et al. [Laryngeal leiomyosarcoma]. Acta Otorrinolaringol Esp 2007;58(9):445–8. Leiomiosarcoma laringeo.

79. Abbas A, Ikram M, Yaqoob N. Leiomyosarcoma of the larynx: a case report. Ear Nose Throat J 2005;84(7):435–6, 440.

80. Darouassi Y, Bouaity B, Zalagh M, et al. Laryngeal leiomyosarcoma. B-ENT 2005;1(3):145–9.

81. Jain A, Singh SN, Singhal P, et al. A rare case of subglottic embryonal rhabdo-myosarcoma: managed with the aim of organ preservation. J Laryngol Otol 2015;129(1):106–9.
82. Shayah A, Agada FO, Karsai L, et al. Adult laryngeal rhabdomyosarcoma: report of a case and literature review. Ann Afr Med Dec 2007;6(4):190–3.
83. Mungan S, Arslan S, Kucuktulu E, et al. Pleomorphic rhabdomyosarcoma arising from true vocal fold of larynx: report of a rare case and literature review. Case Rep Otolaryngol 2016;2016:8135967.
84. Ruske DR, Glassford N, Costello S, et al. Laryngeal rhabdomyosarcoma in adults. J Laryngol Otol 1998;112(7):670–2.
85. Panda SP, Chinnaswamy G, Vora T, et al. Diagnosis and management of rhab-domyosarcoma in children and adolescents: ICMR consensus document. In-dian J Pediatr 2017;84(5):393–402.
86. Anderson JL, Park A, Akiyama R, et al. Evaluation of In Vitro activity of the class I PI3K inhibitor buparlisib (BKM120) in pediatric bone and soft tissue sarcomas. PLoS One 2015;10(9):e0133610.
87. Chin OY, Dubal PM, Sheikh AB, et al. Laryngeal chondrosarcoma: a systematic review of 592 cases. Laryngoscope 2017;127(2):430–9.
88. Gu J, Zuo Z, Sun L, et al. Prognostic factors for laryngeal sarcoma and nomo-gram development for prediction: a retrospective study based on SEER data-base. Ann Transl Med 2020;8(8):545.
89. Thompson LD, Gannon FH. Chondrosarcoma of the larynx: a clinicopathologic study of 111 cases with a review of the literature. Am J Surg Pathol 2002;26(7):836–51.
90. Casiraghi O, Martinez-Madrigal F, Pineda-Daboin K, et al. Chondroid tumors of the larynx: a clinicopathologic study of 19 cases, including two dedifferentiated chondrosarcomas. Ann Diagn Pathol 2004;8(4):189–97.
91. Lewis JE, Olsen KD, Inwards CY. Cartilaginous tumors of the larynx: clinicopath-ologic review of 47 cases. Ann Otol Rhinol Laryngol 1997;106(2):94–100.
92. Adeola JO, Patel JS, Povolotskiy R, et al. Clinicopathologic characteristics of laryngeal chondrosarcoma: an analysis of the National Cancer Database. Auris Nasus Larynx 2021;48(5):956–62.
93. Wang Q, Chen H, Zhou S. Chondrosarcoma of the larynx: report of two cases and review of the literature. Int J Clin Exp Pathol 2015;8(2):2068–73.
94. Oliveira JF, Branquinho FA, Monteiro AR, et al. Laryngeal chondrosarcoma–ten years of experience. Braz J Otorhinolaryngol 2014;80(4):354–8.
95. Kuba K, Inoue H, Hayashi T, et al. Laryngeal osteosarcoma: case report and literature review. Head Neck 2015;37(2):E26–9.
96. Berge JK, Kapadia SB, Myers EN. Osteosarcoma of the larynx. Arch Otolar-yngol Head Neck Surg 1998;124(2):207–10.
97. Owosho AA, Estilo CL, Huryn JM, et al. A Clinicopathologic Study of Head and Neck Malignant Peripheral Nerve Sheath Tumors. Head Neck Pathol 2018;12(2):151–9.
98. Le Guellec S, Decouvelaere AV, Filleron T, et al. Malignant peripheral nerve sheath tumor is a challenging diagnosis: a systematic pathology review, immu-nohistochemistry, and molecular analysis in 160 patients from the french sar-coma group database. Am J Surg Pathol 2016;40(7):896–908.
99. Miao R, Wang H, Jacobson A, et al. Radiation-induced and neurofibromatosis-associated malignant peripheral nerve sheath tumors (MPNST) have worse out-comes than sporadic MPNST. Radiother Oncol 2019;137:61–70.

100. Okcu MF, Munsell M, Treuner J, et al. Synovial sarcoma of childhood and adolescence: a multicenter, multivariate analysis of outcome. J Clin Oncol 2003;21(8):1602–11.
101. Madabhavi I, Bhardawa V, Modi M, et al. Primary synovial sarcoma (SS) of larynx: an unusual site. Oral Oncol 2018;79:80–2.
102. Shein G, Sandhu G, Potter A, et al. Laryngeal synovial sarcoma: a systematic review of the last 40 years of reported cases. Ear Nose Throat J 2021;100(2):NP93–104.
103. Wushou A, Miao XC. Tumor size predicts prognosis of head and neck synovial cell sarcoma. Oncol Lett 2015;9(1):381–6.
104. Randall RL, Schabel KL, Hitchcock Y, et al. Diagnosis and management of synovial sarcoma. Curr Treat Options Oncol 2005;6(6):449–59.
105. Harb WJ, Luna MA, Patel SR, et al. Survival in patients with synovial sarcoma of the head and neck: association with tumor location, size, and extension. Head Neck 2007;29(8):731–40.
106. Owosho AA, Estilo CL, Rosen EB, et al. A clinicopathologic study on SS18 fusion positive head and neck synovial sarcomas. Oral Oncol 2017;66:46–51.
107. Karkos PD, Dova S, Sotiriou S, et al. Double primary malignant fibrous histiocytoma and squamous cell carcinoma of the larynx treated with laser laryngeal conservation surgery. Ecancermedicalscience 2016;10:636.
108. Anghelina F, Ionita E, Chiutu L, et al. Malignant fibrous histiocytoma of larynx with giant cell: case report and histological-clinical considerations. Rom J Morphol Embryol 2009;50(3):481–5.
109. Guney E, Yigitbasi OG, Balkanli S, et al. Postirradiation malignant fibrous histiocytoma of the larynx: a case report. Am J Otolaryngol 2002;23(5):293–6.
110. Guo J, Cui Q, Liu C, et al. Clinical report on transarterial neoadjuvant chemotherapy of malignant fibrous histiocytoma in soft tissue. Clin Transl Oncol 2013;15(5):370–5.
111. Bradford Bell EJ, Thomas GR, Leibowitz J, et al. Benign and malignant granular cell tumor of the hypopharynx: two faces of a rare entity. Head Neck Pathol 2021;15(1):281–7.
112. Aksoy S, Abali H, Kilickap S, et al. Metastatic granular cell tumor: a case report and review of the literature. Acta Oncol 2006;45(1):91–4.
113. Fanburg-Smith JC, Meis-Kindblom JM, Fante R, et al. Malignant granular cell tumor of soft tissue: diagnostic criteria and clinicopathologic correlation. Am J Surg Pathol 1998;22(7):779–94.
114. Kumar VFN, Abbas A. Robbins & coltran pathologic basis of disease. 7th edition. Philadelphia, PA: Saunders; 2004.
115. Quimby AE, Caulley L, Rodin D, et al. Primary Burkitt lymphoma of the supraglottic larynx: a case report and review of the literature. J Med Case Rep 2017;11(1):65.
116. Rahman B, Bilal J, Sipra QU, et al. All that wheezes is not asthma: a case of diffuse large b-cell lymphoma of the larynx. Case Rep Oncol Med 2017;2017:7072615.
117. Markou K, Goudakos J, Constantinidis J, et al. Primary laryngeal lymphoma: report of 3 cases and review of the literature. Head Neck 2010;32(4):541–9.
118. Nicolai P, Puxeddu R, Cappiello J, et al. Metastatic neoplasms to the larynx: report of three cases. Laryngoscope 1996;106(7):851–5.
119. Grasso RF, Quattrocchi CC, Piciucchi S, et al. Vocal cord metastasis from breast cancer. J Clin Oncol 2007;25(13):1803–5.
120. Becker M, Moulin G, Kurt AM, et al. Non-squamous cell neoplasms of the larynx: radiologic-pathologic correlation. Radiographics 1998;18(5):1189–209.

Voice Restoration and Quality of Life in Larynx Cancer

Jessica A. Tang, MD[a], Liane McCarroll, MS, CCC-SLP/L[b],
Cecelia E. Schmalbach, MD, MSc[c],*

KEYWORDS

- Voice restoration • Electrolarynx • Tracheoesophageal puncture
- Esophageal speech • Quality of life

KEY POINTS

- Over 90% of laryngectomy patients seek voice rehabilitation.
- The three most common restorative techniques are: esophageal speech, artifical larynx, and tracheoesophageal puncture.
- Tracheoesophageal puncture (TEP) is most comparable alternative to pre-laryngectomy voice quality.

INTRODUCTION

Three major modalities currently exist in which voice and speech are restored for total laryngectomy patients: esophageal speech (ES), artificial larynx (electrolarynx [EL]), and tracheoesophageal puncture (TEP). Although a small percentage of the population choose to remain nonvocal following total laryngectomy (8%),[1] most patients adapt to 1 of the 3 options to maintain the ability to communicate verbally.

The choice of restorative technique depends on a variety of factors including level of mental and physical function, support from family and caregivers, access to rehabilitative services, financial capabilities, and motivation. These methods are not mutually exclusive, and many patients learn to use more than one method to communicate verbally. Although the EL was historically the most used technique,[1] TEP has quickly become the gold standard with many surgeons opting to place a primary TEP during the laryngectomy. ES remains the least frequently used

[a] Department of Otolaryngology Head and Neck Surgery, Johns Hopkins Hospital, 601 N. Caroline Street, Baltimore, MD 21287, USA; [b] Fox Chase Cancer Center, 333 Cottman Avenue, Philadelphia, PA 19111, USA; [c] Department of Otolaryngology-HNS, Lewis Katz School of Medicine at Temple University, Temple Head & Neck Institute, Fox Chase Cancer Center, 3440 North Broad Street, Kresge West 309, Philadelphia, PA 19140, USA
* Corresponding author.
E-mail address: Cecelia.Schmalbach@TUHS.Temple.edu

Otolaryngol Clin N Am 56 (2023) 361–370
https://doi.org/10.1016/j.otc.2022.11.003
0030-6665/23/© 2022 Elsevier Inc. All rights reserved.

oto.theclinics.com

technique in developed countries, likely because it is the most difficult to teach and for patients to learn. Each technique with associated benefits and challenges is outlined below. Aspects of patient selection are highlighted, along with the impact on quality of life (QOL).

Esophageal Speech

Despite being the least popular of the 3 modalities for voice restoration following laryngectomy in developed countries, ES is the most economical and requires the least maintenance. ES was the traditional treatment of choice because patients could learn to produce a voice on their own without the constraints of prosthesis maintenance, manual dexterity, or potentially costly devices. It is therefore the most widely used method in developing countries in which financial costs and access to resources may be prohibitive.[2]

In ES, patients are taught to produce a voice by swallowing air and releasing this air back through the esophagus in a controlled manner. The vibrations created along the mucosa of the esophagus and pharynx create the sound source, and patients learn to use the structures of the oral cavity and pharynx to modulate this voice into understandable speech.

Because additional surgery is not required, risks of surgery and additional procedural complications are mitigated. Unfortunately, instances exist in which ES may not work well or instances in which patients are initially able to use ES but subsequently experience loss of voice. From an anatomic standpoint, spasms or stenosis of the cricopharyngeus muscle may make it difficult for patients to mechanically propagate the vibratory waves up through the pharynx and into the oral cavity.[3] Surgeons must be diligent in releasing all visible muscle fibers when performing cricopharyngeal myotomy during a laryngectomy in order to reduce the chances of this complication. If a cricopharyngeal myotomy is performed at a later stage, patients should be aware that there are risks to this additional procedure to include perforation and recurrence of cricopharyngeal stenosis. If cricopharyngeal spasms are the main cause of cricopharyngeal narrowing that inhibit the ability to produce ES, botulinum toxin injection into the cricopharyngeus can be used. However, these results typically only last 4 to 6 months and would require repeat procedures to maintain continued effects.

For patients choosing to pursue ES as their primary rehabilitative option, motivation and persistence is paramount. ES is a steep learning curve, and patients should be prepared to put in a substantial effort with daily practice and regular sessions with speech language pathologists (SLPs). ES can sometimes take up to half a year to learn. Interestingly, although only a small subset of patients chooses to use ES, those that learn the technique often use an alternative method of voice rehabilitation as their primary means of communication.[4]

Of course, that access to these rehabilitative services to learn ES is paramount. There is a paucity of speech therapists trained to teach this very specific method of voice restoration. Even for those that are specialized in teaching ES, there remains the inherent difficulty for a speech pathologist who has an existing larynx to demonstrate ES to a patient without a larynx; attempting to allow air to pass through an existing larynx is intrinsically different to replicate.

Artificial Larynx (Electrolarynx)

The EL is an electronic battery-powered device used to replicate voice for laryngectomy patients (**Fig. 1**). Speech is produced through transmission of the vibrations from this device, which are applied either externally on the neck or cheek or intraorally

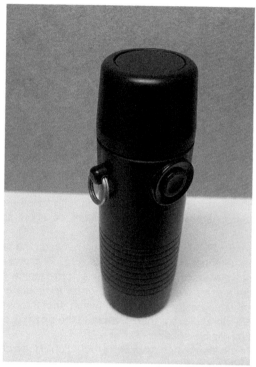

Fig. 1. The EL is a handheld electronic battery-powered device that emits vibrations that are transmitted to the external neck skin (or intraorally through a plastic tube, not pictured) that patients can then use to produce speech by shaping their oral cavity and pharyngeal structures.

through a plastic tube in the oral cavity. Patients must learn to move the structures of their oral cavity and pharynx to shape words and produce understandable speech.

Mastery of the EL takes practice. Although there is still a learning component to articulating speech with this apparatus, it is still easier to learn than ES. There is also the added advantage that electrolaryngeal speech is easier to discriminate in background noise compared with ES.[5]

The choice of the EL does not preclude the ability to use other forms of voice restoration. These devices can be used to bridge the gap until ES or TEP is achieved. Such delays occur either in the postoperative period (because the EL can be used immediately after surgery), or in backup scenarios when other means are temporarily unavailable or inaccessible due to illness, cancer recurrence, or prosthetic malfunction. It can therefore be beneficial to know how to use an EL even if it is not the chosen primary method of verbal communication.

Despite these favorable aspects of the EL, there are several reasons why laryngectomy patients may not choose to use this apparatus. The most conspicuous drawback is the artificial and "robotic" sound quality inherent to these devices, which may be unappealing in drawing unwanted attention to the laryngectomy patient. Speaking also requires the use of at least one hand to hold the device against the cervical skin or intraoral mucosa and thus necessitates manual dexterity and prevents the user from using both hands when attempting to speak. There have been recent developments of a hands-free EL device using an electromyography transducer to provide vibration to the strap muscles[6] but the classic hand-held EL device is still the most popular option.

Finally, the cost of the device may be prohibitive to low-income populations because devices are not always covered by insurance. Durable medical equipment benefits are required for coverage, and without these benefits, patients may have to purchase devices out-of-pocket. Additionally, insurance benefits may limit how frequently a patient can replace their device, which can be problematic when these time parameters are longer than warranties. Patients without coverage may have success obtaining a device through local or national laryngectomy support groups.

Tracheoesophogeal Puncture

Of the 3 options for voice restoration following laryngectomy, TEP has been described as the most comparable alternative to normal laryngeal speech[7] with patients being the most satisfied in the quality of communication with those around them.[8] After all, voice can be produced with the least amount of effort and with the most spontaneity.

As its name suggests, a TEP creates an opening between the trachea and esophagus in which a one-directional valve prosthesis (**Fig. 2**) allows air to be shunted from the trachea into the esophagus. The laryngectomy stoma must be occluded either digitally or with a valve over the stoma in order to create a pressure gradient to activate the one-way prosthetic valve between the trachea and esophagus (**Fig. 3**). Similar to ES, vibrations are then created in the pharynx and oral cavity that can be shaped into intelligible speech.

Digital occlusion of the stoma during speech production is the most intuitive method but requires one hand to be free. Alternatively, a breathing valve can permit hands-free voice production but the difficulty in maintaining a seal can sometimes be frustrating and cumbersome. The breathing valve is manufactured to remain open until there is an increase in airflow when patients exhale forcefully to produce speech. These valves can attach either to the skin around the stoma or just within the lumen of the trachea. Consequently, poor adhesive attachment and irregular stoma contour often preclude the ability to maintain a durable seal.

TEP can be performed either during the primary laryngectomy procedure or as a secondary procedure at a later stage. The benefits of primary TEP include a shorter time to commence voice rehabilitation and the avoidance of the added logistical steps and morbidity of a second operation. Some surgeons who have the resources and expertise may prefer to perform secondary TEP in clinic under local anesthesia.

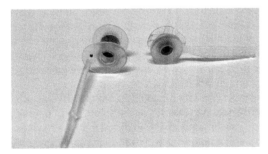

Fig. 2. Two examples of TEP prostheses. The prosthesis is a one-way valve that only allows air to be communicated from the trachea into the esophagus. By occluding the laryngectomy stoma, a pressure gradient is created to shunt air from the trachea into the esophagus to provide speech through the structures of the oral cavity and pharynx.

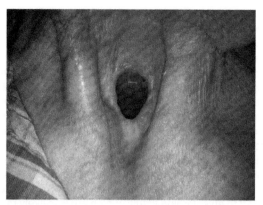

Fig. 3. Example of a TEP prosthesis within a laryngectomy stoma.

For patients in whom there are concerns for wound healing, secondary TEP has previously been preferred especially in the postradiated, salvage laryngectomy patient population in which pharyngocutaneous fistula is a higher risk.[9] However, the concern that secondary TEP may interfere with healing in this patient population is not unequivocally supported, and there are data demonstrating no significant differences in complication rates between primary and secondary TEP even in patients who have previously undergone radiation therapy.[10] Furthermore, microvascular free flap reconstruction is frequently used in the salvage laryngectomy population in order to reduce the incidence of pharyngocutaneous fistulas but undergoing a vascularized free tissue transfer should not serve as a contraindication for simultaneous placement of TEP.[11]

When performed primarily, TEP allows direct access to the esophageal lumen, which is already exposed during a laryngectomy. It is important for the peristomal area to be shallow and flat in order to facilitate ease of accessing the prosthesis. This can be achieved by dividing the sternal heads of the sternocleidomastoid muscles. A right angle instrument is inserted into the esophageal lumen approximately 1 cm below the free edge and the tip of the clamp is directed with force anteriorly to tent up the posterior tracheal wall. A scalpel blade is then used to make an incision over the tip of the clamp along the posterior tracheal wall. A catheter can then be threaded through this surgically created fistula to allow placement of the prosthesis. Alternatively, if there is concern about wound healing, a catheter can be placed as a spacer while the tract matures. It is then changed to a prosthesis at a later date in the office. Regardless, it is important to ensure that the location of this fistula is not too low within the trachea when creating the puncture in order to facilitate care and exchange of the prosthesis in the future.

In more recent years, some surgeons have adopted the practice of performing secondary TEP in clinic[12,13] using transnasal esophagoscopy and local anesthesia. Alternatively, when performed in the operating room, secondary TEP involves advancing an esophagoscope until it can be palpated through the tracheostoma and subsequently using an 18-gauge needle to puncture the back wall of the trachea into the esophageal lumen under direct visualization. Medical device companies have also developed novel introducer kits to simplify seamless insertion of the voice prosthesis.

Using TEP as a primary means of voice restoration after laryngectomy can be tremendously appealing given its advantages in permitting spontaneous, higher quality speech without much effort. Unfortunately, TEP may not be the best modality for all patients, and certain medical comorbidities (such as poor pulmonary function, history of aspiration pneumonia, poor dexterity, and visual limitations), access to rehabilitative services, and ongoing prosthetic maintenance are factors for which patients should be educated that may make TEP less ideal.

Gastroesophageal reflux disease (GERD) is a known culprit for prosthetic failure often due to leakage around the prosthesis.[14] Those with known reflux have higher rates of TEP complications, and treatment with proton pump inhibitors have been shown to decrease leakage around the prosthesis.[15] In addition, postoperative radiation had also been shown to correlate with the risk of GERD and prosthetic failure.[16]

Patients should be counseled of the lifelong need for regular visits with trained specialists at institutions familiar with caring for TEP. The average time of TEP prostheses replacement is approximately every 2 months.[17] This can become a financial burden if the patients insurance does not cover the cost of the prosthesis. TEP prostheses are not without mechanical problems as well. Leakage around TEP prostheses may be attributed to an enlarging fistula, which are less likely related to prosthetic dimensions or timing of prosthetic placement[18] as much as other underlying causes such as *Candida* growth. Certain factors need to be considered in understanding the manifestation of an ill-fitting prosthesis due to an enlarging fistula. Tumor recurrence surrounding the prosthesis and stoma may be associated with an enlarged TEP site.[19] Postoperative stricture, poor nutritional status, radiation therapy, and more extensive resections may also contribute to enlarging fistulas.[19,20] Enlarged TEP should be taken seriously because these can carry a high risk of pneumonia or even aspiration of the prosthesis. Conservative management including temporary removal with intentional fistula contracture, replacement with a prosthesis that has a larger flange, or puncture site injection with a bulking agent can successfully manage this issue.[21,22]

Patient Selection

Although many regard tracheoesophageal speech (TES) as the gold standard, there is no single best option for all patients following total laryngectomy. Patient education and counseling regarding the advantages and limitations of the 3 main modalities: EL speech, ES, and TES should begin preoperatively. When helping the patient decide the best voicing modality for them, numerous factors should be considered to include, but are not limited to, manual dexterity, visual acuity, access to a support system, comorbidities, motivation, financial status, sufficient anatomy, swallowing function, risk factors for leakage around, social support, and the ability to provide self-care.[23–25]

Conversations surrounding TEP candidacy are complex as a universally accepted consensus statement on candidacy is lacking and practice patterns vary widely across facilities and providers. Many head and neck surgeons cite factors such as stoma size, type and extent of reconstruction (ie, free tissue transfer), and risk for postoperative complications such as fistula and poor wound healing as important factors in patient selection for a TEP. In addition, SLPs cite swallowing function, compliance with recommendations, ability to provide self-care and risk factors for leakage as important factors.[17,18,23] These differences highlight the importance of group discussion, with a joint decision being made by all parties involved to include the patient.

When discussing voicing modality options with patients, it is important to consider the entire clinical picture; no patient is going to be a perfect candidate. It has been reported that approximately 80% of patients who receive a TEP achieve TES,[24] and only 26% of patients who are able to complete ES are able to be functional for everyday communication.[4] Creating an environment of realistic voice rehabilitation expectations is paramount. Additionally, patients do not have to choose just one technique, with many opting to learn multiple modalities. Patient selection should be a joint decision-making process with education and counseling provided across the continuum of care.

Quality of Life

Treatment of head and neck cancer can affect structures vital to speech and swallowing. In doing so, it can have a negative influence on a patient's psychosocial well-being and associated QOL. QOL encompasses many aspects, including emotional, physical, spiritual, financial, and social well-being.[26] This is particularly salient when working with patients who have undergone total laryngectomy as aphonia can affect all of these areas. How an individual views their QOL is both unique and multidimensional. Although research on QOL following total laryngectomy is sparse, there is evidence to support that all aspects of QOL may be negatively affected following surgery.[27]

QOL should be assessed from the patient's perspective. This is supported by the World Health Organization who defines QOL as "an individual's perception of their position in life, in the context of the culture and value systems in their life, and in relation to their goals, expectations, standards and concerns."[28] Patients need time to learn and adapt to their new communication method after total laryngectomy. They may think as though they have become inefficient communicators and struggle to accept their new voice.[29]

Prompt and effective voice restoration postoperatively is paramount for this population, with many patients reporting the inability to speak as they once did and communicate their needs in the hospital as their greatest challenge following surgery.[30] Irrespective of their chosen communication method, patients report the following challenges following laryngectomy: difficulty identifying with their new voice, loss of spontaneity in their communication, negative perceptions by others, not being understood by communication partners, and communication difficulties in loud environments. These challenges lead some to avoid social situations.[31] Danker and colleagues[32] interviewed 218 patients after total laryngectomy and found that more than 80% of participants were aware of stigma associated with their voice and that more than 40% experienced social withdrawal due to communication changes.

Making broad statements about voice-related QOL after total laryngectomy is difficult secondary to variability in which aspects of QOL are assessed and patient reported outcomes are used. Although TES is often described as the most natural sounding and closest to laryngeal voicing with the best QOL,[7] these differences are not always statistically significant. de Silva and colleagues reported on 34 patients who completed 3 QOL questionnaires. This study demonstrated that all patients had lower QOL compared with the general population. Although those using TES had the highest QOL followed by those using ES and then the nonvocal group, the findings were not statistically significant. This study did identify a statistically significant difference with higher physical functioning capacity for the ES group compared with the other 2 groups.[33]

In a study by Moukarbel and colleagues,[8] 75 patients completed the Voice-Related Quality of Life questionnaire. A statistically significant difference was not identified between the TES group and the ES group. Both groups performed significantly better than the EL speech group. These findings suggest that TES and ES have comparable QOL. In contrast, in Robertson and colleagues,[34] overall voice-related QOL for EL speech was better than for ES, whereas Evans and colleagues[35] looked at overall voice-related QOL between TES users and non-TES users (ES, EL speech, or other) and found no significant differences.

Communication method after total laryngectomy is not the only factor affecting QOL. One must consider demographics such as age, gender, access to a support system and employment status. Furthermore, a history of radiation or chemotherapy has been shown to negatively affect voice-related QOL.[29,36] Ultimately, how a patient perceives their QOL after total laryngectomy will vary based on the individual. Although initiation of speech therapy to address alaryngeal communication is known to be beneficial, with improvement in intelligibility regardless of voicing modality, other ancillary providers should be consulted as indicated. For example, interventions targeted at addressing anxiety, depression, and stress associated with communication challenges and feelings of social isolation should be offered in addition to alaryngeal voice therapy.[37]

SUMMARY

Voice restoration following laryngectomy has a significant influence on QOL. Three main techniques exist to provide voice: ES, artificial larynx (EL), and TEP. TEP has quickly become the gold standard technique, replacing the traditional EL due to both the potential hands-free nature of the device and the more natural voice quality. ES remains the least frequently used technique in developed countries, likely because it is the most difficult to teach and for patients to learn. Technique selection must be made on an individual basis, considering the patient's cancer history and comorbidities. Ultimately, the choice in voice-restoration technique requires joint decision-making with the surgeon, speech pathologist, and patient.

CLINICS CARE POINTS

- Tracheoesophageal speech can be optimized by creating a shallow and flap peristomal area which is achieved by dividing the sternal attachments of the sternocleidomastoid muscles.
- Mental and physicial capabilities, social support, and patient motivation must all be considered when selecting the optimal vocal restorative technique.
- Patients electing for tracheoesophageal puncture must understand that it is a lifelong commitment, requiring routine visits every 8 to 12 weeks for prosthesis change.

DISCLOSURE

The authors have no commercial or financial conflicts of interest; no funding sources were used for this article.

REFERENCES

1. Hillman RE, Walsh MJ, Wolf GT, et al. Functional outcomes following treatment for advanced laryngeal cancer. Part I--Voice preservation in advanced laryngeal cancer. Part II–Laryngectomy rehabilitation: the state of the art in the VA System. Research Speech-Language Pathologists. Department of Veterans Affairs Laryngeal Cancer Study Group. Ann Otol Rhinol Laryngol Suppl 1998;172:1–27.
2. Xi S. Effectiveness of voice rehabilitation on vocalisation in postlaryngectomy patients: a systematic review. Int J Evid Based Healthc 2010;8(4):256–8.
3. Tang CG, Sinclair CF. Voice Restoration After Total Laryngectomy. Otolaryngol Clin North Am 2015;48(4):687–702.

4. Gates GA, Ryan W, Cooper JC Jr, et al. Current status of laryngectomee rehabilitation: I. Results of therapy. Am J Otolaryngol 1982;3(1):1–7.
5. Babin E, Beynier D, Le Gall D, et al. Psychosocial quality of life in patients after total laryngectomy. Rev Laryngol Otol Rhinol (Bord) 2009;130(1):29–34.
6. Goldstein EA, Heaton JT, Stepp CE, et al. Training effects on speech production using a hands-free electromyographically controlled electrolarynx. J Speech Lang Hear Res 2007;50(2):335–51.
7. Robbins J. Acoustic differentiation of laryngeal, esophageal, and tracheoesophageal speech. J Speech Hear Res 1984;27(4):577–85.
8. Moukarbel RV, Doyle PC, Yoo JH, et al. Voice-related quality of life (V-RQOL) outcomes in laryngectomees. Head Neck 2011;33(1):31–6.
9. Emerick KS, Tomycz L, Bradford CR, et al. Primary versus secondary tracheoesophageal puncture in salvage total laryngectomy following chemoradiation. Otolaryngol Head Neck Surg 2009;140(3):386–90.
10. Cheng E, Ho M, Ganz C, et al. Outcomes of primary and secondary tracheoesophageal puncture: a 16-year retrospective analysis. Ear Nose Throat J 2006; 85(4):264–7.
11. Sinclair CF, Rosenthal EL, McColloch NL, et al. Primary versus delayed tracheoesophageal puncture for laryngopharyngectomy with free flap reconstruction. Laryngoscope 2011;121(7):1436–40.
12. Bach KK, Postma GN, Koufman JA. In-office tracheoesophageal puncture using transnasal esophagoscopy. Laryngoscope 2003;113(1):173–6.
13. Desyatnikova S, Caro JJ, Andersen PE, et al. Tracheoesophageal puncture in the office setting with local anesthesia. Ann Otol Rhinol Laryngol 2001;110(7 Pt 1): 613–6.
14. Cocuzza S, Bonfiglio M, Chiaramonte R, et al. Gastroesophageal reflux disease and postlaryngectomy tracheoesophageal fistula. Eur Arch Otorhinolaryngol 2012;269(5):1483–8.
15. Lorenz KJ, Grieser L, Ehrhart T, et al. The management of periprosthetic leakage in the presence of supra-oesophageal reflux after prosthetic voice rehabilitation. Eur Arch Otorhinolaryngol 2011;268(5):695–702.
16. Cocuzza S, Bonfiglio M, Chiaramonte R, et al. Relationship between radiotherapy and gastroesophageal reflux disease in causing tracheoesophageal voice rehabilitation failure. J Voice 2014;28(2):245–9.
17. Lewin JS, Baumgart LM, Barrow MP, et al. Device Life of the Tracheoesophageal Voice Prosthesis Revisited. JAMA Otolaryngol Head Neck Surg 2017;143(1): 65–71.
18. Hutcheson KA, Lewin JS, Sturgis EM, et al. Enlarged tracheoesophageal puncture after total laryngectomy: a systematic review and meta-analysis. Head Neck 2011;33(1):20–30.
19. Hutcheson KA, Lewin JS, Sturgis EM, et al. Multivariable analysis of risk factors for enlargement of the tracheoesophageal puncture after total laryngectomy. Head Neck 2012;34(4):557–67.
20. Op de Coul BM, Hilgers FJ, Balm AJ, et al. A decade of postlaryngectomy vocal rehabilitation in 318 patients: a single Institution's experience with consistent application of provox indwelling voice prostheses. Arch Otolaryngol Head Neck Surg 2000;126(11):1320–8.
21. Hutcheson KA, Lewin JS, Sturgis EM, et al. Outcomes and adverse events of enlarged tracheoesophageal puncture after total laryngectomy. Laryngoscope 2011;121(7):1455–61.

22. Lorincz BB, Lichtenberger G, Bihari A, et al. Therapy of periprosthetical leakage with tissue augmentation using Bioplastique around the implanted voice prosthesis. Eur Arch Otorhinolaryngol 2005;262(1):32–4.

23. Zenga J, Goldsmith T, Bunting G, et al. State of the art: Rehabilitation of speech and swallowing after total laryngectomy. Oral Oncol 2018;86:38–47.

24. Pou AM. Tracheoesophageal voice restoration with total laryngectomy. Otolaryngol Clin North Am 2004;37(3):531–45.

25. Gress CD. Preoperative evaluation for tracheoesophageal voice restoration. Otolaryngol Clin North Am 2004;37(3):519–30.

26. Murphy BA, Ridner S, Wells N, et al. Quality of life research in head and neck cancer: a review of the current state of the science. Crit Rev Oncol Hematol 2007; 62(3):251–67.

27. Maclean J, Cotton S, Perry A. Dysphagia following a total laryngectomy: the effect on quality of life, functioning, and psychological well-being. Dysphagia 2009;24(3):314–21.

28. World Health Organziation. WHOQOL: measuring quality of life. Available at: who.int/tools/whoqol. Accessed December 15, 2022.

29. Sharpe G, Camoes Costa V, Doube W, et al. Communication changes with laryngectomy and impact on quality of life: a review. Qual Life Res 2019;28(4):863–77.

30. Dooks P, McQuestion M, Goldstein D, et al. Experiences of patients with laryngectomies as they reintegrate into their community. Support Care Cancer 2012; 20(3):489–98.

31. Bickford J, Coveney J, Baker J, et al. Living with the altered self: a qualitative study of life after total laryngectomy. Int J Speech Lang Pathol 2013;15(3): 324–33.

32. Danker H, Wollbruck D, Singer S, et al. Social withdrawal after laryngectomy. Eur Arch Otorhinolaryngol 2010;267(4):593–600.

33. Pereira da Silva A, Feliciano T, Vaz Freitas S, et al. Quality of life in patients submitted to total laryngectomy. J Voice 2015;29(3):382–8.

34. Robertson SM, Yeo JC, Dunnet C, et al. Voice, swallowing, and quality of life after total laryngectomy: results of the west of Scotland laryngectomy audit. Head Neck 2012;34(1):59–65.

35. Evans E, Carding P, Drinnan M. The voice handicap index with post-laryngectomy male voices. Int J Lang Commun Disord 2009;44(5):575–86.

36. Kazi R, De Cordova J, Singh A, et al. Voice-related Quality of Life in laryngectomees: assessment using the VHI and V-RQOL symptom scales. J Voice 2007; 21(6):728–34.

37. Perry A, Casey E, Cotton S. Quality of life after total laryngectomy: functioning, psychological well-being and self-efficacy. Int J Lang Commun Disord 2015; 50(4):467–75.

Swallowing Function After Treatment of Laryngeal Cancer

Maude Brisson-McKenna, MSc(A), S-LP[a],*,
Gina D. Jefferson, MD, MPH[b], Sana H. Siddiqui, MD[c],
Sarah Adams, MS, CCC-SLP[d], Sofia Afanasieva (Sonia), MHSc, S-LP[a],
Aïda Chérid, MHSc, S-LP[a], Jesse Burns, MSc, S-LP(C)[a],
Carla Di Gironimo, MS, S-LP(C), CCC-SLP[a], Leila J. Mady, MD, PhD, MPH[c,e]

KEYWORDS

- Laryngeal cancer • Dysphagia • Swallowing therapy • Radiation therapy
- Chemoradiation • Organ preservation • Laryngeal surgery • Laryngectomy

KEY POINTS

- Changes to the anatomy or physiology of the larynx secondary to a tumor and following treatment of laryngeal cancer commonly affects swallowing safety and efficiency.
- The likelihood, nature, and severity of dysphagia depends on initial tumor stage, as well as treatment modality and intensity.
- Both surgical and nonsurgical treatment of laryngeal carcinoma may significantly affect swallow function. The effect of surgical management is typically acute, whereas the effects of nonsurgical therapy (ie, radiation ± chemotherapy) continue to evolve over time.
- Swallowing evaluation and therapy with a Speech-Language Pathologist benefits patients undergoing laryngeal cancer treatment. Individualized treatment approaches may involve coping strategies, including compensatory swallowing and exercise maneuvers, management of treatment-related sequelae, and surgical interventions.

 Video content accompanies this article at http://www.oto.theclinics.com.

---

[a] Department of Speech-Language Pathology, McGill University Health Centre, Glen site, D04. 7510-1001 boul. Décarie, Montréal, QC, H4A 3J1, Canada; [b] Department of Otolaryngology-Head and Neck Surgery, University of Mississippi Medical Center, 2500 N. State St.Jackson, MS 39216-4505, USA; [c] Head & Neck Surgery, Thomas Jefferson University Hospitals, 925 Chestnut Street, 6th Floor, Philadelphia, PA 19107, USA; [d] Voice and Swallowing Center, Thomas Jefferson University Hospitals, 925 Chestnut Street, 6th Floor, Philadelphia, PA 19107, USA; [e] Cancer Risk and Control Program of Excellence, Sidney Kimmel Cancer Center, 233 S 10th Street, Philadelphia, PA 19107, USA
* Corresponding author. D04.7510-1001 boul. Décarie, Montréal, QC, H4A 3J1.
E-mail address: maude.brisson-mckenna@muhc.mcgill.ca

Otolaryngol Clin N Am 56 (2023) 371–388
https://doi.org/10.1016/j.otc.2022.11.004
0030-6665/23/© 2022 Elsevier Inc. All rights reserved.

INTRODUCTION

The process of swallowing is divided into 3 main phases: the oral phase, pharyngeal phase, and esophageal phase.[1,2] Each phase involves multiple structures and mechanisms, which can make the pinpoint identification for the cause of dysphagia complex.

The oral phase involves the mastication of food in combination with saliva to form a bolus that is then propelled posteriorly into the oropharynx.[1,2] Muscles of facial expression help keep food within the oral cavity, whereas muscles of mastication are involved in the chewing of food. Tongue musculature involuntarily work to thrust food along the teeth. The bolus is then propelled by the force of the tongue retracting and rising to contact the palate, which also elevates to close off the velopharyngeal port. This phase involves cranial nerves V (muscles of mastication), VII (motor function to the lips, taste to the anterior two-thirds of the tongue), IX (general sensation and taste to the posterior one-third of the tongue), X (innervation to the soft palate), and XII (innervation to the musculature of the tongue).[1,2]

Once the bolus is formed in the oral cavity and moved into the oropharynx, it enters the pharyngeal phase. This phase involves the space between the base of tongue, valleculae, and the posterior pharyngeal wall, above the upper esophageal sphincter. The 2 crucial functions of this phase include generating pressure to squeeze the bolus through the pharynx and protecting the airway from bolus material. The valleculae temporarily stores the food bolus, as multiple mechanisms simultaneously occur to promote passage of food into the esophagus. The vocal folds adduct, and the laryngeal complex is protected by the inversion of the epiglottis over the laryngeal orifice. The larynx elevates superiorly and anteriorly with aid of the lateral pharyngeal and suprahyoid musculature to open the UES, whereas the pharyngeal constrictors squeeze against the base of tongue to propel food toward the relaxed UES. Cranial nerves IX and X have crucial roles in controlling much of this musculature, but this phase is largely involuntary through a reflex arc involving all the cranial nerves mentioned previously. The involuntary esophageal phase is then provoked with peristaltic waves moving food through the esophagus into the stomach.[1,2]

Disruptions in normal laryngeal function resulting from laryngeal cancer or its treatments may prevent the larynx from completing its 2 primary swallowing functions: protecting the airway and contributing to clearance of a food bolus through the pharynx and into the esophagus (**Fig. 1**). During normal swallow, laryngeal elevation and anterior excursion, epiglottic retroflexion over the laryngeal orifice, and intralaryngeal closure protect the airway from aspiration by sealing off the airway as the bolus transits through the pharynx. Postswallow, subglottic pressure generated via laryngeal valving may clear pharyngeal residue or any material that has entered the upper airway by coughing or throat clearing.[3] Laryngeal cancer treatment modalities, whether involving total laryngectomy (TL) or organ preservation, cause changes to the anatomy or physiology of the larynx and its surrounding structures, resulting in dysphagia or swallowing difficulty.[2]

Rates of Dysphagia

Patients with laryngeal cancer may present with pretreatment swallowing deficits due to the presence of tumor causing structural or functional anomalies.[2,4] The likelihood and severity of dysphagia following treatments for laryngeal cancer depends on initial tumor stage, pretreatment swallow function, as well as treatment modality and intensity.[2,5–7] In a population-based study of 8002 patients with head and neck cancer (HNC), 40% having laryngeal cancer, 40% experienced dysphagia within 3 years of

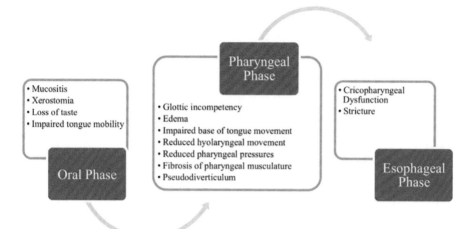

- Mucositis
- Xerostomia
- Loss of taste
- Impaired tongue mobility

Oral Phase

Pharyngeal Phase

- Glottic incompetency
- Edema
- Impaired base of tongue movement
- Reduced hyolaryngeal movement
- Reduced pharyngeal pressures
- Fibrosis of pharyngeal musculature
- Pseudodiverticulum

- Cricopharyngeal Dysfunction
- Stricture

Esophageal Phase

Fig. 1. Contributors to dysphagia by phase of swallow in patients treated by surgery and/or chemoradiation for laryngeal carcinoma.

treatment, with similar rates among those with laryngeal cancer. Higher rates were found among patients who underwent (chemo)radiotherapy [(C)RT] relative to surgery alone.[7] Further, a 2015 retrospective longitudinal study including 2370 elderly patients diagnosed with laryngeal cancer between 2004 and 2007 found that almost 20% of subjects experienced dysphagia 5 years after treatment.[8]

Consequences of Dysphagia

Dysphagia may have significant impacts on posttreatment quality of life (QOL) and survival. Possible medical conditions stemming from dysphagia include malnutrition, weight loss, dehydration, and aspiration-related respiratory infections or complications.[9] QOL is affected when choices in food and liquids are restricted for safety, swallowing efficiency, or comfort. Further, patients may need to use compensatory swallowing strategies or maneuvers that could affect social interactions typically associated with eating and drinking.[10–13]

Assessment and Outcome Measures

Speech-language pathologists (SLPs) are involved in patient care before, during, and after laryngeal cancer treatment and work to mitigate the effects of treatments on swallowing and voice. **Table 1** provides an overview of types of swallowing assessments performed by SLPs.[14] In the literature, multiple swallowing outcome metrics are used to document the impact of HNC treatments on swallow function. These metrics include specific results of instrumental swallowing assessments (eg, aspiration rates or pharyngoesophageal stricture); rates of aspiration pneumonia; and nutritional outcomes such as tube feeding dependency and malnutrition, weight loss, reported diet changes, and self-report patient questionnaires.[5,15,16]

DISCUSSION
Acute and Chronic Swallow Outcomes After Treatment of Laryngeal Cancer

Laryngeal cancer managed with either surgery or radiation results in both acute and chronic swallowing function consequences. Furthermore, as mentioned earlier, dysphagia is often present before treatment due to tumor size that affects mobility

Table 1
Swallowing assessments, benefits, and challenges

Type of Swallowing Assessment	Description	Benefits	Challenges
Videofluoroscopic swallowing study (VFSS) or modified barium swallow (MBS)	Videofluoroscopic examination by recording successive images under fluoroscopy. Patients are provided a series of boluses of varied viscosity mixed with contrast (barium) to swallow.[17]	1. Allows view of oral and esophageal phases of swallowing.[18–20] 2. Availability of standardized protocols such as MBSImp.[18] 3. High sensitivity for aspiration.[9] 4. Noninvasive.[20]	1. Radiation exposure and carcinogenesis limit examination time.[9,20,21] 2. Requires transporting patients to radiology unit.[20] 3. Information may be lost in between swallows when imaging is paused.[20]
Fiberoptic endoscopic evaluation of swallowing (FEES)	Patients are provided with a series of boluses of varied viscosity to swallow during nasoendoscopy with a fiber-optic scope.[22]	1. Can be done at bedside in certain facilities.[23] 2. More sensitive to detecting presence of a bolus.[22] 3. High sensitivity to residue, penetration, and aspiration.[24] 4. Allows visualization of secretion status and lateralization before the assessment and testing of laryngeal sensation.[23] 5. Allows for evaluation of laryngeal and pharyngeal structures.[20]	1. Lack of visibility of the oral and esophageal phases of the swallow.[23] 2. Clinician must make inferences about laryngeal penetration or aspiration during the swallow due to brief whiteout period obstructing view.[20] 3. Rare but occasionally reported discomfort and complications in the patient.[22,23]
Clinical assessment ("bedside")	A clinician observes a patient swallow a series of boluses of varied viscosity, making recommendations based on objective and subjective data.[25]	1. Can identify patients at risk of aspiration.[26] 2. Can guide the administration of an instrumental swallowing assessment.[19,27] 3. Can be performed repeatedly.[27] 4. Noninvasive and most natural swallowing context.[25]	1. Lack of sensitivity.[19,25] 2. Cannot rule out silent aspiration.[26,28]
Less commonly used techniques	• Scintigraphy[29] • Manometry[30,31] • Ultrasonography[32,33]		

of structures, local invasion of participatory structures of swallow, and neurologic impact of tumor causing impaired sensation. Patients who present with dysphagia at diagnosis are at greater risk for long-term swallow dysfunction following treatment.[34,35] Also, median age at diagnosis for laryngeal cancer is 66 years. Increased age may have an associated baseline swallowing dysfunction or *presbyphagia*.[35,36]

Surgery involves transection of muscles and nerves that participate in swallowing, impairment of sensation, and formation of fibrous scar tissue. These surgical changes collectively affect normal swallow. Surgical factors that directly influence swallow are the extent of surgery as dictated by tumor size and reconstruction when necessary.[37,38]

For patients with early-stage laryngeal cancer, and some T3 tumors, surgical intervention may involve transoral laser microsurgery, transoral robotic surgery using a laser or electrocautery, or open partial laryngectomy, which can lead to glottic incompetency and concerns for aspiration and swallowing dysfunction. In the acute setting following surgery, transoral approaches have demonstrated quicker recovery of swallow in comparison to open approaches. Saraniti and colleagues retrospectively showed by Fiberoptic Endoscopic Evaluation of Swallowing (FEES) and Videofluoroscopic Swallow Study (VFSS) that patients who underwent transoral approaches at 3 months postoperatively demonstrated less laryngeal penetration or aspiration than patients who underwent open surgery. At 12 months after surgery, repeat FEES and VFSS demonstrated no difference in swallow function for patients who underwent transoral versus an open approach to partial laryngectomy. The investigators concluded that patients undergoing transoral approaches recovered swallow earlier because of reduced invasiveness, fewer sutures, no violation of strap muscles or thyroid cartilage, and less utilization of tracheostomy.[39]

A study by DiSanto and colleagues evaluated patient swallow function a minimum of 3 years after undergoing supracricoid laryngectomy and reported more than 30% of patients had chronic aspiration on both clinical and instrumental assessment. Patients were assessed by FEES and the M. D. Anderson Dysphagia Inventory (MDADI) for dysphagia-related QOL. Comparisons were made to patient demographic, tumor-related and treatment factors. Younger age at surgery was the only factor that significantly correlated with no aspiration. Type of supracricoid laryngectomy reconstruction, adjuvant radiation, and compliance with speech therapy did not significantly correlate with aspiration. Furthermore, the common prevalence of aspiration in this cohort did not result in increased incidence of late pulmonary complications of pneumonia, reportedly at 12%. It seems that when appropriately selected, patients undergoing open partial laryngectomy often do chronically aspirate but retain adequate pulmonary reserve, intact cough reflex and pharyngoesophageal sensation to not suffer late pulmonary complications. Oral intake is expected and for most patients remains safe.[40]

Swallow function for patients who have undergone TL warrants separate discussion. The anatomy after TL is significantly different secondary to complete separation of the upper airway from the digestive tract. There is a resultant change in swallowing pressure to push a bolus through the neopharyngoesophageal segment. Reconstruction method of the neopharynx also plays a role. Documented pathophysiological changes that compromise swallow include pseudodiverticulum, fistula formation, stricture, fibrosis, impaired pharyngeal propulsion, reflux, and leakage of voice prosthesis.[37,41]

A recent subjective study of 221 postlaryngectomy patients found significantly worse scores on the Swallowing Outcomes After Laryngectomy (SOAL) questionnaire for patients who underwent CRT, either prelaryngectomy or postlaryngectomy, or had a jejunum free flap neopharyngeal reconstruction.[37] Of note, on univariate analysis, primary closure resulted in significantly better swallow in comparison to each individual type of flap performed; this may have contributed to lack of significance in the regression model. Use of flaps for repair of the pharyngoesophageal segment is shown elsewhere to predispose to stricture formation and dysphagia.[38]

Another recent study evaluated TL patients' swallowing by simultaneous VFSS and FEES. Patients included were 3 or more months status postlaryngectomy. This study demonstrated that bolus residue of all consistencies is seen commonly in postlaryngectomy patients.[41] The degree of dysphagia associated with the objective assessment by VFSS and FEES, however, is not quantified. This study and the previously described patient self-assessment of dysphagia using SOAL illustrate the potential benefit of evaluating laryngectomy patients using a combined patient self-assessment tool and instrumental examination.

Before the landmark Veteran's Administration Laryngeal Cancer Study Group clinical trial in 1991, TL with or without adjuvant radiation was the preferred modality of treatment of advanced T3 and T4 laryngeal cancers.[42] Results from this trial demonstrated similar survival to TL with organ preservation strategies (radiation with or without chemotherapy), marking a paradigm shift in the treatment of advanced laryngeal carcinoma.[42,43] Although organ preservation techniques for advanced disease circumvent morbidities that are undesirable to patients, such as loss of phonatory ability and permanent tracheostoma, impact on QOL is mixed, with minimal differences in swallowing outcomes and feeding tube dependence noted in subsequent studies, including in follow-up of the VA Laryngeal Cancer Study Group.[44–47] The lack of difference in swallowing outcomes may be attributed to both acute and chronic effects of nonsurgical modalities, particularly radiation treatment.

Radiation therapy to the head and neck affects swallow function even in this era of intensity modulated radiation therapy (IMRT). The acute impact of radiation on swallow results from xerostomia and mucositis. Despite IMRT treatment plans that largely spare the parotid glands limiting the dose to £ 26 Gy,[48,49] xerostomia still occurs in 25% to 50% of patients with HNC.[49,50] Dry mouth, or xerostomia, typically results in sore throat and altered taste. Early mucosal injuries are attributed to cell death and associated inflammation. Reactive oxygen species result in impaired cell proliferation and epithelial denudation. From a pathologic perspective, these biomolecular features manifest as edema, erythema, tissue infiltration by leukocytes, vasodilation, vascular leakage contributing to more edema, and hypoplasia. These molecular and pathologic features seem clinically as xerostomia, dysgeusia, mucositis, and inflammation.[51] The pathologic tissue changes of xerostomia may result in subjective dysphagia that does not correlate with significant abnormality on objective instrumental assessment.[52] Furthermore, mucositis correlates with cofactors of smoking, infection, oral hygiene, and nutritional status.[53] See Videos 1 and 2 for a FEES comparison between a normal swallow and an impaired swallow in the acute phase of CRT.

Chronic radiation-induced dysphagia is categorized into "consequential late effects" and "generic late effects." Consequential late effects result from a delay in reepithelialization because radiation reduces the cellular barrier function. Severe mucositis may result in necrosis and delayed ulcer formation. Generic late effects are due to direct radiation effect on target tissue, influenced by fractionation schedule, enhanced by concomitant chemotherapy, and do not correspond to the intensity of early damage. Normal cellular behavior disruption leads to nonspecific fibrosis and organ dysfunction. Radiation-induced neuropathies also represent generic late effects and contribute to muscle dysfunction and loss of sensation. Pathologically there is an increase in fibroblast growth rate and increased collagen content. However, the collagen is not organized in a linear fashion; there is hypovascularity that clinically corresponds to tissue fibrosis and atrophy.[51] Comprehensively, the clinical picture is that of reduced retraction of the base of tongue, poor epiglottic retroflexion, reduced laryngeal elevation, delay in pharyngeal transit, and poor coordination of swallowing musculature. Radiation-induced fibrosis may also cause pharyngoesophageal stricture in approximately 20%.[54] Patients experience pain with swallow, malnutrition, and weight loss. The fatigue associated with attempts to swallow may lead to decreased motivation to eat and depression.[53,55]

Months and years beyond completion of radiation treatment, patients may continue to develop significant worsening of their dysphagia even if acute effects subside (**Fig. 2**).[56,57] Late-onset dysphagia is a phenomenon that can develop long after treatment with primary or adjuvant radiation therapy; this means that the safety and efficiency of the swallow may decline overtime, and patients may develop new-onset dysphagia years after therapy.[56] A meta-analysis studying the kinetics of various radiation toxicities, including oral mucosal toxicity, laryngeal edema, and dysphagia, found that there is an initial steep increase in the percentage of symptomatic patients up until 12 to 18 months, followed by a gradual exponential increase that lasts at least several years.[58] This continued gradual increase describes the progressive nature of this phenomenon, coined chronic or delayed radiation-induced injury, which[51] is thought to be secondary to chronic hypoxia and oxidative stress,[59] resulting in a perpetuation of tissue damage and increased fibrosis, possibly due to autocrine hyperstimulation of transforming growth beta 1.[51,56]

Management of Dysphagia

History and physical examination
Determining the cause of dysphagia in a patient following treatment of laryngeal carcinoma may be complex, as there are several contributors at play. Patients can present with a variety of concerns and of paramount importance is obtaining a detailed history that includes age, other co-morbidities associated with dysphagia, presence of recurrent pneumonias, frequency and progression of symptoms, and changes in diet and unintentional weight loss. In a systematic review of oropharyngeal dysphagia following TL, longer meal times and need for fluids to help pass a food bolus, pain,

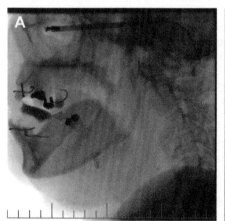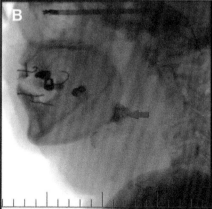

Fig. 2. VFSS 5 years post-CRT for laryngeal carcinoma. (*A*) Arrow pointing to puree bolus in oral cavity before swallow initiation. (*B*) Top arrow pointing to mild-to-moderate vallecular residue. Bottom arrow pointing to aspirated material postswallow.

regurgitation, reflux, coughing, and the sensation of food getting stuck in the throat were most commonly reported.[60] Oral cavity examination should include evaluation of dentition; mucosal tissue quality (eg, mucositis, xerostomia); and strength, range of motion, and sensory assessment for buccal, lingual, labial, palatal, and jaw function. Neck examination may reveal increased lymphedema, fibrosis, neuropathy/sensory changes, or range of motion restriction that may suggest similar findings in the pharynx. Flexible laryngoscopy can be used to augment physical examination to evaluate for presence of aspiration, pharyngeal residue, laryngeal sensation, lymphedema, vocal fold mobility, and glottic closure (depending on the primary modality of treatment).[23,27]

Speech therapy

Swallowing management by the SLP includes implementation of compensatory strategies (**Table 2**) and treatment via prophylactic and rehabilitative swallowing exercises (**Table 3**).[61] In acute stages of (C)RT, assessments and interventions aim to maximize patients' swallowing comfort and safety. Interprofessional collaboration with registered dieticians is important in maintaining adequate, safe nutrition, while minimizing the effects of (C)RT on the swallow.[62] Reinforcing oral care helps minimize the effects of mucositis and mitigate episodes of aspiration.[63] Bolus modifications to overcome odynophagia and improve swallow safety may be indicated, including consideration of an alternate feeding route should swallow safety and efficiency be compromised.[64]

Reduction in swallowing frequency due to dysfunction, discomfort, or use of an alternate feeding route promotes the development of disuse atrophy of the swallowing musculature, subsequent fibrosis, and atrophic changes, which can exacerbate dysphagia in the long-term.[65,66] MD Anderson uses a 2-fold "use it or lose it" program to minimize chronic effects of (C)RT on the swallow. This program encourages patients to keep the oropharyngeal musculature active during treatment by (1) encouraging and facilitating oral intake and (2) following a prophylactic exercise program (see **Table 3**).[67,68] Although compliance with home programs in this patient population is challenging to estimate,[69] it is usually low,[70] with only 38% of patients complying with a provided exercise program after 6 weeks of treatment.[71] Deconditioning, physical weakness, pain, and psychosocial factors such as depression or lack of support may make it difficult for a patient to adhere to swallowing exercise regimens as their treatment progresses.[72,73] However, those who follow prescribed exercise programs receive higher QOL scores and are less likely to modify their diet, use a feeding tube, or develop stenosis.[68,74] SLPs therefore support implementation of a prophylactic exercise program in addressing postradiation dysphagia,[75–79] but further research is needed for optimization.[66,80–83]

For patients undergoing organ-preserving surgery, early swallowing rehabilitation to improve airway protection usually consists of postural techniques such as tilting the chin or turning the head and are helpful in combination with swallowing maneuvers involving a breath hold (see **Table 2**).[84,85] Once initial postoperative swelling is resolved, an exercise program to compensate for reduced airway closure and improve bolus propulsion is implemented (see **Table 3**).[84,86] Bolus modification in both acute and chronic phases to reduce the risk of aspiration and improve bolus transit is beneficial (see **Table 2**).[63,85]

Although TL patients are protected against aspiration, studies have shown that dysphagia is common and can have a negative impact on their QOL, with increased perceived disability and distress.[87–89] Neopharyngeal bolus transit is improved by bolus modification, alternating liquids and solids, and strengthening the tongue base (see **Tables 2** and **3**).[85,90] A recent study revealed that a combination of

Table 2
Compensatory strategies

	Compensatory Strategy	Impairment Targeted
Swallowing maneuvers	Super-supraglottic swallow	Reduced or late vocal fold closure, delayed pharyngeal swallow[92]
	Supraglottic swallow	Reduced closure of airway entrance[92]
	Effortful or hard swallow	Pharyngeal weakness[93,94]
Postural techniques	Head postural adjustment (chin-tuck, head tilt, head rotation)	Delay in triggering the pharyngeal swallow; unilateral laryngeal dysfunction; unilateral pharyngeal dysfunction; cricopharyngeal dysfunction[93,95,96]
	Body postural adjustments (lying down, side-lying)	Unilateral pharyngeal weakness[93,94]
Bolus modifications	Bolus viscosity modification	Delay in triggering the pharyngeal swallow; reduced closure of airway entrance; decreased UES opening/sphincter weakness[97]
	Bolus temperature modification	Delay in triggering the pharyngeal swallow; reduced sensation[98]
	Bolus taste modification	Delay in triggering the pharyngeal swallow; reduced sensation[99]
	Bolus volume modification	Pharyngeal weakness, decreased UES opening/sphincter weakness, reduced pharyngeal and laryngeal sensation, reduced base of tongue retraction[97]

Table 3
Prophylactic and rehabilitative swallowing exercises

Exercise	Rationale
Mendelsohn	Enhance opening of the cricopharyngeal segment by increasing the extent and duration of laryngeal elevation.[100]
Masako	Enhance pharyngeal clearance pressures by increasing contact between the base of tongue and the posterior pharyngeal wall.[101,102]
Effortful or hard swallow	Increase posterior movement of the base of tongue and/or increase oropharyngeal pressure.[93,94]
Shaker (isometric/isotonic exercise)	Enhance opening of the cricopharyngeal segment by strengthening suprahyoid muscles.[94]
Effortful pitch glide	Enhance laryngeal elevation and pharyngeal shortening by strengthening the longitudinal pharyngeal muscles.[103]
Tongue resistance training	Enhance hyolaryngeal excursion by strengthening the tongue and suprahyoid muscles.[104]
Use of TheraBite	Enhance hyolaryngeal excursion by strengthening the suprahyoid muscles.[105,106] Treat trismus.[107]
Surface electrical stimulation (NMES), thermal application at the anterior faucial pillars	Recover motor control of weak muscles by stimulating intact peripheral motor nerves.[94]

strengthening exercises, postural techniques, and nutritional intervention can improve swallowing function, nutritional status, and patient QOL.[91]

Lymphedema and fibrosis management

Two therapies that may improve the tissue changes resulting from the effects of surgery or radiation are lymphedema therapy, or complete decongestive therapy (CDT), and myofascial release (MFR). The pathologic changes that result from treatment include edema and fibrosis. CDT may address lymphedema, whereas MFR may serve to ameliorate fibrosis.

Edema that persists as a consequential late effect of acute reactions to radiation may clinically manifest as internal edema of mucosa and external edema of the skin and subcutaneous tissues. Patients may experience a sensation of globus accompanying an impaired ability to swallow, pain with swallow, and dysphonia. Manual lymphatic drainage and compression are the mainstay of CDT. A model used by MD Anderson Department of Head and Neck Surgery combines an outpatient treatment phase and an aggressive home-based treatment regimen used by the patient or caregiver. MD Anderson prescribes daily use of a home therapy component from the initiation of treatment. Decongestive therapy begins in the supraclavicular region and progresses to the trunk, neck, and face. Depending on the patient's cancer treatment, emphasis on anterior lymphatic drainage pathways or posterior lymphatic drainage patterns is used. Radiation therapy alone often benefits from improvement in anterior drainage pathways, whereas surgical patients often benefit from techniques to improve both anterior and posterior lymphatic drainage pathways.[108]

Complete decongestive therapy includes use of compression garments that provides flat and even application of pressure to promote lymphatic drainage. The MD Anderson protocol differs from traditional CDT by using compression before and after manual decongestion in an attempt to improve skin elasticity and pliability to improve efficacy of manual therapy.[108]

For patients experiencing dysphagia as a result of (C)RT, there is an excessive production of extracellular matrix proteins creating fibrosis. Fibrosis causes reduced mobility of tissues and decreased function of peripheral nerves. Manual therapy represents a variety of techniques including passive and active stretching, light and deep soft tissue mobilization, and joint manipulation. This spectrum of therapy may mitigate the wound healing process and reduce fibrosis-associated dysphagia. There is a dearth of publications focused on manual therapy for dysphagia management. The biological basis for interest in manual therapy MFR to address chronic dysphagia related to fibrosis is apparent.[109] Prospective studies are needed to identify appropriate treatment regimens, assessment of treatment outcomes, efficacy, side effects, and associated morbidity.

Surgical management

Stenosis typically occurs at the anastomotic sites in the neopharynx for patients undergoing TL or within the radiation treatment field for patients undergoing primary or adjuvant (C)RT.[60,110,111] The management of pharyngoesophageal stricture may also involve dilation of stenotic segments. Dilation success at improving dysphagia ranges from 40% to 100%. The improvement is often transient, necessitating multiple trips to the operating room for improved swallow.[112,113] Complications occur reportedly 10% of the time in irradiated patients including bleeding and perforation; this is greater than for patients undergoing dilation for benign stricture.[113]

Cricopharyngeal dysfunction can also develop following treatment of laryngeal carcinoma.[114] Cricopharyngeal bar, prominence of the cricopharyngeal muscle observed on lateral view of a radiograph or as part of VFSS examination, or elevated UES pressures on manometry suggest cricopharyngeal dysfunction. Possibly due to fibrosis of this muscle, this may be treated with dilation, botulinum toxin injection, or in refractory or nonresponsive cases, surgical myotomy with varying success.[112]

FUTURE DIRECTIONS

Most of the current research for improving swallowing dysfunction following treatment of HNC is focused on IMRT. There is some evidence of improved swallow markers at least for patients with oropharyngeal primaries treated with IMRT technology compared with conventional wide-field radiation therapy.[115–117] The literature for use of IMRT in laryngeal carcinoma is limited, focused primarily on early glottic cancers without note on the functional benefit received.[118–120]

Areas of other evolving research in this patient population include use of prophylactic swallow therapy before and during cancer treatment, impact of reconstruction technique for primary and salvage laryngectomy, and influence of early enteral access on swallowing outcomes.[72,114] The importance of maintaining crucial functions of daily life, like swallowing, in patients with laryngeal carcinoma is of increased interest.

SUMMARY

The breadth of modalities used in treating patients with laryngeal cancer either solitarily or in combination are based largely on tumor characteristics. The primary aim is to achieve cure while maintaining the function of the organ when possible. Swallowing is a critical function of daily life, and a dysfunctional swallow can have significant impact on a patient's nutritional and psychosocial well-being. However, both the disease itself and treatment contribute to swallow dysfunction. A multidisciplinary approach involving the oncologists, speech language pathologists, and dieticians is necessary to maintain safe swallow and prevent malnutrition. Ideally, a swallowing therapy program is instituted before onset of treatment, continued throughout and into the post-treatment phase to best mitigate disuse atrophy and further dysfunction. Posttreatment remedies of lymphedema therapy and myofascial release are likely beneficial but in need of further investigation. Early recognition and intervention are key to reducing the impact of dysphagia on QOL for patients following treatment of laryngeal carcinoma.

CLINICS CARE POINTS

- Patients who undergo laryngeal cancer treatment experience dysphagia more than 40% of the time.
- Dysphagia may significantly affect QOL when food choices are modified for safety, and swallowing becomes inefficient and uncomfortable.
- FEES and VFSS are comparable studies for detecting laryngeal aspiration, pharyngeal residue, and delayed initiation of a swallow. In deciding which study to use first, consider VFSS to evaluate the entire oropharyngeal swallow and FEES to detect structural abnormalities in the pharynx.
- Dysphagia affects survivorship mainly secondary to aspiration-related complications of infections, dehydration, malnutrition, and depression.
- Multidisciplinary approaches to evaluation, pretreatment of dysphagia, and continuation of dysphagia therapy throughout and after treatment are necessary to optimize patient function.

DISCLOSURE

There are no conflicts with the content of this material.

SUPPLEMENTARY DATA

Supplementary data related to this article can be found online at https://doi.org/10.1016/j.otc.2022.11.004.

REFERENCES

1. Servagi-Vernat S, Ali D, Roubieu C, et al. Dysphagia after radiotherapy: State of the art and prevention. Eur Ann Otorhinolaryngol Head Neck Dis 2015; 132(1):25–9.
2. Granell J, Garrido L, Millas T, et al. Management of Oropharyngeal Dysphagia in Laryngeal and Hypopharyngeal Cancer. Int J Otolaryngol 2012;2012. https://doi.org/10.1155/2012/157630.
3. Logemann J. Dysphagia: Evaluation and Treatment. Logop 1995;47:140–64.
4. Starmer HH, Gourin CG, Lua LL, et al. Pretreatment swallowing assessment in head and neck cancer patients. Laryngoscope 2011;121(6):1208–11.
5. Hutcheson KA, Lewin JS. Functional outcomes after chemoradiotherapy of laryngeal and pharyngeal cancers. Curr Oncol Rep 2012;14(2):158–65.
6. Baijens LWJ, Walshe M, Aaltonen LM, et al. European white paper: oropharyngeal dysphagia in head and neck cancer. Eur Arch Otorhinolaryngol 2021; 278(2):577–616.
7. Francis DO, Weymuller EA, Parvathaneni U, et al. Dysphagia, stricture, and pneumonia in head and neck cancer patients: Does treatment modality matter? Ann Otol Rhinol Laryngol 2010;119(6):391–7.
8. Gourin CG, Starmer HM, Herbert RJ, et al. Short-and long-term outcomes of laryngeal cancer care in the elderly. Laryngoscope 2015;125(4):924–33.
9. Denaro N, Merlano MC, Russi EG. Dysphagia in Head and Neck Cancer Patients: Pretreatment Evaluation, Predictive Factors, and Assessment during Radio-Chemotherapy, Recommendations. Clin Exp Otorhinolaryngol 2013; 6(3):117–26.
10. Szuecs M, Kuhnt T, Punke C, et al. Subjective voice quality, communicative ability and swallowing after definitive radio(chemo)therapy, laryngectomy plus radio(chemo)therapy, or organ conservation surgery plus radio(chemo)therapy for laryngeal and hypopharyngeal cancer. Radiat Res 2014;56(1):159–68.
11. Mcquestion M, Fitch M, Howell D. The changed meaning of food: Physical, social and emotional loss for patients having received radiation treatment for head and neck cancer. Eur J Oncol Nurs 2011;15(2):145–51.
12. Patterson JM, Lu L, Watson LJ, et al. Associations between markers of social functioning and depression and quality of life in survivors of head and neck cancer: Findings from the Head and Neck Cancer 5000 study. Psychooncology 2022;31(3):478–85.
13. Nund RL, Ward EC, Scarinci NA, et al. The lived experience of dysphagia following non-surgical treatment for head and neck cancer. Int J Speech Lang Pathol 2014;16(3):282–9.
14. American Speech-Language-Hearing Association (ASHA). Adult Dysphagia (Practice Portal). Available at: www.asha.org www.asha.org/Practice-Portal/Clinical-Topics/Adult-Dysphagia/. Accessed September 11, 2022.

15. Hassan SJ, Weymuller EA. Assessment of quality of life in head and neck cancer patients. Head Neck 1993;15(6):485–96.
16. Kolator M, Kolator P, Zatoński T. Assessment of quality of life in patients with laryngeal cancer: A review of articles. Adv Clin Exp Med 2018;27(5):711–5.
17. Martin-Harris B, Canon CL, Bonilha HS, et al. Best Practices in Modified Barium Swallow Studies. Am J Speech Lang Pathol 2020;29:1078–93.
18. Martin-Harris B, Jones B. The Videofluorographic Swallowing Study. Phys Med Rehabil Clin N Am 2008;19(4):769–85.
19. Ouyoung L. Videofluoroscopy Swallow Study: Technique and Protocol. In: Thankappan K, Iyer S, Menon JR, editors. Dysphagia management in head and neck cancers. 1st edition. Singapore: Springer; 2018. p. 67–72.
20. Brady S, Donzelli J. The Modified Barium Swallow and the Functional Endoscopic Evaluation of Swallowing. Otolaryngol Clin North Am 2013;46(6):1009–22.
21. Ingleby HR, Bonilha HS, Steele CM. A Tutorial on Diagnostic Benefit and Radiation Risk in Videofluoroscopic Swallowing Studies. Dysphagia 2021;1–26. https://doi.org/10.1007/s00455-021-10335-y.
22. Langmore SE. History of Fiberoptic Endoscopic Evaluation of Swallowing for Evaluation and Management of Pharyngeal Dysphagia: Changes over the Years. Dysphagia 2017;32(1):27–38.
23. Menon UK. Flexible Endoscopic Evaluation of Swallowing (FEES): Technique and Interpretation. In: Thankappan K, Iyer S, Menon JR, editors. Dysphagia management in head and neck cancers. 1st edition. Singapore: Springer; 2018. p. 73–81.
24. Giraldo-Cadavid LF, Leal-Leaño LR, Leon-Basantes GA, et al. Accuracy of endoscopic and videofluoroscopic evaluations of swallowing for oropharyngeal dysphagia. Laryngoscope 2017;127(9):2002–10.
25. O'Horo JC, Rogus-Pulia N, Garcia-Arguello L, et al. Bedside diagnosis of dysphagia: a systematic review. J Hosp Med 2015;10(4):256–65.
26. Hassan HE, Aboloyoun AI. The value of bedside tests in dysphagia evaluation. Egypt J Ear, Nose, Throat Allied Sci 2014;15(3):197–203.
27. Villegas BC. Clinical Swallow Evaluation in Head and Neck Cancer. In: Thankappan K, Iyer S, Menon JR, editors. Dysphagia management in head and neck cancers. Singapore: Springer; 2018. p. 55–65.
28. Langerman A, MacCracken E, Kasza K, et al. Aspiration in chemoradiated patients with head and neck cancer. Arch Otolaryngol Head Neck Surg 2007;133(12):1289–95.
29. Sundaram PS, Subramanyam P. Scintigraphic evaluation of swallowing. In: Thankappan K, Iyer S, Menon JR, editors. Dysphagia management in head and neck cancers. Singapore: Springer; 2018. p. 89–100.
30. Winiker K, Gillman A, Guiu Hernandez E, et al. A systematic review of current methodology of high resolution pharyngeal manometry with and without impedance. Eur Arch Oto-Rhino-Laryngology. 2019;276(3):631–45.
31. Ryu JS, Park D, Kang JY. Application and interpretation of high-resolution manometry for pharyngeal dysphagia. J Neurogastroenterol Motil 2015;21(2):283–7.
32. Allen JE, Clunie GM, Winiker K. Ultrasound: an emerging modality for the dysphagia assessment toolkit? Curr Opin Otolaryngol Head Neck Surg 2021;29(3):213–8.
33. Hsiao MY, Wahyuni LK, Wang TG. Ultrasonography in Assessing Oropharyngeal Dysphagia. J Med Ultrasound 2013;21(4):181–8.

34. Nguyen NP, Vos P, Moltz CC, et al. Analysis of the factors influencing dysphagia severity upon diagnosis of head and neck cancer. Br J Radiol 2008;81(969): 706–10.
35. Raber-Durlacher JE, Brennan MT, Verdonck-De Leeuw IM, et al. Swallowing dysfunction in cancer patients. Support Care Cancer 2011;20:433–43.
36. Martin-Harris B, Brodsky MB, Michel Y, et al. Breathing and Swallowing Dynamics Across the Adult Lifespan. Arch Otolaryngol Head Neck Surg 2005; 131(9):762–70.
37. Lee MT, Govender R, Roy PJ, et al. Factors affecting swallowing outcomes after total laryngectomy: Participant self-report using the swallowing outcomes after laryngectomy questionnaire. Head Neck 2020;42(8):1963–9.
38. Mahalingam S, Srinivasan R, Spielmann P. Quality-of-life and functional outcomes following pharyngolaryngectomy: a systematic review of literature. Clin Otolaryngol 2016;41(1):25–43.
39. Saraniti C, Ciodaro F, Galletti C, et al. Swallowing Outcomes in Open Partial Horizontal Laryngectomy Type I and Endoscopic Supraglottic Laryngectomy: A Comparative Study. Int J Environ Res Public Health 2022;19(13):1–9.
40. di Santo D, Bondi S, Giordano L, et al. Long-term Swallowing Function, Pulmonary Complications, and Quality of Life after Supracricoid Laryngectomy. Otolaryngol Head Neck Surg 2019;161(2):307–14.
41. Coffey MM, Tolley N, Howard D, et al. An Investigation of the Post-laryngectomy Swallow Using Videofluoroscopy and Fiberoptic Endoscopic Evaluation of Swallowing (FEES). Dysphagia 2018;33:369–79.
42. The Department of Veterans Affairs Laryngeal Cancer Study, Wolf GT, Fisher SG, et al. Induction Chemotherapy plus Radiation Compared with Surgery plus Radiation in Patients with Advanced Laryngeal Cancer. Engl J Med 2010;324(24): 1685–90.
43. Forastiere AA, Weber RS, Trotti A. Organ Preservation for Advanced Larynx Cancer: Issues and Outcomes. J Clin Oncol 2015;33(29):3262.
44. Terrell JE, Fisher SG, Wolf GT. Long-term quality of life after treatment of laryngeal cancer. The Veterans Affairs Laryngeal Cancer Study Group. Arch Otolaryngol Head Neck Surg 1998;124(9):964–71.
45. Lee MY, Belfiglio M, Zeng J, et al. Primary Total Laryngectomy versus Organ Preservation for Locally Advanced T3/T4a Laryngeal Cancer. Laryngoscope 2022;0(0):1–10.
46. Rieger JM, Zalmanowitz JG, Wolfaardt JF. Functional outcomes after organ preservation treatment in head and neck cancer: a critical review of the literature. Int J Oral Maxillofac Surg 2006;35(7):581–7.
47. Fung K, Lyden TH, Lee J, et al. Voice and swallowing outcomes of an organ-preservation trial for advanced laryngeal cancer. Int J Radiat Oncol Biol Phys 2005;63(5):1395–9.
48. Grégoire V, Jeraj R, Aldo Lee J. Radiotherapy for head and neck tumours in 2012 and beyond: conformal, tailored, and adaptive? Rev Lancet Oncol 2012; 13:292–300.
49. Nutting CM, Morden JP, Harrington KJ, et al. Parotid-sparing intensity modulated versus conventional radiotherapy in head and neck cancer (PARSPORT): a phase 3 multicentre randomised controlled trial. Lancet Oncol 2011;12(2): 127–63.
50. Muzumder S, Srikantia N, Udayashankar AH, et al. Patients and Methods Study design and setting Burden of acute toxicities in head-and-neck radiation therapy: A single-institutional experience. South Asian J Cancer 2019;8:120–3.

51. King SN, Dunlap NE, Tennant PA, et al. Pathophysiology of Radiation-Induced Dysphagia in Head and Neck Cancer. Dysphagia 2016;31(3):339–51.

52. Vainshtein JM, Samuels S, Tao Y, et al. Impact of xerostomia on dysphagia after chemotherapy–intensity-modulated radiotherapy for oropharyngeal cancer: Prospective longitudinal study. Head Neck 2016;38(S1):E1605–12.

53. Denham JW, Peters LJ, Johansen J, et al. Do acute mucosal reactions lead to consequential late reactions in patients with head and neck cancer? Radiother Oncol 1999;52:157–64.

54. Nguyen NP, Moltz CC, Frank C, et al. Dysphagia following chemoradiation for locally advanced head and neck cancer. Ann Oncol 2004;15(3):383–8.

55. Denham JW, Hauer-Jensen M. The radiotherapeutic injury-a complex "wound. Radiother Oncol 2002;63(2):129–45.

56. Nguyen NP, Moltz CC, Frank C, et al. Evolution of chronic dysphagia following treatment for head and neck cancer. Oral Oncol 2006;42(4):374–80.

57. Hutcheson KA, Nurgalieva Z, Zhao H, et al. Two-year prevalence of dysphagia and related outcomes in head and neck cancer survivors: An updated SEER-Medicare analysis. Head Neck 2019;41(2):479–87.

58. Jung H, Beck-Bornholdt HP, Svoboda V, et al. Quantification of late complications after radiation therapy. Radiother Oncol 2001;61(3):233–46.

59. Murphy BA, Gilbert J. Dysphagia in Head and Neck Cancer Patients Treated With Radiation: Assessment, Sequelae, and Rehabilitation. Semin Radiat Oncol 2009;19(1):35–42.

60. Terlingen LT, Pilz W, Kuijer M, et al. Diagnosis and treatment of oropharyngeal dysphagia after total laryngectomy with or without pharyngoesophageal reconstruction: Systematic review. Head Neck 2018;40(12):2733–48.

61. Riffat F, Gunaratne DA, Palme CE. Swallowing assessment and management pre and post head and neck cancer treatment. Curr Opin Otolaryngol Head Neck Surg 2015;23(6):440–7.

62. Talwar B, Donnelly R, Skelly R, et al. Nutritional management in head and neck cancer: United Kingdom National Multidisciplinary Guidelines. J Laryngol Otol 2016;130(S2):S32–40.

63. Pauloski BR. Rehabilitation of Dysphagia Following Head and Neck Cancer. Phys Med Rehabil Clin N Am 2008;19(4):889–x.

64. Rosenthal DI, Lewin JS, Eisbruch A. Prevention and treatment of dysphagia and aspiration after chemoradiation for head and neck cancer. J Clin Oncol 2006; 24(17):2636–43.

65. Delanian S, Lefaix JL. The radiation-induced fibroatrophic process: therapeutic perspective via the antioxidant pathway. Radiother Oncol 2004;73(2):119–31.

66. Carnaby-Mann G, Crary MA, Schmalfuss I, et al. "Pharyngocise": Randomized Controlled Trial of Preventative Exercises to Maintain Muscle Structure and Swallowing Function During Head-and-Neck Chemoradiotherapy Radiation Oncology. Int J Radiat Oncol Biol Phys 2012;83(1):210–9.

67. Hutcheson KA, Lewin JS, Barringer DA, et al. Late dysphagia after radiotherapy-based treatment of head and neck cancer. Cancer 2012;118(23):5793–9.

68. Hutcheson KA, Bhayani MK, Beadle BM, et al. Eat and exercise during radiotherapy or chemoradiotherapy for pharyngeal cancers: use it or lose it. JAMA otolaryngology–head neck Surg 2013;139(11):1127–34.

69. Wells M, King E. Patient adherence to swallowing exercises in head and neck cancer. Curr 2017;25(3):175–81.

70. Mortensen HR, Jensen K, Aksglæde K, et al. Prophylactic Swallowing Exercises in Head and Neck Cancer Radiotherapy. Dysphagia 2015;30(3):304–14.

71. Cnossen IC, van Uden-Kraan CF, Witte BI, et al. Prophylactic exercises among head and neck cancer patients during and after swallowing sparing intensity modulated radiation: adherence and exercise performance levels of a 12-week guided home-based program. Eur Arch Otorhinolaryngol 2017;274(2): 1129–38.

72. Paleri V, Roe JWG, Strojan P, et al. Strategies to reduce long-term postchemoradiation dysphagia in patients with head and neck cancer: An evidence-based review. Head Neck 2014;36(3):431–43.

73. Baudelet M, Duprez F, van den Steen L, et al. Increasing Adherence to Prophylactic Swallowing Exercises During Head and Neck Radiotherapy: The Multicenter, Randomized Controlled PRESTO-Trial. Dysphagia 2022;1:1–10.

74. Duarte VM, Chhetri DK, Liu YF, et al. Swallow preservation exercises during chemoradiation therapy maintains swallow function. Otolaryngol Head Neck Surg 2013;149(6):878–84.

75. Krisciunas GP, Sokoloff W, Stepas K, et al. Survey of usual practice: Dysphagia therapy in head and neck cancer patients. Dysphagia 2012;27(4):538–49.

76. Banda KJ, Chu H, Kao CC, et al. Swallowing exercises for head and neck cancer patients: A systematic review and meta-analysis of randomized control trials. Int J Nurs Stud 2021;114:103827.

77. Ciucci M, Jones CA, Malandraki GA, et al. Dysphagia Practice in 2035: Beyond Fluorography, Thickener, and Electrical Stimulation. Semin Speech Lang 2016; 37(3):201–18.

78. Virani A, Kunduk M, Fink DS, et al. Effects of 2 different swallowing exercise regimens during organ-preservation therapies for head and neck cancers on swallowing function. Head Neck 2015;37(2):162–70.

79. Langmore S, Krisciunas GP, Miloro KV, et al. Does PEG use cause dysphagia in head and neck cancer patients? Dysphagia 2012;27(2):251–9.

80. Kraaijenga SA, van der Molen L, Jacobi I, et al. Prospective clinical study on long-term swallowing function and voice quality in advanced head and neck cancer patients treated with concurrent chemoradiotherapy and preventive swallowing exercises. Eur Arch Otorhinolaryngol 2015;272(11):3521–31.

81. Perry A, Lee SH, Cotton S, et al. Therapeutic exercises for affecting post-treatment swallowing in people treated for advanced-stage head and neck cancers. Cochrane Database Syst Rev 2016;8:CD011112.

82. Kotz T, Federman AD, Kao J, et al. Prophylactic swallowing exercises in patients with head and neck cancer undergoing chemoradiation: a randomized trial. Arch Otolaryngol Head Neck Surg 2012;138(4):376–82.

83. Yang W, Nie W, Zhou X, et al. Review of prophylactic swallowing interventions for head and neck cancer. Int J Nurs Stud 2021;123:104074.

84. Rademaker AW, Logemann JA, Pauloski BR, et al. Recovery of postoperative swallowing in patients undergoing partial laryngectomy. Head Neck 1993; 15(4):325–34.

85. Subramaniam N, Nikitha Av, Thankappan K. Dysphagia After Laryngeal Surgery. In: Thankappan K, Iyer S, Menon JR, editors. Dysphagia management in head and neck cancers. 1st ed. Springer Singapore; 2018. p. 257–75.

86. Logemann JA, Gibbons P, Rademaker AW, et al. Mechanisms of recovery of swallow after supraglottic laryngectomy. J Speech Hear Res 1994;37(5):965–74.

87. Ward EC, Bishop B, Frisby J, et al. Swallowing Outcomes Following Laryngectomy and Pharyngolaryngectomy. Arch Otolaryngol Head Neck Surg 2002;128: 181–6.

88. Wulff NB, Dalton SO, Wessel I, et al. Health-Related Quality of Life, Dysphagia, Voice Problems, Depression, and Anxiety After Total Laryngectomy. Laryngoscope 2022;132(5):980–8.

89. MacLean J, Cotton S, Perry A. Dysphagia Following a Total Laryngectomy: The Effect on Quality of Life, Functioning, and Psychological Well-Being. Dysphagia 2009;24(3):314–21.

90. Zenga J, Goldsmith T, Bunting G, et al. State of the art: Rehabilitation of speech and swallowing after total laryngectomy. Oral Oncol 2018;86:38–47.

91. Zhu X, Liu D, Zong M, et al. Effect of swallowing training combined with nutritional intervention on the nutritional status and quality of life of laryngeal cancer patients with dysphagia after operation and radiotherapy. J Oral Rehabil 2022; 49(7):729–33.

92. Logemann JA, Pauloski BR, Rademaker AW, et al. Super-supraglottic swallow in irradiated head and neck cancer patients. Head Neck 1997;19(6):535–40.

93. Logemann JA. Behavioral Management for Oropharyngeal Dysphagia. Folia Phoniatr Logop 1999;51(4–5):199–212.

94. Speyer R. Behavioral treatment of oropharyngeal dysphagia. In: Ekberg O, editor. Dysphagia med radiol.vol. 0 Cham: Springer; 2017. p. 669–86.

95. Logemann JA, Kahrilas PJ, Kobara M, et al. The benefit of head rotation on pharyngoesophageal dysphagia. Arch Phys Med Rehabil 1989;70(10):767–71.

96. Alghadir AH, Zafar H, Al-Eisa ES, et al. Effect of posture on swallowing. Afr Health Sci 2017;17(1):133–7.

97. Ferris L, Doeltgen S, Cock C, et al. Modulation of pharyngeal swallowing by bolus volume and viscosity. Am J Physiology-Gastrointestinal Liver Physiol 2021;320(1):G43–53.

98. Bisch EM, Logemann JA, Rademaker AW, et al. Pharyngeal effects of bolus volume, viscosity, and temperature in patients with dysphagia resulting from neurologic impairment and in normal subjects. J Speech Hear Res 1994;37(5):1041–9.

99. Pauloski BR, Logemann JA, Rademaker AW, et al. Effects of enhanced bolus flavors on oropharyngeal swallow in patients treated for head and neck cancer. Head Neck 2013;35(8):1124–31.

100. Inamoto Y, Saitoh E, Ito Y, et al. The Mendelsohn Maneuver and its Effects on Swallowing: Kinematic Analysis in Three Dimensions Using Dynamic Area Detector CT. Dysphagia 2018;33(4):419–30.

101. Fujiu-Kurachi M, Fujiwara S, Tamine KI, et al. Tongue pressure generation during tongue-hold swallows in young healthy adults measured with different tongue positions. Dysphagia 2014;29(1):17–24.

102. Lazarus C. Mendelson Maneuver and Masako Maneuver. In: Shaker R, Easterling C, Belafsky PC, et al, editors. Manual of diagnostic and therapeutic techniques for disorders of deglutition. New York: Springer; 2013. p. 269–80.

103. Miloro KV, Pearson WG, Langmore SE. Effortful pitch glide: A potential new exercise evaluated by dynamic MRI. J Speech Lang Hear Res 2014;57(4):1243–50.

104. Namiki C, Hara K, Tohara H, et al. Tongue-pressure resistance training improves tongue and suprahyoid muscle functions simultaneously. Clin Interv Aging 2019; 14:601–8.

105. Roe JWG, Ashforth KM. Prophylactic swallowing exercises for patients receiving radiotherapy for head and neck cancer. Curr Opin Otolaryngol Head Neck Surg 2011;19(3):144–9.

106. Matsubara M, Tohara H, Hara K, et al. High-speed jaw-opening exercise in training suprahyoid fast-twitch muscle fibers. Clin Interv Aging 2018;13:125–31.

107. Kamstra JI, Roodenburg JLN, Beurskens CHG, et al. TheraBite exercises to treat trismus secondary to head and neck cancer. Support Care Cancer 2013; 21(4):951–7.

108. Smith BG, Lewin JS. The Role of Lymphedema Management in Head and Neck Cancer. Curr Opin Otolaryngol Head Neck Surg 2010;18(3):153–8.

109. Krisciunas GP, Vakharia A, Lazarus C, et al. Application of Manual Therapy for Dysphagia in Head and Neck Cancer Patients: A Preliminary National Survey of Treatment Trends and Adverse Events. Glob Adv Health Med 2019;8:1–8.

110. Sweeny L, Golden JB, White HN, et al. Incidence and outcomes of stricture formation postlaryngectomy. Otolaryngol - Head Neck Surg 2012;146(3):395–402.

111. Sullivan CA, Goguen LA, Norris CM, et al. Endoscopic Management of Hypopharyngeal Stenosis after Organ Sparing Therapy for Head and Neck Cancer. Laryngoscope 2004;114(11):1924–31.

112. Abu-Ghanem S, Sung CK, Junlapan A, et al. Endoscopic Management of Postradiation Dysphagia in Head and Neck Cancer Patients: A Systematic Review. Ann Otol Rhinol Laryngol 2019;128(8):767–73.

113. Moss WJ, Pang J, Orosco RK, et al. Esophageal dilation in head and neck cancer patients: A systematic review and meta-analysis. Laryngoscope 2018; 128(1):111–7.

114. Perkins KA, Hancock KL, Ward EC. Speech and Swallowing Following Laryngeal and Hypopharyngeal Cancer. In: Ward EC, van As-Brooks CJ, editors. Head and neck cancer: treatment, rehabilitation, and outcomes. 2nd edition. Plural Publishing; 2014. p. 173–240.

115. Eisbruch A, Schwartz M, Rasch C, et al. Dysphagia and aspiration after chemoradiotherapy for head-and-neck cancer: which anatomic structures are affected and can they be spared by IMRT? Int J Radiat Oncol Biol Phys 2004;60(5): 1425–39.

116. Pauloski BR, Rademaker AW, Logemann JA, et al. Comparison of swallowing function after intensity-modulated radiation therapy and conventional radiotherapy for head and neck cancer. Head Neck 2015;37(11):1575–82.

117. Eisbruch A, Levendag PC, Feng FY, et al. Can IMRT or Brachytherapy Reduce Dysphagia Associated With Chemoradiotherapy of Head and Neck Cancer? The Michigan and Rotterdam Experiences. Int J Radiat Oncol Biol Phys 2007; 69(2):S40–2.

118. Janssen S, Glanzmann C, Huber G, et al. Risk-adapted partial larynx and/or carotid artery sparing modulated radiation therapy of glottic cancer. Radiat Oncol 2014;9(136):1–8.

119. Zumsteg ZS, Riaz N, Jaffery S, et al. Carotid sparing intensity-modulated radiation therapy achieves comparable locoregional control to conventional radiotherapy in T1-2N0 laryngeal carcinoma. Oral Oncol 2015;51(7):716–23.

120. Gomez D, Cahlon O, Mechalakos J, et al. An investigation of intensity-modulated radiation therapy versus conventional two-dimensional and 3D-conformal radiation therapy for early stage larynx cancer. Radiat Oncol 2010; 5(74):1–9.

Prognosis

Chihun Han, MD[a], Nayel I. Khan, MD[a], Leila J. Mady, MD, PhD, MPH[b],*

KEYWORDS

- Larynx • Laryngeal cancer • Squamous cell carcinoma • Prognosis • Survival

KEY POINTS

- Prognosis of laryngeal cancer is multifactorial and influenced by a combination of patient and tumor factors.
- Overall prognosis of laryngeal cancer has not improved over the past few decades.
- Patient factors include age, sex, performance status, comorbidities, nutritional status, and social factors.
- Tumor factors include subsite, staging, histology, and tumor markers.
- Utilization of novel markers and emerging molecular technologies hold the potential to improve the prognostication of laryngeal cancers.

INTRODUCTION

The diagnosis and treatment of laryngeal cancer have evolved over several decades, with treatment goals focused on optimizing functional and oncologic outcomes. However, the overall prognosis of laryngeal cancer has not correlated with such evolution in diagnostic and treatment paradigms.[1] Currently, the 5-year overall survival rate for patients with early-stage laryngeal cancer is 80% to 90%.[2,3] For patients with more advanced stage disease, it remains less than 50%.[4] This is further seen when examining published relative survival rates for patients diagnosed with laryngeal cancer from the Surveillance, Epidemiology, and End Results (SEER) database[5] (**Fig. 1**). There are multiple factors that affect the survival and prognosis of patients with laryngeal cancer. These factors can be classified into the patient, disease, and treatment factors (**Fig. 2**). Patient factors include age, sex, performance status (PS), comorbidities, nutritional status, and social determinants of health. Tumor factors, previously limited to tumor subsite and tumor, nodes, and metastases (TNM) staging, now include novel markers based on emerging molecular technologies and improved understanding of

[a] Department of Otolaryngology – Head & Neck Surgery, Thomas Jefferson University Hospitals, 925 Chestnut Street, 6th Floor, Philadelphia, PA 19107, USA; [b] Department of Otolaryngology - Head & Neck Surgery, The Johns Hopkins University School of Medicine, 601 North Caroline Street, 6th Floor, Baltimore, MD 21287, USA
* Corresponding author:
E-mail address: lmady1@jh.edu

Otolaryngol Clin N Am 56 (2023) 389–402
https://doi.org/10.1016/j.otc.2022.12.005
0030-6665/23/© 2022 Elsevier Inc. All rights reserved.

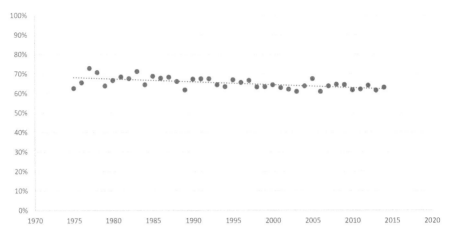

Fig. 1. Laryngeal cancer 5-year relative survival trends for each year from 1975 to 2014 as adapted from data from the SEER 8 database.

the tumor microenvironment (TME). Lastly, different treatment approaches and modalities can impact the prognosis and survival of patients with laryngeal cancer.

PATIENT FACTORS
Age

Increasing chronologic age is an adverse prognostic marker for cancer overall, given the higher prevalence of frailty and other comorbid conditions, including other cancers, with aging.[6] It is important to note that frailty is a syndrome, distinct from age, comorbidity, or disability alone, which describes decreased physiologic reserve and resistance to stressors.[7] However there is limited quality data on the impact of age on the prognosis of patients with laryngeal cancer, given that elderly patients have frequently been under-represented in clinical trials.[8] Furthermore, significant patient characteristics such as nutritional or functional status are often unreported in retrospective studies, limiting our ability to independently assess and understand the

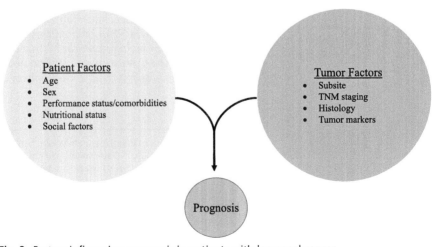

Fig. 2. Factors influencing prognosis in patients with laryngeal cancer.

interplay between chronologic age and decreased physiologic reserve on cancer survivorship. It follows that with the continued increases in average life expectancy, the number of patients with cancer aged 65 years and older will become more common. In a population-based study investigating the effect of age on laryngeal cancer survivorship using the SEER database from 1995 to 2009, wherein most patients (57%) received radiation only, improved survival was demonstrated with younger age.[2] A pooled analysis, including 4759 head and neck cancer (HNC) patients from five studies within the International Head and Neck Cancer Epidemiology (INHANCE) Consortium, also showed that increasing age at diagnosis was a negative prognostic factor for cancer of the oropharynx and larynx.[9]

Sex

There are significant sex-based differences that have been reported in the incidence and survival of laryngeal cancer. Although more than 80% of patients with laryngeal cancer are males,[10] in recent years, there has been a progressive and significant increase in laryngeal cancer incidence among females. This is possibly due to proportional increases in alcohol use and smoking in this population.[10,11] Interestingly, the subsite of laryngeal cancer also varies according to sex. Previous studies have shown that males predominantly present with glottic cancer, whereas higher rates of supraglottic carcinomas are observed in females.[12,13] Despite the overall worse survival generally associated with supraglottic cancers compared with glottic cancers, studies have shown improved laryngeal cancer survival in females compared with their male counterparts. Female patients with laryngeal cancer had better 1-, 3- and 5-year cancer specific and overall survival than males with laryngeal cancer even in an unmatched group. These differences were magnified when the groups were matched for race, site, grade, age, and year of diagnosis.[13] Among 10 cancers with the highest male-to-female age-adjusted mortality rate ratios (MRR), laryngeal cancer ranks second (MRR 5.37, 95% confidence interval [CI]: 5.29 to 5.45), though it is notable that these sex differences have decreased with time over the last 30 years.[14] Lastly, compared with males, female patients with laryngeal cancer appear to have a reduced risk of cancer recurrence.[15] One theory suggests that endogenous sex hormones, specifically estrogen, may lead to these differences and is further supported by the observed inverse association of hormone replacement use with HNC incidence[13,16] This is also shown by the more aggressive behavior of cancers including colon cancer, gliomas, skin cancer, head and neck squamous cell carcinoma (HNSCC), esophageal cancer, and non-small cell lung cancer in post-menopausal compared with premenopausal females.[17] No prospective study to date has explored the hormonal effect on survival in HNSCC.

Performance Status and Comorbidities

PS refers to an individual's ability to care for themselves and perform physical and other daily activities.[18] The ECOG PS Scale (scored 0 to 5, with higher scores representing worse PS) and the Karnofsky PS Scale (scored 0 to 100, with higher scores describing better PS) are two widely used methods to assess a patient's functional status.[19] Though there is no universally accepted definition of "comorbidity", the term is used to describe chronic conditions that impact survival outcomes, especially long-term survival.[20] The Charlson Comorbidity Index (CCI; weighted score of 19 conditions with higher scores indicating more severe conditions) and the Adult Comorbidity Evaluation-27 (ACE-27; index of 26 ailments with overall scores of 0 to 3, wherein higher scores represent more severe disease) are two widely validated comorbidity indices used in the HNC population.[21–23] Behavioral mechanisms, including cigarette smoking and alcohol consumption which are established risk factors for laryngeal cancer, can also increase the likelihood of poor PS and coexisting medical problems, including cardiovascular disease, lung disease, liver disease, and other cancers.[24–26] Therefore, understanding the interplay and impact of PS and comorbid medical problems is essential in accurate disease prognostication.

Examination of survival outcomes suggests that non-cancer-related death is a significant hazard for patients with high comorbidity burden, contributing to increased susceptibility to competing causes of morbidity and mortality. In a retrospective review of 548 patients with previously untreated T3 or T4 laryngeal SCC, higher CCI scores (P = .01), age-adjusted CCI scores >3 (P = .0001), and worse ECOG PS (P = .001) were all associated with worse overall survival.[27] However, age-adjusted CCI score > 3 was not associated with differences in disease-specific survival at 5- and 10-year (69% vs 59% and 64% vs 64%, respectively, P = .60). Irrespective of treatment modality, nodal status was the only independent factor associated with cancer-related mortality. In patients with increased comorbidities the risk of non-cancer-related death exceeded the risk of cancer-specific years after treatment.[27] These findings highlight the importance of holistic and patient-specific discussions surrounding prognosis, with an emphasis on shared-decision making regarding treatment recommendations.

Nutritional Status

Laryngeal cancer, as with other malignancies of the upper aerodigestive system, can result in significant symptoms affecting oral food intake, including dysphagia and odynophagia.[28] This, is often compounded by treatment-related toxicities and cachexia secondary to tumor-induced systemic inflammation.[29–31] Malnutrition is highly prevalent and is associated with poorer outcomes in this disease group.[32–35] There are several methods to assess nutritional status, among which the body mass index (BMI) is one of the most frequently used in clinical practice. BMI is defined as a person's weight in kilograms divided by the square of the person's height in meters (kg/m^2) and can be categorized according to cutoff points proposed by the World Health Organization (underweight <18.5, healthy weight 18.5 to 24.9, overweight 25 to 29.9, and obese >30). In a retrospective review of 243 patients who underwent total laryngectomy, malnutrition as assessed by BMI was a significant prognosticator in patients with HNSCC of the larynx.[34] In this analysis, the hazard ratio of death was significantly lower among individuals with a higher BMI (hazard ratio [HR] 0.93, 95% CI: 0.90 to 0.97, P = .0008).[34] However, BMI is an imperfect measure as it does not reflect changes in fluid volume status or body composition such as decreased skeletal muscle mass and increased adiposity associated with aging.[36] Other methods used to assess nutritional deficits including the Geriatric Nutritional Risk Index, the Nutritional Risk Index, and the Global Leadership Initiative on Malnutrition have been developed to overcome the shortcomings of BMI. A retrospective review of 144 patients found to be malnourished per the Nutritional Risk Index showed that 64% of these patients had normal or overweight/obese BMI at the time of the diagnosis.[37]

Analysis of weight loss has been another modality used for monitoring malnutrition, wherein a 5% loss over 6 months has been associated with adverse outcomes including increased medical and surgical complications, length of hospitalization, and hospital-related costs in HNC patients.[34] Like other nutritional assessments, weight loss has been shown as an independent predictor of survival in patients with cancer, further reinforcing the role nutritional status plays in the prognosis for these patients.[35] Although nutritional metrics have been shown to provide useful prognostic information in HNC, isolated use in laryngeal malignancies have not been investigated.[38] Regardless of the method used to assess nutritional status, malnutrition is a modifiable risk factor that may be targeted to improve the treatment outcomes of patients with malignancies of the upper aerodigestive system.

Social Determinants of Health

Previous studies have identified a disproportionate burden of HNC among historically underrepresented and lower-income groups.[39–41] In an SEER database study of 24,069 patients with HNSCC of the larynx, black patients were more likely to have advanced disease at the time of diagnosis.[42] Furthermore, black race was found to be an independent prognostic factor for inferior overall survival in patients with laryngeal cancer.[42] This phenomenon may be a result of systemic differences in health care access among historically underrepresented populations. A retrospective review of 1128 patients (N = 478 black, 650 white) showed that after controlling for other variables, insurance status was the only element that had a significant effect on survival in black patients.[43] Such disparities in disease presentation and outcomes cannot be explained by a single factor; rather they represent the complexities of multiple social determinants of health. In a retrospective review of 72,472 patients with laryngeal cancer in the United States, there were significant correlations between advanced stage at diagnosis and Medicaid insurance, lack of insurance, female sex, older age, black race, and certain states of residence. The strongest predictor of advanced stage was lack of insurance (OR 2.2, 95% CI: 2.03 to 2.40, $P < .001$).[39] The impact of equitable access to care is highlighted by the Veterans Health Administration, which is the largest integrated health care network in the United States. In a study of patients with laryngeal cancer treated at a tertiary Veterans Affairs Medical Center, there were no statistically significant differences in cancer stage at presentation, disease-free survival, and overall survival between individuals of black and white race, highlighting the critical importance and impact of equity in health care access in achieving superior oncologic outcomes.[40] Though increased benefit options may reduce the proportion of patients without insurance and decrease the time to diagnosis and treatment, as shown by Medicaid expansion under the Affordable Care Act, the implications of such expansions specifically in laryngeal cancer populations remain an area in need of investigation.[41,44]

DISEASE FACTORS
Subsites

Laryngeal cancer has varying survival rates based on its anatomic subsites: glottic, supraglottic, and subglottic. Glottic cancer is the most common HNSCC of the larynx and has the best 5-year relative survival rates, approximately 77%, among all subsites. In comparison, 5-year relative survival for patients with supraglottic and subglottic malignancies are approximately 46% and 53%, respectively.[45] Such differences may be in part to earlier disease presentation with glottic tumors, as even small glottic lesions can cause significant dysphonia. Additionally, the glottis is surrounded by dense connective tissues and has sparse lymphatic drainage that act as anatomic barriers to the regional spread of disease. Thus, a large proportion of patients with glottic cancer present with localized disease (83%), leading to overall improved survival.[45] On the contrary, the supraglottic subsite has an abundant lymphatic drainage pathway and typically requires a larger tumor volume before eliciting any symptoms. Thus, a significant proportion of patients with supraglottic tumors present with more extensive tumor volume, nodal disease, and advanced stage, all associated with decreased survival.[46] Among patients with supraglottic tumors, 55% will have clinical evidence of nodal metastasis at the time of the diagnosis, and 16% will have contralateral neck disease as compared with the rare presence of nodal disease in glottic tumors.[47]

Even when matched by T and N stages, supraglottic tumors are generally associated with inferior overall survival and disease-free survival compared with glottic cancers, in addition to higher rates of recurrence and post-treatment distant metastasis.[48–51] Underlying biological differences between glottic and supraglottic tumors may contribute to variances observed in survival. Previous studies have shown significant differences in protein expression patterns between tumors of these two subsites. For example, increased expression of carbonic anhydrase IX and cyclin D-retinoid X receptor alpha have been identified in glottic tumors compared with those of the subglottis, although the prognostic significance of this difference has not been elucidated at this time.[48,52] However, many of these molecules, such as retinoid X receptor alpha, play a significant role in regulation of physiologic processes such as embryonic development, cellular differentiation, apoptosis, proliferation, and homeostasis. Such differential protein expression may suggest distinct biologic mechanisms between these tumor sites which require disease-specific diagnostic and therapeutic approaches.[53]

Compared with primary malignancies of the glottis and supraglottis, subglottic tumors are rare and most literature on this entity exists in small series with variable survival outcomes.[54] Nevertheless, disease involving this subsite is generally considered aggressive, typically presenting with cartilage invasion and metastasis to prelaryngeal (delphian), pretracheal, and paratracheal nodal basins, often with extranodal extension.[55,56] The largest review of subglottic carcinoma from the SEER database identified 889 cases, representing 1.5% of all queried cases of HNSCC of the larynx. In this study, subglottic disease was associated with a 5-year disease-specific survival of 54%.[57]

TNM Staging

The TNM staging system by the American Joint Committee on Cancer provides a unified prognostic classification scheme based on a tumor's anatomic location and size (T) and presence of regional (N) or distant (M) tumor involvement. It is widely used to guide the treatment of laryngeal cancer. As would be expected, decreased survival is observed with increasing T, N, and M stage. Of the TNM factors, nodal metastasis is often considered to be the most significant negative prognosticator. The presence of nodal disease in laryngeal cancer can decrease long-term survival by up to 50%.[58,59] In a large retrospective review of 1840 patients with untreated HNSCC of the larynx, patients with node-negative disease (N0) showed superior disease-specific survival (75% vs 48%, $P = .001$) and fewer recurrences (26% vs 36%; $P = .001$) compared with those with nodal disease.[60] In this analysis, there was a three-fold increase in the risk of distant metastasis for laryngeal malignancies with nodal disease compared with patients without nodal disease. Up to a 9-fold increase in the risk of distant metastasis has been observed for laryngeal carcinoma with extranodal disease.[61]

Although TNM staging is a useful prognosticator at the population level, it is not without its limitations, particularly at the individual level given the lack of incorporation of individual patient's factors and tumor factors discussed in this article.[62] As a result, several alternatives have been proposed to the TNM system to incorporate age, sex, and margin status, but these have not been validated in larger populations nor accepted into mainstream practice.[46,63,64]

Histologic Grading

The vast majority (95%) of laryngeal cancers are squamous cell carcinomas and can be graded as well differentiated (G1), moderately differentiated (G2), or poorly differentiated (G3).[65,66] Tumors of the glottis are more commonly well differentiated, whereas those of the supraglottis are more often poorly differentiated.[49,59] Other commonly documented histologic findings include pleomorphism, mitotic activity index, keratinization, necrosis, lymphatic invasion, and blood vessel invasion. Currently, no clear association exists between the clinical/pathologic stage and the histologic grade of laryngeal malignancy. Although some studies have suggested that poorly differentiated cancers may have a higher rate of metastatic disease when compared with well-differentiated cancers, other studies showed that histologic grading is not a significant predictor of survival or recurrence.[67]

Tumor Markers

With emerging technologies improving our understanding of tumor biology and the TME, novel molecular markers are being explored to improve early detection, increase survival outcomes, and accurately predict treatment outcomes in laryngeal cancer. Though there is increasing recognition that this ecosystem is crucial to tumorigenesis and tumor progression, the application of this knowledge remains largely investigational. Still, a few promising biomarkers with prognostic implications are worth highlighting.

Tumor microenvironment: programmed death-1/programmed cell death Ligand-1, tumor infiltrating lymphocytes

The TME refers to the ecosystem surrounding tumor cells and is composed of various immune cells such as cytotoxic CD8+ T cells, fibroblasts, and other cells, including normal keratinocytes. There is a complex interplay between immune cell surveillance and tumor cell immune evasion. Briefly, under normal conditions, immune checkpoints, including the PD-1/PD-L1 pathway, induce and maintain peripheral immune tolerance and prevent excessive tissue inflammation and autoimmune diseases. In the oncologic setting, the tumor leverages this system to inhibit the host antitumor response. One such mechanism is through the expression of PD-L1 which interacts with PD-1 expressed on tumor-infiltrating lymphocytes (TILs) promoting tumor immune escape by inhibiting TIL activation and subsequent tumor death.[68]

The prognostic significance of PD-L1 expression was shown in three randomized phase III trials using immune checkpoint inhibitors against PD-L1 (pembrolizumab) and PD-1 (nivolumab).[69–71] Overall, the studies showed higher efficacy of immune checkpoint inhibitors (nivolumab, pembrolizumab) against tumors expressing PD-L1 than non-PD-L1 expressing tumors as assessed by the combined positive score (CPS), which is a percentage of the number of tumor cells, lymphocytes, macrophages that express PD-L1 per total number of viable tumor cells.[69–71] Based on this, a CPS score >1 has been defined as a predictive marker for response to immune checkpoint inhibitor therapy in HNSCC. Only one study has focused on the prognostic role of PD-L1 expression exclusively in laryngeal HNSCC, wherein increased PD-L1 expression was associated with improved disease-free survival (HR 0.0532; 95% CI: 0.301 to 0.941; P = .030) and overall survival (HR 0.570; 95% CI: 0.333 to 0.973; P = .039).[72]

Infiltration of the tumor by lymphocytes has been shown to be a favorable prognostic factor in colorectal cancer and melanoma, secondary to a presumed improved host anti-tumor immune response.[73,74] In a meta-analysis of 11 studies evaluating the association between TILs and cancer survival, which included 1398 patients with HNSCC of the larynx, there was a positive correlation between TIL density and overall survival. This relationship was shown regardless of the infiltrating lymphocyte cell types (CD4+, CD3+, or CD8+).[75] A meta-analysis of studies investigating the TIL infiltration in laryngeal HNSCC also showed that high level of stromal TIL was associated with improved overall survival (HR 0.57; 95% CI 0.36 to 0.91, P = .02) and disease-free survival (0.56; 95% CI 0.34 to 0.94, $P = .03$).[72] Additionally, another immune check-point molecule, B7-H3, has shown significant overexpression in laryngeal cancer compared with normal tissue, and its expression is negatively correlated with TIL density and overall survival.[76]

MicroRNA

MicroRNA (miRNAs) are endogenous, small non-coding RNAs with an average length of 20 to 22 nucleotides that regulate post-transcriptional gene expression. They can have tumor-suppressing or oncogenic roles and are, also, found to have heavy dysregulation in cancer cells.[77] They are highly stable and readily harvested from all biological fluids, allowing for quick noninvasive detection and monitoring. In a meta-analysis of 36 studies with 5037 patients with laryngeal cancer, 24 miRNAs were examined to evaluate the association between miRNA expression levels and patient survival outcomes.[78] Among these studies, 10 miRNAs were upregulated, whereas 14 miRNAs were downregulated. Six miRNAs (miRNA-34a, miRNA-195, miRNA-100, miRNA-21, miRNA-155 and miRNA-let-7) were found to have significant prognostic value. For example, miRNA-195 expression was associated with improved survival (HR 0.33, 95% CI 0.20 to 0.55, $P < .05$), whereas miRNA-21 (HR 1.78, 95% CI 1.23 to 2.57, $P < .05$), miRNA-155 (HR 1.26, 95% CI 1.09 to 1.45, $P < .05$), and miRNA-let-7 (HR 2.74, 95% CI 1.94 to 3.86, $P < .05$) overexpression were found to be associated with poor survival.

Circulating tumor DNA

Circulating tumor DNA (ctDNA) is tumor-derived fragmented DNA with around 200 nucleotides that can be detected in bodily fluids, most commonly from the saliva or blood in the context of head and neck tumors.[79] Of note, anatomic tumor location can play a role in the sensitivity of ctDNA detection in various bodily fluids. In an analysis of 47 patients with HNSCC, ctDNA was found in 100% of saliva samples from patients with oral cavity cancers compared with 47% to 70% of saliva samples from the oropharynx, larynx, and hypopharynx. In contrast, ctDNA was detected in the plasma of 80% of patients with oral cavity primaries, compared with 86% to 100% of patients with cancers of the other subsites. These findings highlight that saliva is preferentially enriched for tumor-specific DNA from the oral cavity, whereas plasma is preferentially enriched for tumor-derived DNA from other sites.[79] A possible biological mechanism for these findings can be explained by the differential release of tumor DNA based on the polarity of epithelial cells: tumor DNA released from the basal surface of epithelial cells into the lymphatics or venous system can be detected in plasma whereas DNA release on the apical side is harbored in saliva.

Two current methods of detecting ctDNA include targeted and untargeted approaches based on searching for known tumor mutations. Mutations of the tumor protein 53 (TP53) tumor suppressor gene represent the most frequent somatic genomic alterations in HNSCC and the presence of p53 mutations has been associated, though not significantly, with decreased survival in laryngeal cancer in pooled analyses (HR 1.87 95% CI, 1.00 to 3.51).[80,81] In an examination of the utility of ctDNA in screening for TP53 mutations, plasma and oral rinses from 12 patients with laryngeal cancer showed that only 17% and 25%, respectively, had detectable ctDNA. In this study, there was no difference in overall survival in cases with identified mutations to those without.[82]

Human papilloma virus

Human papilloma virus (HPV) infection has been suggested to play a role in benign and malignant pathologies of the larynx. Among laryngeal cancer patients, the prevalence of high-risk HPV types 16 and 18 is reported between 20% and 30%.[83] Though the frequent co-occurrence of HPV infection and laryngeal cancer have been identified, evidence of its prognostic role remains mixed at this time. In a large meta-analysis, including 9793 patients with laryngeal cancer, HPV-positive tumors had improved overall survival (HR: 0.71; 95% CI, 0.54 to 0.92, $P = .009$).[84] However, other studies have reported no association between HPV status and overall survival in laryngeal cancer.[85,86] Thus, more work is needed to determine the clinical and prognostic relevance of HPV status in laryngeal cancer.

Additional markers
Other molecular makers that have been previously implicated with a negative prognosis of laryngeal HNSCC are listed here. High levels of Epidermal Growth Factor Receptor (EGFR) have been associated with shorter survival and increased tumor recurrence.[87] Decreased expression of E-Cadherin has been linked with the presence of nodal disease, and worse prognosis.[88] In addition to p53 discussed previously, cyclin-1, B-cell lymphoma 2 (BCl-2), cyclooxygenase-2 (COX-2) and P300 levels also have been correlated with negative prognosis, treatment failure, and increased relapse rates.[89–92]

SUMMARY

The detection and management of laryngeal cancer is evolving. Patient factors such as age, sex, PS, comorbidities, nutrition, and even social factors are increasingly recognized as key determinants of prognosis and treatment response in patients with laryngeal HNC. There is a strong need for the identification of modifiable factors that can improve prognosis. Further, emerging technologies and novel biomarkers hold the potential for earlier cancer detection, a more molecularly precise diagnosis, and improved prognosis. However, there are no gold standard biomarkers that have been identified which can reliably predict survival and treatment responses at this time. Prospective trials looking at these biomarkers will be key in improving upon the currently stagnant prognosis in these patients. In summary, physicians must consider the patient and disease factors to engage in shared decision-making when assessing therapeutic options for patients with laryngeal cancers.

CLINICS CARE POINTS

- Patient factors such as older age, female sex, poor performance status, presence of comorbidities, malnutrition, and poor access to health care are all poor prognostic factors.
- Tumor factors such as advanced stage and supraglottic subsites are known as poor prognostic factors.
- Molecular tumor markers including programmed cell death ligand-1 status, presence of tumor-infiltrating lymphocytes, and presence of certain microRNAs are evolving markers in the initial phases of use in more precisely prognosticating patients with laryngeal cancer.
- At this time, the prognosis of patients with laryngeal cancer has not improved significantly over the past 30 years with 5-year relative survival remaining at 65% to 70%.

DISCLOSURE

The authors above have no commercial or financial disclosures.

REFERENCES

1. Li MM, Zhao S, Eskander A, et al. Stage migration and survival trends in laryngeal cancer. Ann Surg Oncol 2021;28(12):7300–9.
2. Misono S, Marmor S, Yueh B, et al. Treatment and survival in 10,429 patients with localized laryngeal cancer: a population-based analysis. Cancer 2014;120(12):1810–7.
3. Adeel M, Faisal M, Rashid A, et al. Outcomes of definitive radiotherapy for early laryngeal cancer in terms of survival and patterns of failure. Journal of Laryngology & Otology 2019;133(12):1087–91.
4. Timmermans AJ, van Dijk BA, Overbeek LI, et al. Trends in treatment and survival for advanced laryngeal cancer: a 20-year population-based study in The Netherlands. Head Neck 2016;38(Suppl 1):E1247–55.
5. Cancer stat facts: laryngeal cancer. Available at: https://seer.cancer.gov/statfacts/html/laryn.html. Accessed 08 December, 2022..
6. Atakul E, Akyar I. Frailty prevalence and characteristics in older adults with hematologic cancer: a descriptive study. Asia Pac J Oncol Nurs 2019;6(1):43–9.
7. Fried LP, Ferrucci L, Darer J, et al. Untangling the concepts of disability, frailty, and comorbidity: implications for improved targeting and care. J Gerontol A Biol Sci Med Sci 2004;59(3):255–63.
8. Horiot J-C. Radiation therapy and the geriatric oncology patient. Journal of Clinical Oncology 2007;25(14):1930–5.
9. Giraldi L, Leoncini E, Pastorino R, et al. Alcohol and cigarette consumption predict mortality in patients with head and neck cancer: a pooled analysis within the International Head and Neck Cancer Epidemiology (INHANCE) Consortium. Ann Oncol 2017;28(11):2843–51.
10. Nocini R, Molteni G, Mattiuzzi C, et al. Updates on larynx cancer epidemiology. Chin J Cancer Res 2020;32(1):18–25.
11. Brandstorp-Boesen J, Falk RS, Boysen M, et al. Long-term trends in gender, T-stage, subsite and treatment for laryngeal cancer at a single center. Eur Arch Otorhinolaryngol 2014;271(12):3233–9.
12. Stephenson WT, Barnes DE, Holmes FF, Norris hW. Gender influences subsite of origin of laryngeal carcinoma. Archives of Otolaryngology–Head & Neck Surgery 1991;117(7):774–8.
13. Wang N, Lv H, Huang M. Impact of gender on survival in patients with laryngeal squamous cell carcinoma: a propensity score matching analysis. Int J Clin Exp Pathol 2020;13(3):573–81.
14. Cook MB, McGlynn KA, Devesa SS, et al. Sex disparities in cancer mortality and survival. Cancer Epidemiology, Biomarkers & Prevention 2011;20(8):1629–37.
15. Leoncini E, Vukovic V, Cadoni G, et al. Tumour stage and gender predict recurrence and second primary malignancies in head and neck cancer: a multicentre study within the INHANCE consortium. European Journal of Epidemiology 2018;33(12):1205–18.
16. Hashim D, Sartori S, La Vecchia C, et al. Hormone factors play a favorable role in female head and neck cancer risk. Cancer Med 2017;6(8):1998–2007.
17. Clocchiatti A, Cora E, Zhang Y, et al. Sexual dimorphism in cancer. Nature Reviews Cancer 2016;16(5):330–9.
18. West H, Jin JO. Performance Status in Patients With Cancer. JAMA Oncology 2015;1(7):998.
19. ECOG Performance Status Scale. Available at: https://ecog-acrin.org/resources/ecog-performance-status/. Accessed 08 June, 2022.

20. Charlson ME, Carrozzino D, Guidi J, et al. Charlson comorbidity index: a critical review of clinimetric properties. Psychother Psychosom 2022;91(1):8–35.
21. Hu M, Ampil F, Clark C, et al. Comorbid predictors of poor response to chemo-radiotherapy for laryngeal squamous cell carcinoma. The Laryngoscope 2012; 122(3):565–71.
22. Paleri V, Wight RG, Silver CE, et al. Comorbidity in head and neck cancer: a critical appraisal and recommendations for practice. Oral Oncology 2010;46(10): 712–9.
23. Singh B, Bhaya M, Stern J, et al. Validation of the Charlson comorbidity index in patients with head and neck cancer: a multi-institutional study. The Laryngoscope 1997;107(11):1469–75.
24. Menach P, Oburra HO, Patel A. Cigarette smoking and alcohol ingestion as risk factors for laryngeal squamous cell carcinoma at kenyatta national hospital, kenya. Clin Med Insights Ear Nose Throat 2012;5:17–24.
25. Piano MR. Alcohol's effects on the cardiovascular system. Alcohol Res 2017; 38(2):219–41.
26. Warren GW, Alberg AJ, Kraft AS, et al. The 2014 surgeon general's report: "The health consequences of smoking–50 years of progress": a paradigm shift in cancer care. Cancer 2014;120(13):1914–6.
27. Group MLCW, Mulcahy CF, Mohamed ASR, et al. Age-adjusted comorbidity and survival in locally advanced laryngeal cancer. Head & Neck 2018;40(9):2060–9.
28. Alshadwi A, Nadershah M, Carlson ER, et al. Nutritional considerations for head and neck cancer patients: a review of the literature. Journal of Oral and Maxillofacial Surgery 2013;71(11):1853–60.
29. Gorenc M, Kozjek NR, Strojan P. Malnutrition and cachexia in patients with head and neck cancer treated with (chemo)radiotherapy. Rep Pract Oncol Radiother 2015;20(4):249–58.
30. O'Neill CB, O'Neill JP, Atoria CL, et al. Treatment complications and survival in advanced laryngeal cancer: a population-based analysis. The Laryngoscope 2014;124(12):2707–13.
31. Mäkitie AA, Alabi RO, Orell H, et al. Managing cachexia in head and neck cancer: a systematic scoping review. Advances in Therapy 2022;39(4):1502–23.
32. Steer B, Loeliger J, Edbrooke L, et al. Malnutrition prevalence according to the GLIM Criteria in head and neck cancer patients undergoing cancer treatment. Nutrients 2020;12(11).
33. van Bokhorst-de van der Schueren MA, van Leeuwen PA, Kuik DJ, et al. The impact of nutritional status on the prognoses of patients with advanced head and neck cancer. Cancer 1999;86(3):519–27.
34. Santos A, Santos IC, dos Reis PF, et al. Impact of nutritional status on survival in head and neck cancer patients after total laryngectomy. Nutrition and Cancer 2022;74(4):1252–60.
35. Gourin CG, Couch ME, Johnson JT. Effect of weight loss on short-term outcomes and costs of care after head and neck cancer surgery. Ann Otol Rhinol Laryngol 2014;123(2):101–10.
36. Hobday S, Armache M, Paquin R, et al. The body mass index paradox in head and neck cancer: a systematic review and meta-analysis. Nutrition and Cancer 2022;1–13.
37. Magnano M, Mola P, Machetta G, et al. The nutritional assessment of head and neck cancer patients. European Archives of Oto-Rhino-Laryngology 2015; 272(12):3793–9.

38. Przekop Z, Szostak-Węgierek D, Milewska M, et al. Efficacy of the nutritional risk index, geriatric nutritional risk index, BMI, and GLIM-defined malnutrition in predicting survival of patients with head and neck cancer patients qualified for home enteral nutrition. Nutrients 2022;14(6).

39. Shin JY, Truong MT. Racial disparities in laryngeal cancer treatment and outcome: a population-based analysis of 24,069 patients. The Laryngoscope 2015;125(7): 1667–74.

40. Gourin CG, Podolsky RH. Racial disparities in patients with head and neck squamous cell carcinoma. Laryngoscope 2006;116(7):1093–106.

41. Lebo NL, Khalil D, Balram A, et al. Influence of socioeconomic status on stage at presentation of laryngeal cancer in the United States. Otolaryngol Head Neck Surg 2019;161(5):800–6.

42. Sandulache VC, Kubik MW, Skinner HD, et al. Impact of race/ethnicity on laryngeal cancer in patients treated at a Veterans Affairs Medical Center. Laryngoscope 2013;123(9):2170–5.

43. Sineshaw HM, Ellis MA, Yabroff KR, et al. Association of medicaid expansion under the affordable care act with stage at diagnosis and time to treatment initiation for patients with head and neck squamous cell carcinoma. JAMA Otolaryngology Head & Neck Surgery 2020;146(3):247–55.

44. Cannon RB, Shepherd HM, McCrary H, et al. Association of the patient protection and affordable care act with insurance coverage for head and neck cancer in the SEER database. JAMA Otolaryngology–Head & Neck Surgery 2018;144(11): 1052–7.

45. Survival rates for laryngeal and hypopharyngeal cancers. Available at: https://www.cancer.org/cancer/laryngeal-and-hypopharyngeal-cancer/detection-diagnosis-staging/survival-rates.html#references. Accessed 08 Jan, 2022.

46. Issa MR, Samuels SE, Bellile E, et al. Tumor volumes and prognosis in laryngeal cancer. Cancers (Basel) 2015;7(4):2236–61.

47. Koroulakis A, Agarwal M. Laryngeal cancer. Treasure Island (FL): StatPearls Publishing; 2022. StatPearls.

48. Wachters JE, Kop E, Slagter-Menkema L, et al. Distinct biomarker profiles and clinical characteristics in T1-T2 glottic and supraglottic carcinomas. Laryngoscope 2020;130(12):2825–32.

49. Hirvikoski P, Virtaniemi J, Kumpulainen E, et al. Supraglottic and glottic carcinomas: clinically and biologically distinct entities? European Journal of Cancer 2002;38(13):1717–23.

50. Brandstorp-Boesen J, Sørum Falk R, Folkvard Evensen J, et al. Risk of recurrence in laryngeal cancer. PLoS One 2016;11(10):e0164068.

51. Ferlito A, Haigentz M Jr, Bradley PJ, et al. Causes of death of patients with laryngeal cancer. Eur Arch Otorhinolaryngol 2014;271(3):425–34.

52. Kourelis K, Papadas T, Vandoros G, et al. Glottic versus supraglottic tumors: differential molecular profile. Eur Arch Otorhinolaryngol 2008;265(1):79–84.

53. Evans Ronald M, Mangelsdorf David J. Nuclear receptors, RXR, and the Big Bang. Cell 2014;157(1):255–66.

54. Coskun H, Mendenhall WM, Rinaldo A, et al. Prognosis of subglottic carcinoma: is it really worse? Head & Neck 2019;41(2):511–21.

55. Kurita S, Hirano M, Matsuoka H, et al. A histopathological study of carcinoma of the larynx. Auris Nasus Larynx 1985;12(Suppl 2):S172–7.

56. Plaat RE, de Bree R, Kuik DJ, et al. Prognostic importance of paratracheal lymph node metastases. The Laryngoscope 2005;115(5):894–8.

57. Marchiano E, Patel DM, Patel TD, et al. Subglottic squamous cell carcinoma: a population-based study of 889 cases. Otolaryngology–Head and Neck Surgery 2015;154(2):315–21.

58. Gogna S, Kashyap S, Gupta N. Neck cancer resection and dissection. Treasure Island (FL): StatPearls Publishing; 2022. StatPearls.

59. STELL PM. Prognosis in laryngeal carcinoma: tumour factors. Clinical Otolaryngology & Allied Sciences 1990;15(1):69–81.

60. Layland MK, Sessions DG, Lenox J. The influence of lymph node metastasis in the treatment of squamous cell carcinoma of the oral cavity, oropharynx, larynx, and hypopharynx: N0 versus N+. Laryngoscope 2005;115(4):629–39.

61. Oosterkamp S, de Jong JM, Van den Ende PL, et al. Predictive value of lymph node metastases and extracapsular extension for the risk of distant metastases in laryngeal carcinoma. Laryngoscope 2006;116(11):2067–70.

62. Burke HB, Henson DE. Criteria for prognostic factors and for an enhanced prognostic system. Cancer 1993;72(10):3131–5.

63. Petersen JF, Stuiver MM, Timmermans AJ, et al. Development and external validation of a risk-prediction model to predict 5-year overall survival in advanced larynx cancer. Laryngoscope 2018;128(5):1140–5.

64. Ganly I, Amit M, Kou L, et al. Nomograms for predicting survival and recurrence in patients with adenoid cystic carcinoma. An international collaborative study. Eur J Cancer 2015;51(18):2768–76.

65. Marioni G, Marchese-Ragona R, Cartei G, et al. Current opinion in diagnosis and treatment of laryngeal carcinoma. Cancer Treat Rev 2006;32(7):504–15.

66. Chu EA, Kim YJ. Laryngeal cancer: diagnosis and preoperative work-up. Otolaryngologic Clinics of North America 2008;41(4):673–95.

67. Jakobsson PA. Histologic grading of malignancy and prognosis in glottic carcinoma of the larynx. Can J Otolaryngol 1975;4(5):885–92.

68. Akinleye A, Rasool Z. Immune checkpoint inhibitors of PD-L1 as cancer therapeutics. Journal of Hematology & Oncology 2019;12(1):92.

69. Ferris RL, Blumenschein G Jr, Fayette J, et al. Nivolumab for recurrent squamous-cell carcinoma of the head and neck. N Engl J Med 2016;375:1856–67.

70. Bauml J, Seiwert TY, Pfister DG, et al. Pembrolizumab for platinum- and cetuximab-refractory head and neck cancer: results from a single-arm, phase II study. J Clin Oncol 2017;35(14):1542–9.

71. Chow LQM, Haddad R, Gupta S, et al. Antitumor activity of pembrolizumab in biomarker-unselected patients with recurrent and/or metastatic head and neck squamous cell carcinoma: results from the phase Ib KEYNOTE-012 expansion cohort. J Clin Oncol 2016;34(32):3838–45.

72. Vassilakopoulou M, Avgeris M, Velcheti V, et al. Evaluation of PD-L1 expression and associated tumor-infiltrating lymphocytes in laryngeal squamous cell carcinoma. Clinical Cancer Research 2016;22(3):704–13.

73. Maibach F, Sadozai H, Seyed Jafari SM, et al. Tumor-infiltrating lymphocytes and their prognostic value in cutaneous melanoma. Front Immunol 2020;11:2105.

74. Idos GE, Kwok J, Bonthala N, et al. The prognostic implications of tumor infiltrating lymphocytes in colorectal cancer: a systematic review and meta-analysis. Scientific Reports 2020;10(1):3360.

75. Rodrigo JP, Sánchez-Canteli M, López F, et al. Tumor-infiltrating lymphocytes in the tumor microenvironment of laryngeal squamous cell carcinoma: systematic review and meta-analysis. Biomedicines 2021;9(5):486.

76. Li Y, Cai Q, Shen X, Chen X, Guan Z. Overexpression of B7-H3 Is Associated With Poor Prognosis in Laryngeal Cancer. Front Oncol 2021;11:759528.

77. Di Leva G, Garofalo M, Croce CM. MicroRNAs in cancer. Annu Rev Pathol 2014;9: 287–314.
78. Huang Y, Gu M, Tang Y, et al. Systematic review and meta-analysis of prognostic microRNA biomarkers for survival outcome in laryngeal squamous cell cancer. Cancer Cell Int 2021;21(1):316.
79. Wang Y, Springer S, Mulvey CL, et al. Detection of somatic mutations and HPV in the saliva and plasma of patients with head and neck squamous cell carcinomas. Science Translational Medicine 2015;7(293). 293ra104-293ra104.
80. Kogo R, Manako T, Iwaya T, et al. Individualized circulating tumor DNA monitoring in head and neck squamous cell carcinoma. Cancer Medicine.n/a(n/a).
81. Tandon S, Tudur-Smith C, Riley RD, et al. A Systematic Review of p53 as a Prognostic Factor of Survival in Squamous Cell Carcinoma of the Four Main Anatomical Subsites of the Head and Neck. Cancer Epidemiology, Biomarkers & Prevention 2010;19(2):574–87.
82. Perdomo S, Avogbe PH, Foll M, et al. Circulating tumor DNA detection in head and neck cancer: evaluation of two different detection approaches. Oncotarget 2017;8(42):72621–32.
83. Li X, Gao L, Li H, et al. Human papillomavirus infection and laryngeal cancer risk: a systematic review and meta-analysis. J Infect Dis 2013;207(3):479–88.
84. Sahovaler A, Kim MH, Mendez A, et al. Survival outcomes in human papillomavirus-associated nonoropharyngeal squamous cell carcinomas: a systematic review and meta-analysis. JAMA Otolaryngol Head Neck Surg 2020;146(12): 1158–66.
85. Fakhry C, Westra WH, Wang SJ, et al. The prognostic role of sex, race, and human papillomavirus in oropharyngeal and nonoropharyngeal head and neck squamous cell cancer. Cancer 2017;123(9):1566–75.
86. Hernandez BY, Goodman MT, Lynch CF, et al. Human papillomavirus prevalence in invasive laryngeal cancer in the United States. PLoS One 2014;9(12):e115931.
87. Jiang M, Zhang H, Xiao H, et al. High expression of c-Met and EGFR is associated with poor survival of patients with glottic laryngeal squamous cell carcinoma. Oncol Lett 2018;15(1):931–9.
88. Re M, Gioacchini FM, Scarpa A, et al. The prognostic significance of E-cadherin expression in laryngeal squamous-cell carcinoma: a systematic review. Acta Otorhinolaryngol Ital 2018;38(6):504–10.
89. Jovanovic IP, Radosavljevic GD, Simovic-Markovic BJ, et al. Clinical significance of Cyclin D1, FGF3 and p21 protein expression in laryngeal squamous cell carcinoma. J Buon 2014;19(4):944–52.
90. Du J, Feng J, Luo D, et al. Prognostic and clinical significance of COX-2 overexpression in laryngeal cancer: a meta-analysis. Front Oncol 2022;12:854946.
91. Chen YF, Luo RZ, Li Y, et al. High expression levels of COX-2 and P300 are associated with unfavorable survival in laryngeal squamous cell carcinoma. Eur Arch Otorhinolaryngol 2013;270(3):1009–17.
92. Nix P, Cawkwell L, Patmore H, et al. Bcl-2 expression predicts radiotherapy failure in laryngeal cancer. Br J Cancer 2005;92(12):2185–9.

Laryngeal Cancer and the End of Life (As We Know It)

Monica H. Bodd, MTS[a], Susan D. McCammon, MD, PhD, FAAHPM[b],*

KEYWORDS

- Laryngectomee • Psychosocial needs • Suffering • Personhood • Disability
- Palliative care

KEY POINTS

- Patients suffering from laryngeal cancer undergo life-changing interventions that affect their well-being.
- The symptom burden at the end of life originates earlier in the course of illness, in forms such as societal shame, poor mental health, and disproportionate outcomes based on gender and race.
- For patients with advanced laryngeal cancer, surgical palliative care provides a helpful paradigm for caregiver support, goals-of-care conversations, and treatment counseling.

INTRODUCTION

There are some things that are worse than death. To deny one's own integrity of personality in the presence of the human challenge is one of those things.[1]
                                                                    Reverend Howard Thurman

Laryngeal cancer is statistically rare: 0.7% (12,470) of all new cancer cases in the United States in 2022 and 0.6% (3820) of all deaths.[2] This disease is, however, disproportionately alarming to patients, to caregivers, and to the public. The threat to voice and swallow, the prospect of being a "neck breather," is a threshold risk that many people find intolerable or even unthinkable. The 5-year relative survival for patients with laryngeal cancer is 61% ranging from 78.3% for early disease to 33% for disease diagnosed when there are already distant metastases. Thus, although it is a life-threatening disease, and many people die from it, it is also a survivable disease, and many people live in the aftermath of its treatment for many years. This disease occupies a unique place in the narrative of twentieth-century cancer care, as a disease for which surgical and nonsurgical treatments were at one time found to have

[a] Duke University, School of Medicine, Durham, NC, USA; [b] Department of Otolaryngology, Heersink School of Medicine, 1155 Faculty Office Tower, 510 20th Street South, Birmingham, AL 35233, USA
* Corresponding author.
E-mail address: smccammon@uabmc.edu

Otolaryngol Clin N Am 56 (2023) 403–412
https://doi.org/10.1016/j.otc.2022.11.005
0030-6665/23/© 2022 Elsevier Inc. All rights reserved.

equivalent survival outcomes, and thus preference-sensitive treatment decisions were based on perceived and predicted quality of life.

Preferences were and are very strong. The prospect of a total laryngectomy is one that is still often met with the reaction: "Never; I could never live like that; I would rather be dead." This disgust and rejection of a potentially curative treatment option is largely based on the necessity of a permanent stoma for breathing and the changes to vocal communication. This article addresses issues that face patients with laryngeal cancer as they face biological death, the literal end of their lives. We will also focus on the suffering and loss of identity that can precede that: a kind of social death. Change in body image and loss of self-expression affect self-identity and adjustment, and the necessary reframing is dramatically influenced by the reactions of others, including physicians and health care professionals. Although there are many things that can be done upstream to improve outcomes and decrease treatment burdens for patients with laryngeal cancer, there are currently too many missed opportunities to attend to their human and social needs with a respect that does not primarily see them as mutilated or monstrous. We argue here for a radical re-envisioning of the experience of people who prospectively think "I could never live like that" or retrospectively feel that they are "social outcasts."

Patients suffering from laryngeal cancer undergo life-changing interventions that impact how they interact with the world. In our society, these patients are often cast outside of the norm for their (dis)abilities, appearance, and overall functional status. Practices of exclusion are particularly dominant against patients who have advanced-stage disease, large ablative surgeries and reconstructions, or recurrent disease near the end of their life. Within the hospital, these patients may also undergo a significant shift in orientation from cure/restitution to symptom management/supportive care. Although this nexus has been identified as a significant care gap,[3] there remains a lack of in-depth characterization of the multidimensional symptom burden faced by patients with laryngeal cancer at the end of life (EOL).

An understanding of needs is prerequisite to caring for persons with laryngeal cancer at EOL; this can then allow us to ask: *What role, if any, does the surgeon have in restoring human dignity to patients facing total laryngectomy? What might it mean for these patients to live/flourish, both inside and outside the walls of the hospital?*

DEFINITIONS

Although the instinctual contrast to life/living is death/dying, we thicken this distinction by claiming that physical death is an insufficient descriptor of EOL. Death is at once physical and social, threaded through the entire, engaged life of humans. As philosophers ranging from Plato to Montaigne to Heidegger argue, death is understood metaphorically as separation from the common *bios* (social death) or from the resources and goods that would allow an even subsistence level of *zoe* (economic death). [4] Of note, the incidence of social and economic death is higher than physical death. Within our society that defines the "good death" as one that is medically attended to and in the presence of loving family, to be alone and poor is to face a "bad death." This American stereotype of EOL continues to value individual self-determination and to expect individuals to define and then achieve what they want, including their own "good death." Such individualistic emphasis turns a deliberately blind eye to the social determinants of existence that limit what someone even has access to—pain medication, food, shelter, reassurance of what will happen to their body after death, and so on. EOL reveals the edges of humanity—our "sacred universe of moral obligation"[5]—bringing to light the societal and individual priorities, relationships, and abilities that matter. As the artist in residence at MD Anderson Cancer Center, Professor Marcia Brennan, would say, "the end-of-life is about life itself."

Dying—and living—are multidimensional. It follows, then, that care at EOL must alleviate all forms of suffering. Dr Eric Cassell, a physician who deeply influenced medical scholarship on suffering, defines suffering as "pain without meaning, or existential threat to the self or person."[6] Specific to laryngeal cancer, this threat to self may range from postsurgical disability (loss of voice, eating) to societal isolation (disfigured appearance, electrolarynx). As this threat to self endures throughout time and community, we must ask: *What forms of flourishing constitute this patient's enduring sense of personal identity? To which communities and values does this patient belong? And, how are these threatened in their course of illness?*

This article first characterizes the psychosocial suffering experienced by patients with laryngeal cancer, including societal shame, poor mental health, and disproportionate outcomes based on gender and race. The authors then suggest opportunities to provide upstream and postsurgical care, including attention to narrative paradigms embedded in treatment counseling.[7,8] (Upstream care refers to care during the earliest stages of illness, including prevention, immediately after diagnosis, and before surgical intervention.)

SOCIETAL LOSS

In addition to communication difficulties, total laryngectomees are reduced by media to a cautionary tale; they have been the subject of antismoking advertisements, which depict a clear before- and after-cancer image to warn viewers about tobacco misuse. Sharon, a 37-year-old mother with recurrent laryngeal cancer, emphasized the sudden and drastic change after diagnosis: "I had two children, made the kids lunches, took them to school, was on the PTA...Life was going to change for me pretty quick."[9] Terrie, a 40-year-old laryngectomee, described moments of daily life taken away from her, including eating and talking at the same time, smelling a cake in the oven, brewing coffee, and her natural voice: "I never recorded my voice for [my grandson]...this is the only voice he knows."[10,11] The voice of Ronaldo, a 30-year-old laryngectomee, was part of an audio message campaign shared over 5000 times, "scary enough" to prompt numerous New Yorkers to quit smoking.[12] And, Debi, a 42-year-old laryngectomee, described the dangers of nicotine addiction by her persistent cigarette use via stoma: "They say nicotine isn't addictive. How could they say that?"[13] Patients who are portrayed equally as surgical specimens or artifacts in these advertisements are given a voice insofar as they express self-blame and guilt for their cancer. The uncanny timbre of the prosthetic voice literally embodies the overt warning: to have laryngeal cancer is to lose something essentially human.

The stories of patients with laryngeal cancer have become admonishments—images of loss, blame, and guilt meant to be seared into viewers' minds. In contrast, patients with human papillomavirus-related oropharyngeal cancer are often portrayed as well-preserved images of (hetero)sexually active, young adults.[14,15] These news reports focus on the patients' surprise and underlying innocence. As seen in these advertisements, patients with laryngeal cancer fall outside the range of normalcy, cast as guilty and responsible for their own suffering. This stigma has been well studied in other "vice"-related cancers, such as lung and liver.[16–20] The public portrayal of laryngeal cancer undoubtedly impedes reintegration into communal life.

INTERPERSONAL LOSS

Patients with laryngeal cancer experience significant embarrassment related to their appearance and activities of daily living. In a study by Graboyes and colleagues,[21] patients with head and neck cancer experienced an increase in body image disturbance from 11% preoperatively to 25% (1 month) and 27% (3 months) postoperatively. Those with pT3/4 tumors were nearly 9 times more likely to experience body image disturbance. Other risk factors included female sex, baseline shame/stigma and social isolation, and depression.[21] A qualitative analysis of postlaryngectomy patients showed that more than 40% of them withdrew from conversation and only one-third participated in social activities. Two patterns of withdrawal were identified: (1) depression related to poor speech intelligibility (87% perceived stigma due to voice changes) and (2) anxiety with perceived stigmatization (50% felt embarrassed because of their tracheal stoma).[22] Unfortunately, it is no surprise that surgical interventions that affect critical daily functions result in profound social losses.

Qualitative research by Bickford and colleagues[23] has categorized reframing patterns of patients with laryngectomies as destabilized, resigned, resolute, and transformed. As defined by Cassell,[6] stigma often presents in "daily life filled from the first to the last second with intentions and purposes," in the self that "is injured in illness and lost in suffering." Although the stigma about the stoma is overwhelmingly most powerful, misconceptions about voice come next, even despite alternate communication options and total laryngectomees in the public eye (eg, Dr Itzhak Brook). Pain of the loss of social eating is the most unexpected for these patients. These ordinary, communal acts of living are interrupted and too often neglected during cancer treatment.

PSYCHOSOCIAL LOSS

For patients with laryngeal cancer, physical symptoms are often followed by mental health exacerbations. In a study of total laryngectomees, increase in symptom burden, assessed by the MD Anderson Dysphagia Inventory, and the Hospital Anxiety and Depression Scale (HADS-anxiety and HADS-depression) correlated with a decrease of 2.7 and 3.0 points, respectively.[24] Depression has been reported in up to 40% of patients with head and neck cancer, heightened within 3 months of diagnosis.[25] The risk of suicide in head and neck cancer is twice that of other cancers,[26] and it is the highest in cancers of the hypopharynx and larynx (64.7 per 100,000 person-years).[27] Noting these trends, Lydiatt and colleagues[28,29] conducted a trial of antidepressants (citalopram or escitalopram) in patients diagnosed with head and neck cancer. Prophylactic antidepressants were correlated with decreased rates of depression and improved global mood and quality of life.[28,29] Although these findings are unsurprising given medicine's widely applauded use of antidepressants, it is worth questioning why these patients are depressed—and if there are ways in which our oncologic community has failed to heal. *Might there be other interventions besides broad prescription of antidepressants? Is our impulse to treat depression a pathologizing of the human condition, or our resistance to witnessing despair in our patients?* Psychosocial symptom management remains a care gap for the field of head and neck oncologic surgery.

INEQUITABLE LOSS

The incidence of head and neck cancer falls disproportionately on minority populations and has wide-reaching socioeconomic effects. Although not yet studied independently, laryngeal cancer is a disruptive, resource-intensive subset of head and neck cancer. Survival outcomes differ based on race and gender; in one study, black female patients with nonoropharyngeal head and neck cancer had poorer survival than their white or Hispanic male counterparts.[30] In addition, head and neck cancer is more prevalent among minorities and those with lower education status, poverty, and medical comorbidities. This disenfranchised group of patients is further disadvantaged by high medical expenses in head and neck cancer versus other cancers.[31]

Those in medicine are mandated to devote themselves to the sick, and in the setting of disproportionate head and neck cancer incidence: the poorest of our patients. *As the late Dr Paul Farmer asks of us healers—will we "make an option—a choice—for the poor, to work on their behalf?"*[32] Drawing near to these patients suffering from life-changing, threatening, destabilizing diagnoses is our ethical imperative as surgeon-leaders. This is embodied resistance against the inequitable violence of disease; this is healing justice, and we have the privilege of creative participation in it. *Will we choose to enter in?*

DISCUSSION: A WAY FORWARD

Whole-person healing addresses "unconquerable loneliness–a loneliness over which many have preferred death."[6] Loneliness takes on new meaning and significance when patients are *literally* devoid of speech, eating, and prior appearance after laryngeal cancer treatment. Head and neck surgery may address this care gap by integrating with palliative care. As a form of accompaniment, specialized palliative care aims to alleviate the multidimensional burden of suffering through targeted interventions and discussions in the face of serious illness. Surgical palliative care is "the treatment of suffering and promotion of quality of life for seriously ill patients undergoing surgical care"[33]; it has been implemented in numerous other surgical disciplines (eg, trauma and critical care, general surgery) but remains largely unintegrated in standard head and neck cancer care.[3,34] For patients with advanced laryngeal cancer, surgical palliative care provides a helpful paradigm for caregiver support, goals-of-care conversations, and treatment counseling.

First, involvement of palliative care for head and neck cancer has been shown to improve family-perceived care and symptom distress at the time of patient death.[35] One of our patients' greatest fears is being a burden or embarrassment for their loved ones. As patients with laryngeal cancer endure a totalizing loss of physical capacity at EOL, their caregivers are magnified in discussions of survival and palliative practices (ie, symptom management, communication, advanced care planning).[36] Caregiver support provides a scaffolding that humanizes caregivers and sufferers.

Next, the art of goals-of-care conversations with patients who receive a recommendation for total laryngectomy relies on an understanding of the patient's story and clear description of outcomes. Within the treatment paradigm of laryngeal cancer—"all other things being equal"—extensive preoperative counseling is necessary given the sudden and distressing loss of communicative ability.[3] The high risk of recurrence despite salvage therapy and tumultuous, symptom-laden course of death by head and neck cancer places the responsibility on surgeons to provide clear communication. These conversations should include both health and experiential outcomes: *How might we accurately convey these expected outcomes given variable disease and patient factors?* Outside of survival curves and standardized patient-reported outcomes research, the field of disability studies offers a promising addition.

By thickening reality, disability studies move us past the "clinical gaze"—the face-to-face (or face-to-stoma)—of surgeon and cancerous patient. ("Thick Description"[37] documents the experience of persons beyond what meets the eye; it sees life as *lived*—socially embedded, influenced (and excluded) by cultural norms.) The "clinical gaze"[38,39] is a longstanding form of dominance that recalibrates actors into an existing power dynamic. (For Foucault, the panopticon is a metaphor for this dominating act, which enforces a narrowing vision of health in accordance with the society's need for order.) In doing so, this narrows possibilities in the encounter to cure and "normal"— negating the spectrum of flourishing for patients with laryngeal cancer. Patients' existence is not limited to their medical viability, but rather should include the communities that choose to uphold, humanize, and personalize them even, and especially, in their disabilities. The surgical reduction of patient to statistic is just one way that the surgical ideology slips into public eye; it provides a framework of normalcy that is forcibly internalized by all within its reach. The surgical encounter asserts surgery as the only viable option—and the subjects of it are left with little option to escape.

However, hospice and palliative care, although popularly considered the "do-nothing," "soft" medicine—is a radical form of resistance. Surgical palliative care widens context through extensive conversation regarding intolerable outcomes, limitations to rescue, and exit opportunities[40-42]; it has the unique opportunity to enter the stories of patients suffering from laryngeal cancer. Its openness to all possibilities challenges "the notion that defective body-minds are undesirable, worthless, disposable, or in need of cure."[43] The support of disfigured patients, in their full embodiment, destabilizes the politics of cure. By attending to physical and psychosocial symptoms, we can mitigate risks of mental health and social isolation.

Last, palliative care includes goal concordance as a core tenet of patient counseling. Goal-concordant care minimizes decisional conflict and regret,[44] emphasizing the need to understand patient priorities during surgical decision making. Such care may also require that treatment options are laden with a mix of palliative and curative intent, contrary to the focus on "doing something versus not doing something."[45] Goal-concordant care conversations most often happen upstream, for example, surgery versus chemoradiation counseling, preparation for total laryngectomy, and understanding of postoperative changes in voice. However, outcomes are not completely understood until experienced by patients themselves. Perhaps, decisional regret is best mitigated by helping patients feel empowered to adjust to their new embodiment without shame, after intervention or at the "end"; this can happen by some serious work and humility on the part of viewers including the surgical team, community members, and family. The imperfection of the stoma and change in voice "wakes [us] up to a body relentlessly subject to the disturbances of desire, illness, and mortality...insisting on [our] notice and holding [us] thrall."[39] As disability/feminist scholar Rosemarie Garland-Thomson describes, this disruptive reality leads to vulnerability on the part of the one who views, gazes upon, and labels the patient as diseased. The destabilization of surgeon-as-prescriber of a laryngectomee's reality temporarily takes away the surgeon's power to write the patient's narrative. Namely, the patient is no longer a specimen for the operation room, but a whole-bodied person who lives in and through limitation.[46] *How might we invite patients' lived realities into our surgical decision making? Could the disciplines of disability studies and medical ethnography more accurately portray prognosis, empowering survivors to live fully beyond surgery?*

As we stated in the introduction, death can be socially constructed. Be it brain death, cardiac death, ontological death, social death, symbolic death, or economic death, the social construction of death changes when one dies without resources or without social standing. Here we ask, *how is our contemporary reception of patients with laryngeal cancer built upon the scaffolding of our construction of social death?*

As EOL has been expanded to include personhood, these conversations about goal-concordant care (and cure) must be ongoing from time of laryngeal cancer diagnosis. "Cure" must be continually leveraged against the cost, violence, and controlled trauma of surgical intervention. In one study, almost one-fifth (18%) of patients with head and neck cancer ranked "being cured" as second or third priority; "living as long as possible" was placed in the top 3 priorities by more than half (56%) of patients. Energy, swallowing, voice, and appearance were ranked in the top 3 priorities by up to 24% of the patients.[47] One landmark study of healthy firemen underscored patient-specific priorities of laryngeal preservation versus survival.[48] We must make room for patients like these: cure and health are nonequivalent. In fact, by considering them as equal,[49] we simply extend Foucauldian biopower—the power to foster life or disallow it to the point of death. The surgical imperative to cure or leave "[commits] damage, routinely turning body-minds into medical objects and creating lies about normal and natural."[43] A myopic vision of health can limit the many forms of flourishing, living, and meaning-making that patients develop in the setting of advanced laryngeal cancer. As key players in laryngeal cancer treatment, we must pause to consider what is broken, what needs fixing, and how we can be in solidarity with patients who inhabit the margins of this framework. Surgical palliative care is a promising guide for our positionality in these narratives: ultimately, our care is political.

SUMMARY

Care at EOL engages life in its barest form. For patients with advanced laryngeal cancer or postlaryngectomy, living is circumscribed by loss in many forms—societal, interpersonal, psychosocial, inequitable. In this article, we ask: *How might we better attend to these patients facing the end of their personhood? How can we help them live (and die) well?* Surgical palliative care is an informative, necessary component to a renewed paradigm of laryngeal cancer care. However, this is not sufficient. We, as surgeons, must ask ourselves how we participate in a narrow definition of cure and "a life well lived," tending to its repercussions ranging from social isolation (eg, medical aid in dying for patients "burdening" the health system as an extreme example) to the loneliness of psychosocial suffering. *To what extent is death "undignified" because we do not imbue the space of dying with dignity?* Our gaze is fraught with clinical power patients see us in their most vulnerable moments, and we have the immense privilege of *seeing* them. We can generate dignity by beholding them, in their depth of suffering.[50–52] We have a part to play, and to heal, in the community of patients living, and flourishing, with advanced laryngeal cancer.

The price is simply too high to live chasing cures, because in doing so, I'm missing living my life. I know only that in chasing to achieve the person I once was, I will miss the person I have become.[53]

Liz Moore

CLINICS CARE POINTS

- For patients with advanced laryngeal cancer, the symptom burden includes societal shame, poor mental health, and disproportionate outcomes based on gender and race.
- Surgical palliative care provides a helpful paradigm for caregiver support, goals-of-care conversations, and treatment counseling.

DISCLOSURES

The authors have no disclosures to report.

AUTHOR CONTRIBUTIONS

Both authors made substantial contributions to conception and design, analysis, and interpretation of data. Both were involved in drafting the article or revising it critically for important intellectual content. Both provided approval of the article and agree to be accountable for all aspects of the work.

REFERENCES

1. Thurman H, Harding V. Jesus and the disinherited. Beacon Press; 1996.
2. Database S. 2022. Available at: https://seer.cancer.gov/statfacts/html/laryn.html. Accessed October 31, 2022.
3. McCammon SD. Concurrent palliative care in the surgical management of head and neck cancer. J Surg Oncol 2019;120(1):78–84.
4. Agamben G. Homo sacer: sovreign power and bare life. Stanford, CA: Stanford University Press; 1998.
5. Rubenstein RL, Roth JK. Approaches to auschwitz: the legacy of the holocaust. SCM Press; 1987.
6. Cassell EJ. Recognizing suffering. Hastings Cent Rep 1991;21(3):24.
7. Aho KA. Heidegger, ontological death, and the healing professions. Med Health Care Philos 2016;19(1):55–63.
8. Ratcliff C, Naik AD, Martin LA, et al. Examining cancer survivorship trajectories: Exploring the intersection between qualitative illness narratives and quantitative screening instruments. Palliat Support Care 2018;16(6):712–8.
9. CDC: Tips From Former Smokers - Sharon A.'s Diagnosed at 37 Story: CDC.
10. CDC: Tips From Former Smokers - Terrie H.'s I Wish Tip: CDC.
11. CDC: Tips From Former Smokers - Terrie H.'s Tip Ad: CDC.
12. The New York Times: Digital and Home Delivery Subscriptions. 2007.
13. Debi Austin "Voicebox" - Tobacco Free CA.
14. Steve's story - oral cancer caused by HPV. Minnesota Department of Health; 2022. Accessed.
15. Kotz D. Michael Douglas blames throat cancer on oral sex: what are risks? 2013.
16. Hamann HA, Williamson TJ, Studts JL, et al. Lung cancer stigma then and now: continued challenges amid a landscape of progress. J Thorac Oncol 2021;16(1): 17–20.
17. Hamann HA, Ver Hoeve ES, Carter-Harris L, et al. Multilevel opportunities to address lung cancer stigma across the cancer control continuum. J Thorac Oncol 2018;13(8):1062–75.
18. Warner ET, Park ER, Luberto CM, et al. Internalized stigma among cancer patients enrolled in a smoking cessation trial: The role of cancer type and associations with psychological distress. Psychooncology 2022;31(5):753–60.
19. Wahlin S, Andersson J. Liver health literacy and social stigma of liver disease: a general population e-survey. Clin Res Hepatol Gastroenterol 2021;45(5):101750.
20. Schomerus G, Leonhard A, Manthey J, et al. The stigma of alcohol-related liver disease and its impact on healthcare. J Hepatol 2022;77(2):516–24.
21. Graboyes EM, Hill EG, Marsh CH, et al. Body image disturbance in surgically treated head and neck cancer patients: a prospective cohort pilot study. Otolaryngol Head Neck Surg 2019;161(1):105–10.

22. Danker H, Wollbrück D, Singer S, et al. Social withdrawal after laryngectomy. Eur Arch Oto-Rhino-Laryngology. 2010;267(4):593–600.
23. Bickford J, Coveney J, Baker J, et al. Validating the changes to self-identity after total laryngectomy. Cancer Nurs 2019;42(4):314–22.
24. Kemps GJ, Krebbers I, Pilz W, et al. Affective symptoms and swallow-specific quality of life in total laryngectomy patients. Head & Neck 2020;42(11):3179–87.
25. Sehlen S, Lenk M, Herschbach P, et al. Depressive symptoms during and after radiotherapy for head and neck cancer. Head & Neck 2003;25(12):1004–18.
26. Osazuwa-Peters N, Simpson MC, Zhao L, et al. Suicide risk among cancer survivors: head and neck versus other cancers. Cancer 2018;124(20):4072–9.
27. Kam D, Salib A, Gorgy G, et al. Incidence of suicide in patients with head and neck cancer. JAMA Otolaryngol Head Neck Surg 2015;141(12):1075–81.
28. Lydiatt WM, Denman D, McNeilly DP, et al. A randomized, placebo-controlled trial of citalopram for the prevention of major depression during treatment for head and neck cancer. Arch Otolaryngol Head Neck Surg 2008;134(5):528–35.
29. Lydiatt WM, Bessette D, Schmid KK, et al. Prevention of depression with escitalopram in patients undergoing treatment for head and neck cancer: randomized, double-blind, placebo-controlled clinical trial. JAMA Otolaryngol Head Neck Surg 2013;139(7):678–86.
30. Mazul AL, Naik AN, Zhan KY, et al. Gender and race interact to influence survival disparities in head and neck cancer. Oral Oncol 2021;112:105093.
31. Massa ST, Osazuwa-Peters N, Adjei Boakye E, et al. Comparison of the financial burden of survivors of head and neck cancer with other cancer survivors. JAMA Otolaryngol Head Neck Surg 2019;145(3):239–49.
32. Farmer P. Pathologies of power: health, human rights, and the new war on the poor, 4. Univ of California Press; 2004.
33. Dunn GP, Johnson AG. Surgical palliative care, 1. OUP Oxford; 2004.
34. Mulvey CL, Smith TJ, Gourin CG. Use of inpatient palliative care services in patients with metastatic incurable head and neck cancer. Head Neck 2016;38(3):355–63.
35. Shuman AG, Yang Y, Taylor JM, et al. End-of-life care among head and neck cancer patients. Otolaryngol Head Neck Surg 2011;144(5):733–9.
36. Esce A, McCammon S. Holding Curative and Palliative Intentions. AMA J Ethics 2021;23(10):E766–71.
37. Geertz C. Thick description: Toward an interpretive theory of culture. In: The cultural geography reader. Routledge; 2008. p. 41–51.
38. Foucault M. The birth of the clinic : an archaeology of medical perception. London: Tavistock; 1973.
39. Garland-Thomson R. Staring: how we look. Oxford University Press; 2009.
40. Shinall MC, Bonnet K, Schlundt D, et al. Integrating specialist palliative care in the liver transplantation evaluation process: a qualitative analysis of hepatologist and palliative care provider views. Liver Transpl 2022;28(4):678–88.
41. Shinall MC, Beskow LM, Karlekar M, et al. Psychosocial stress before major oncologic operations: a qualitative content analysis of palliative care provider documentation. Ann Surg 2021;274(6):e649–50.
42. Shinall MC, Hoskins A, Hawkins AT, et al. A randomized trial of a specialist palliative care intervention for patients undergoing surgery for cancer: rationale and design of the Surgery for Cancer with Option of Palliative Care Expert (SCOPE) Trial. Trials 2019;20(1):713.
43. Clare E. Brilliant imperfection: grappling with cure. Duke University Press; 2017. https://doi.org/10.1215/9780822373520.

44. Shuman AG, Larkin K, Thomas D, et al. Patient Reflections on Decision Making for Laryngeal Cancer Treatment. Otolaryngol Head Neck Surg 2017;156(2):299–304.
45. Davies L, Rhodes LA, Grossman DC, et al. Decision making in head and neck cancer care. Laryngoscope 2010;120(12):2434–45.
46. Vogel E. Rewriting another: discussing ethics and disability through lucy grealy's autobiography of a face and ann patchett's truth and beauty. Transformations 2014;25(2):163–7.
47. List MA, Stracks J, Colangelo L, et al. How Do head and neck cancer patients prioritize treatment outcomes before initiating treatment? J Clin Oncol 2000; 18(4):877–84.
48. McNeil BJ, Weichselbaum R, Pauker SG. Speech and survival: tradeoffs between quality and quantity of life in laryngeal cancer. N Engl J Med 1981;305(17):982–7.
49. Palacios M. Naming Ableism. 2017.
50. Rantanen P, Chochinov HM, Emanuel LL, et al. Existential quality of life and associated factors in cancer patients receiving palliative care. J Pain Symptom Manage 2022;63(1):61–70.
51. Chochinov HM, McClement S, Hack T, et al. Eliciting personhood within clinical practice: effects on patients, families, and health care providers. J Pain Symptom Manage 2015;49(6):974–80.e972.
52. Chochinov HM. Dignity and the eye of the beholder. J Clin Oncol 2004;22(7): 1336–40.
53. Wong A. Disability visibility: first-person stories from the twenty-first century. Vintage; 2020.

Moving?

Make sure your subscription moves with you!

To notify us of your new address, find your **Clinics Account Number** (located on your mailing label above your name), and contact customer service at:

Email: journalscustomerservice-usa@elsevier.com

800-654-2452 (subscribers in the U.S. & Canada)
314-447-8871 (subscribers outside of the U.S. & Canada)

Fax number: 314-447-8029

Elsevier Health Sciences Division
Subscription Customer Service
3251 Riverport Lane
Maryland Heights, MO 63043

*To ensure uninterrupted delivery of your subscription, please notify us at least 4 weeks in advance of move.

Printed and bound by CPI Group (UK) Ltd, Croydon, CR0 4YY

03/10/2024

01040466-0003